Handbook of the Sociology of Medical Education

The *Handbook of the Sociology of Medical Education* provides a contemporary introduction to this classic area of sociology by examining the social origin and implications of the epistemological, organizational and demographic challenges facing medical education in the twenty-first century.

Beginning with reflections on the historical and theoretical foundations of the sociology of medical education, the collection then focuses on current issues affecting medical students, the profession and the faculty, before exploring medical education in different national contexts.

Leading sociologists analyse: the intersection of medical education and social structures such as gender, ethnicity and disability; the effect of changes in medical practice, such as the emergence of evidence-based medicine, on medical education; and the ongoing debates surrounding the form and content of medical curricula. By examining applied problems within a framework which draws from social theorists such as Pierre Bourdieu, this new collection suggests future directions for the sociological study of medical education and for medical education itself.

Caragh Brosnan is a Research Associate in the Centre for Biomedicine and Society at King's College London. While undertaking work on the *Handbook*, she was a Lecturer in Medical Education in the Medical School at Keele University. She completed her doctoral thesis, 'The Sociology of Medical Education: the struggle for legitimate knowledge in two English medical schools', at the University of Cambridge in 2007.

Bryan S. Turner was Professor of Sociology at the University of Cambridge (1998–2005) and at the National University of Singapore (2005–2009). He is currently the Alona Evans Distinguished Visiting Professor of Sociology at Wellesley College, US. He has published *The New Medical Sociology* (2004) and *The Body and Society* (2008).

Handbook of the Sociology of Medical Education

Edited by Caragh Brosnan and Bryan S. Turner

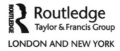

Routledge
Taylor & Francis Group

LONDON AND NEW YORK

First published 2009
by Routledge
2 Park Square, Milton Park, Abingdon, Oxon OX14 4RN

Simultaneously published in the USA and Canada
by Routledge
711 Third Ave, New York, NY 10017

Routledge is an imprint of the Taylor & Francis Group, an informa business

First issued in paperback 2012

Typeset in Times by Wearset Ltd, Boldon, Tyne and Wear

British Library Cataloguing in Publication Data
A catalogue record for this book is available from the British Library

Library of Congress Cataloging-in-Publication Data
Handbook of the sociology of medical education/edited by Caragh
Brosnan and Bryan S. Turner.
p.; cm.
Includes bibliographical references.
1. Medical education–Social aspects. I. Brosnan, Caragh. II. Turner, Bryan
S. III. Title: Sociology of medical education.
[DNLM: 1. Education, Medical. 2. Sociology, Medical. 3. Students,
Medical. W 18 H2365 2009]
R737.H36 2009
362.1–dc22   2008054319

ISBN13: 978-0-415-46044-6 (hbk)
ISBN13: 978-0-203-87563-6 (ebk)
ISBN13: 978-0-415-53418-5 (pbk)

Contents

Illustrations

Figure

Tables

Boxes

Notes on contributors

Jon Adams is Associate Professor and Head of the Discipline of Social Science, School of Population Health, University of Queensland and holds a PHCRED Research Fellowship, Department of Health and Ageing, Australia. Jon has been researching complementary and alternative medicine for over ten years and has published three edited research books, 13 research book chapters and over 70 peer-reviewed journal articles on this healthcare area.

Gary L. Albrecht is Professor Emeritus, University of Illinois at Chicago, Fellow of the Belgian Academy of Science and Arts and Guest Professor of Social Sciences, University of Leuven. His current research is on disabled immigrants in Belgium.

Paul Atkinson is Distinguished Research Professor in Sociology at Cardiff University. He is an Academician of the Academy of the Social Sciences and a Fellow of the Institute of Welsh Affairs.

Jennifer Aylward is a recent graduate of the Health Research Methodology Master's programme at McMaster University. She is also pursuing studies in the McMaster Midwifery Education Program. Her research interests include the choice of place of birth for midwifery clients in Ontario.

Ivy Lynn Bourgeault is a Professor of Health Sciences at the University of Ottawa, the Canadian Institutes of Health Research Chair in Health Human Resource Policy and the Associate Director of the Community Health Research Unit.

Alex Broom is Senior Lecturer in Health Sociology, Faculty of Health Sciences, at the University of Sydney, Australia. His recent books include *Therapeutic Pluralism* (Routledge 2008) and *Men's Health: body, identity and social context* (Wiley 2009). He currently leads research projects in Australia, India, Sri Lanka and Brazil.

Caragh Brosnan is a Research Associate in the Centre for Biomedicine and Society at King's College London. While undertaking work on the *Handbook*, she was a Lecturer in Medical Education in the Medical School at Keele University. She completed her doctoral thesis, 'The Sociology of

Medical Education: the struggle for legitimate knowledge in two English medical schools', at the University of Cambridge in 2007. An earlier version of her chapter (Chapter 4) was presented at the International Sociological Association World Congress in Durban in 2006.

Brian Castellani is an Assistant Professor of Sociology at Kent State University and an Adjunct Professor of Psychiatry at Northeastern Ohio Universities College of Medicine. His research applies the latest advances in complexity science to the study of health and healthcare (see www.personal.kent.edu/~bcastel3/).

Neetu Chawla is a PhD student in the Department of Health Services at the UCLA School of Public Health. She is also affiliated with the Division of Cancer Prevention and Control Research at the UCLA Jonsson Comprehensive Cancer Center.

William C. Cockerham is Distinguished Professor of Sociology at the University of Alabama at Birmingham. He is President of the Research Committee on Health Sociology of the International Sociological Association. His most recent books include *Social Causes of Health and Disease* (Polity 2007) and *Medical Sociology*, 10th edn (Pearson Prentice-Hall 2007).

Oonagh Corrigan is a medical sociologist with an interest in bioethics. Before joining the University of Plymouth she held posts in Sociology at the University of Cambridge and in 2007–2008 was a Leverhulme Visiting Scholar at the Centre for Applied Ethics, University of British Columbia. She is currently a Senior Lecturer in Clinical Education Research at the Peninsula Medical School, University of Plymouth.

Raymond G. De Vries is a member of the Bioethics Program, the Department of Obstetrics and Gynecology and the Department of Medical Education at the Medical School, University of Michigan. He is the author of *A Pleasing Birth: midwifery and maternity care in the Netherlands* (Temple University Press 2005) and co-editor of *The View from Here: bioethics and the social sciences* (Blackwell 2007).

Sara Delamont is Reader in Sociology at Cardiff University. She is an Academician of the Academy of the Social Sciences. She was the first woman to be president of the British Education Research Association.

Michael D. Fetters serves as Associate Professor, Department of Family Medicine and Director, Japanese Family Health Program, University of Michigan Health System. His research interests focus on the interface of culture and medical decision-making.

Frederic W. Hafferty is Professor of Behavioral Sciences at the University of Minnesota Medical School–Duluth. He received his undergraduate degree in Social Relations from Harvard in 1969 and his PhD in Medical Sociology from Yale in 1976.

Carla C. Keirns is a Robert Wood Johnson Clinical Scholar at the University of Michigan. A physician trained in history, sociology and public health, she is completing a book on the history of asthma in the United States.

Heidi Lempp is a Post-Doctoral Research Fellow with Guy's and St Thomas' Foundation Trust/King's College London, National Institute for Health Research, Biomedical Research Centre, Academic Rheumatology, King's College London School of Medicine, and is a Visiting Research Fellow, Institute of Psychiatry, Department of Health Service and Population Research. She completed her PhD (Sociology) in 2004 on undergraduate medical education, University of London.

Margot L. Lyon is an anthropologist at the Australian National University. Her current theoretical interests are primarily focused on the study of social approaches to emotion, particularly in regard to how social–emotional processes constitute a crucial axis in the relationship between social and bodily domains.

Alan Petersen is Professor of Sociology in the School of Political and Social Inquiry, Faculty of Arts, Monash University, Melbourne. He has researched and published extensively in the fields of the sociology of health and illness, the sociology of new technologies and gender and society.

Ian Pinchen is a specialist in the sociology of health and illness with an interest in medical practice and health policy. During the 1990s he worked extensively as a research consultant in health policy before taking up a senior lectureship post at Anglia Ruskin University, Cambridge. He is currently a Lecturer in the Sociology of Health and Illness at the Peninsula Medical School, University of Plymouth.

Samantha Regan de Bere is a Lecturer in Medical Sociology at the Peninsula College of Medicine and Dentistry, Universities of Exeter and Plymouth. A sociologist by background, she has published several research papers and chapters on the role of clinical anatomy in medical education.

Elianne Riska is Professor of Sociology at the Swedish School of Social Science, University of Helsinki, Finland. She has examined the position of women physicians in *Medical Careers and Feminist Agendas: American, Scandinavian and Russian women physicians* (Aldine de Gruyter 2001).

Graham Scambler is Professor of Medical Sociology in the Research Department of Infection and Population Health at University College London. He has been teaching medical students and practitioners for over 30 years, has published widely on the sociology of health and illness and is editor of the textbook *Sociology as Applied to Medicine* (Saunders 2003), now in its sixth edition.

Fred C. J. Stevens is Associate Professor at the Department of Educational Development and Research, Maastricht University, the Netherlands. His interests and the focus of his recent publications include the division of labour of the health professions, healthcare manpower, professionalism and medical careers and the international comparison of healthcare systems.

Stefan Timmermans is Professor of Sociology at the University of California, Los Angeles. His research interests include medical technologies, death and dying and qualitative research methods. He is the author of *Sudden Death and the Myth of CPR* (Temple University Press 1999), *The Gold Standard* (with Marc Berg, Temple University Press 2003), and *Postmortem* (Chicago University Press 2006).

Bryan S. Turner was Professor of Sociology at the University of Cambridge (1998–2005) and at the National University of Singapore (2005–2009). He is currently the Alona Evans Distinguished Visiting Professor of Sociology at Wellesley College, US. He has published *The New Medical Sociology* (W. W. Norton 2004) and *The Body and Society* (Sage 2008).

Acknowledgements

The editors would like to thank Martin Richards and Darin Weinberg for being stimulating and supportive colleagues during their time in the Faculty of Social and Political Sciences at Cambridge.

Caragh Brosnan would like to thank the following bodies for the doctoral funding which enabled her to develop her work on the sociology of medical education: Australian Federation of University Women, Queensland; International Federation of University Women; Cambridge Political Economy Society Trust; Cambridge Board of Graduate Studies; and Magdalene College, Cambridge. She is also grateful for the support of staff at Keele Medical School where she worked from 2008–2009.

1 Introduction

The struggle over medical knowledge

Caragh Brosnan and Bryan S. Turner

Why a sociology of medical education?

> Embodied in the training of any profession are the profession's ideals about
> itself and its relations to the public. Answers to such questions as what work
> is worthwhile, which patients or clients are 'crocks' or 'duds', what treat-
> ment procedures are the best or worst, and how should professional work be
> organized are contained implicitly or explicitly in the training program.
>
> (Light 1980: x)

From the first emergence of medical sociology in the 1950s, medical education
enjoyed a central place on its research agenda (Hafferty 2000: 239), beginning
with the publication of Robert Merton *et al.*'s (1957) *The Student-Physician:
introductory studies in the sociology of medical education*. The sociology of
medical education had emerged, Merton explained, owing to a number of developments within medical education itself: the need to incorporate the expansion
of scientific knowledge within limited curricular time; the renewed focus on
treating 'the patient as a person' and the sense that sociology, though not well
understood within the medical profession, could play a role in developing this
aspect of practice; the development of systematic research into medical education; and innovations in medical curricula. Simultaneously, sociology was beginning to focus on the professions, organizations and adult socialization processes,
and was developing social-scientific research methods (Merton *et al.* 1957). *The
Student-Physician* aimed to showcase some early work applying sociological
methods to the study of medical education.

Howard Becker and his colleagues (1961) quickly followed Merton's team
with their publication of *Boys in White: student culture in medical school*, which
offered a critical interpretation of medical-student socialization to counter Merton's more conservative approach, and a lively theoretical and methodological
debate between the two perspectives ensued. However, despite an auspicious
beginning, in which for example Merton and colleagues were invited to address
the Association of American Medical Colleges (AAMC) (Hafferty 2000: 239),
the sociology of medical education has remained marginal to the discipline as a
whole, managing neither to influence medical education significantly, nor to

keep up with theoretical developments in the broader field of sociology. Hafferty (2007) notes that, 'What once helped to legitimate an emerging academic field (medical sociology) in the 1950s and 1960s has fallen on hard conceptual and analytic times.'

Meanwhile, the social factors which for Merton demanded the creation of a sociology of medical education 50 years ago have each continued to be salient: medical education continues to struggle to keep up with advances in scientific knowledge while at the same time trying to focus on 'the patient as a person'; consequently, medical curricula are in a continual process of transformation and reform. Medical sociology continues to focus on professions and organizational change, among other areas. In addition, since 1957, enormous changes have taken place in the wider society to healthcare and the medical profession, and to higher education. Each of these changes has had an impact on medical education, indicating its continuing relevance as an area of sociological enquiry.

While sociology has neglected medical education as a specific topic of research, medical education has emerged as a distinct discipline in its own right since the late twentieth century with its own journals, international conferences and professorial chairs. Medical schools often now employ dedicated medical education researchers, some of whom are social scientists. This development raises the question as to whether a *sociology* of medical education is actually required at all. There is certainly a considerable amount of overlap between sociology and medical-education studies. However, the strongest analytical focus of such educational studies is on questions surrounding the cognitive processes of learning and the effectiveness of specific educational techniques, with psychometric testing and surveys of medical students being the predominant research methods (although qualitative approaches are increasingly used) (Dimitroff and Davis 1996). Sociology, on the other hand, is orientated critically to consider the full spectrum of social processes shaping medical education, from student socialization to global health-policy changes, and draws from a wide range of theories and methods. Medical educationalists lament the fact that medical-education research tends towards repetition and opportunism (with the vast majority of studies being conducted within the researchers' own institutions) and lacks theoretical grounding, being directed towards users rather than to an academic audience (Albert *et al.* 2007; Schuwirth and van der Vleuten 2006). Furthermore, medicine's philosophical bias towards objectivity is carried through to research on medical education, which favours positivist models and often lacks critical reflexivity (Albert *et al.* 2007; Cribb and Bignold 1999). This is not to say that existing medical-education research cannot contribute towards a sociology of medical education, but that, without a more developed sociology of this area, many important issues will not be fully analysed and the field as a whole will not be developed in terms of a sophisticated theoretical framework.

A sociological approach can help to strengthen medical-education studies which aim to improve medical education; at the same time, medical education warrants sociological analysis for what it can tell us about society. Medical education can be seen as a crucible in which many of the questions central to sociology come to the foreground, involving as it does the socialization of professional groups, the interaction of institutions such as universities, hospitals, the medical profession and the state, the collaboration of different disciplinary groups, the production of knowledge and the construction of professional values. Important sociological work on medical education has in fact been conducted over the last few decades, but it has largely appeared as isolated journal articles or book chapters, rather than in a coherent collection, with the exception in 1988 of a special issue of the *Journal of Health and Social Behavior* (Colombotos 1988) which is still widely cited today. In fact, there have been no full-length research monographs providing an overview of the topic since the initial contribution of Merton and his colleagues in 1957. The studies published since have usually been based on ethnographic inquiries carried out in single medical schools – for example, Atkinson (1981), Becker *et al.* (1961), Hafferty (1991), Sinclair (1997) – which, while often examples of good sociology, have been too disparate to advance a clearly identifiable and coherent sociology of medical education. The *Handbook of the Sociology of Medical Education* aims to re-introduce the field, to demonstrate the distinctiveness of a sociological approach to the study of medical education, to provide an overview of key issues, both classical and contemporary, and to suggest future directions for the sociology of medical education and for medical education itself.

The remainder of this introduction considers the main areas of change since the establishment of a sociology of medical education, examining in turn, first, the need for new theoretical perspectives in the sociology of medical education; second, changes in health, healthcare and the medical profession; and finally, struggles over knowledge in medical curricula.

The need for new theoretical perspectives in the sociology of medical education

The first section of the *Handbook* presents three contributions to the conceptual analysis of medical education as a social process. Although the sociology of medical education was forged within one of the key debates in twentieth-century social theory – between structural functionalism (drawn on in *The Student-Physician*) and symbolic interactionism (developed in *Boys in White*) – it has remained somewhat disconnected from subsequent theoretical developments in sociology.

Functionalism tends to emphasize the importance of stability, asking how various social structures contribute to or function in relation to the maintenance of the whole. As a result, it is seen to presuppose somewhat conservative assumptions. By contrast, interaction looks at how social actors create and construct meaning and order in their everyday lives, and how these meanings constantly change and evolve. It is seen to be a more critical approach than functionalism. When in the 1970s medical sociology turned to a much more critical analysis of macro-level structures in healthcare and the inequalities these perpetuate, Renée Fox (1979: 97) lamented that sociologists had begun to emphasize the significance of medical practice and the constraints under which physicians work, de-emphasizing the 'anticipatory socialization' of the medical school years. Freidson's (1970 and 1972) influential work on the professional dominance of medicine fuelled this trend (Fox 1979), because his work concentrated on the structural organization of medical practice, rather than on medical training, as the key factor in determining physician behaviour. With the exception of a small body of feminist work on medical training around human reproduction (Davis-Floyd 1987; Kapsalis 2001; Scully 1980), the few studies of medical education since the 1970s have tended to defer to Merton *et al.* and Becker *et al.*, while the influence of political economy, post-structuralism and postmodernism has largely bypassed the sociology of medical education. This lack of theoretical development has led to and been perpetuated by a narrow empirical focus, with most studies continuing to centre on student socialization. The consequence has been to limit sociology's ability to unpack contemporary problems in medical education, many of which go well beyond the level of the individual student and involve the whole distribution of power in modern societies.

Chapters 2, 3 and 4 in the *Handbook* attempt to move beyond this impasse, each outlining a different theory of medical education. Fred Hafferty and Brian Castellani (Chapter 2) outline the origins of the theory of the 'hidden curriculum' – one of the most widely used concepts in medical education and the sociology of medical education. This concept refers to the notion that the formal and official curriculum is not the only way in which the student's education is shaped, because there is also an unofficial, hidden curriculum which moulds students' values. The authors critically examine how the concept has been used in medical education and develop a model for mapping the relationship of the hidden curriculum to other concepts in sociology. Both they and Heidi Lempp (Chapter 5) also discuss the utility of Erving Goffman's concepts of the 'presentation of self' and his dramaturgical perspective on social life in analysing medical-student socialization. In Chapter 3, Paul Atkinson and Sara Delamont argue for the application of sociologist of education Basil Bernstein's curricular codes to medical education. Taking the United Kingdom General Medical Council's curricular guidance, *Tomorrow's Doctors* (1993 and 2003), as their focus, they explain how the shifts in medical curricula which this document has attempted to instigate can helpfully be interpreted in Bernstein's terms.

Caragh Brosnan (Chapter 4) discusses how the division between structure and agency in studies of medical education may be overcome by following Pierre Bourdieu's mandate to 'think relationally' about individual practices and institutional politics. She suggests that Bourdieu's concepts of habitus and field, when applied together, point to the co-production of medical students' problematic attitudes towards practice and institutional challenges to curriculum reform. Bourdieu's influential theory of education, class and the reproduction of society, which implicates cultural practices in the perpetuation of power relations, is drawn on as a guiding framework in the *Handbook*. Bourdieu's work has been the major influence on our conceptualization of the medical curriculum as the site of struggles between the medical profession, the state, the public, medical schools, medical students and various academic disciplines. Throughout this collection, medical education is essentially viewed as a competition to legitimate various forms of individual, institutional, professional and political investments which Bourdieu calls 'capital'. In analysing what is at stake in this competition, each chapter considers both medical-educational practices and broader social shifts, and the relationships between them, offering a uniquely sociological perspective on medical education.

Much greater theoretical engagement with mainstream sociology is needed in the sociology of medical education, but these chapters may serve as a springboard for further work.

Changes in health, healthcare and the medical profession

Since Merton's identification of medical education as an important subject, there have been significant changes in the West to the types of illness medical students can expect to encounter, to the composition of professionals involved in healthcare and to the status of the medical profession. Epidemiological transitions, requiring new forms of healthcare, challenge biomedical dominance and create uncertainties in medical knowledge. In particular there have been major demographic changes in the population which have made chronic illness a more significant challenge for medical practice. Professional medicine, driven by high technology, has traditionally ignored these geriatric diseases which are difficult to treat and largely impossible to cure in favour of acute disease. Hence these prevalent but incurable diseases do not appear prominently if at all in the medical curriculum. Similarly disability – increasingly prevalent as the population ages, but affecting people at all stages of the life course – is not something medical students have traditionally been well prepared to deal with. To change this situation, Gary Albrecht (Chapter 7) argues that disabled people must comprise an integral part of the social networks of medical students, in the roles of fellow student, doctor, patient, administrator and so on. He believes that greater incorporation of disability into medical education will not only enable better healthcare for the disabled, but will help to engender holistic perspectives, a team approach and a focus on broad-based patient outcomes among the medical profession.

People suffering from chronic illness and/or disability often turn now to complementary and alternative medicine (CAM). CAM is occasionally in competition with allopathic practice and challenges the traditional medical model in which the patient is treated in isolation from his or her social and cultural environment. Medical practice based on the traditional medical model also tends to be invasive. While the needs of the elderly, the chronically sick and the disabled may be better served by CAM, it has not been fully accepted into medical education. Alex Broom and Jon Adams (Chapter 8) demonstrate that sociology is important in understanding the place of CAM in medical education, and that sociology can simultaneously be used to provide medical students with a critical perspective on the relationship between CAM and biomedicine. Their chapter includes specific recommendations for teaching about CAM in medical curricula.

There are other important changes that have a direct bearing on the context and character of medical education. There has been a significant growth in the number of medical students entering medical faculties in recent decades amid fears of doctor shortages. Another significant change is the feminization of medical education, with women now constituting the majority of medical students in many western countries, and therefore it is clearly time to reanalyse an area of sociology whose most-cited work is ironically called *Boys in White*. In her chapter, Elianne Riska considers the history and implications of increasing female enrolment, how gendered medical knowledge is currently represented in medical education, and the relationship between trainee career choices and gender imbalances both across specialties and across the hierarchy of the profession. A further change has been that the intake into medical schools is more ethnically diverse, reflecting the changing ethnic composition of the population as a whole. However, neither the academic contents of the medical curriculum nor the culture of medical training have changed to reflect or to address these social changes. Medical schools, as Lempp's contribution shows, remain deeply conservative institutions. Drawing on her empirical work in a British medical school, Lempp shows how staff exploited their power over medical students and often taught by a method involving humiliation. The pervasive hidden curriculum catered to white males, and this bias had a negative impact on ethnic minority students who consequently felt excluded and lacked professional role models.

Another important issue is that there has been a democratization of knowledge through the twentieth century with rising literacy, longer periods of schooling, greater access to knowledge through the internet and universal secondary education. As a result there is also a greater emphasis on access, transparency and openness. Patients are better informed about their conditions (particularly about chronic illnesses) and increasingly proactive. Hence the hierarchy between doctor and patient has been flattened. But at the same time, knowledge/information has expanded, becoming at the same time more fragmented. Therefore doctors must struggle to keep up with this explosion of knowledge. Clearly medicine has had to respond to increased demands from patients and patient-centredness is now part of many medical-school curricula.

These epidemiological and social changes have contributed to a reduction in the status of the medical profession. It has been argued that, while much of the twentieth century can be accurately described as a 'golden age of doctoring', in which the medical profession enjoyed almost unquestioned prestige and trust, this situation has now come to an end, owing to biomedicine's inability to cope with contemporary health problems, competition from CAM, the public's greater access to information and demands for better healthcare, and resource shortages in the health services (McKinlay and Marceau 2002; Turner 2004: 118). In the United Kingdom, a series of medical scandals at the turn of the twenty-first century, most notably the serial murders of General Practitioner Harold Shipman, raised doubts about the profession's ability to monitor itself. These events have seen a decrease in trust and an erosion of the autonomy of the medical profession, as evidenced, for example, by the advent of the British 'clinical governance' agenda and the rise of managed care in the United States. A characteristic of modern society more generally is the emphasis on accountability and hence on measurement. These changes are often described under the notion of 'the audit society' (Power 1997) which we can see reflected in changes to medical governance. The growth of evidence-based medicine (EBM) is an important part of these developments. In Chapter 9, Stefan Timmermans and Neetu Chawla review the literature to examine how and to what degree EBM has been integrated into medical education, how it has affected values surrounding uncertainty and autonomy in medical training and whether its place in medical curricula has actually resulted in better outcomes for patients.

Medical education is deeply involved in these social changes and in the challenges to medicine's status. Medicine's 'golden age' began with Abraham Flexner's famous report on the state of medical schools in the United States and Canada (Flexner 1910) which fuelled the worldwide proliferation of the science-based and research-driven medical curriculum. This curriculum was a key element in professional medicine's rise to power. Doctors were able to lay claim to an esoteric body of knowledge, one of the central requirements of professionalism, and on this basis they successfully gained state support and public trust (Freidson 1972). Just as medical education was instrumental in cementing the status of the medical profession, it has also been affected by the changes in medical governance. For example, the recent focus on 'competencies' and outcomes in medical education cross-nationally reflects attempts to render the profession more accountable. In Chapter 14, William Cockerham discusses the historical and current directions of medical education in the context of the evolving American healthcare system. Managed care is now the dominant style of practice in American healthcare centres associated with medical schools and teaching is no longer these schools' primary mission. Oonagh Corrigan and Ian Pinchen (Chapter 15) examine how challenges to the medical profession are manifested in changes to undergraduate and post-graduate medical education in the United Kingdom. Recent controversial attempts to standardize post-graduate training in the United Kingdom are an interesting example of struggles between the state and the profession over what training should consist of.

These chapters show how the changing field of medical practice, knowledge and institutions is having an impact on medical education. However, despite these changes, medical faculties are conservative and they have explicitly, and more frequently implicitly, resisted these changes. Medical students are taught in faculties that have to compete with natural science for funding and where academic status is rewarded by pure research activity. Medical faculties are therefore resistant to embracing social psychology, anthropology or sociology as disciplines that might have useful contributions to offer students. The implicit norms of 'heroic medicine' still inform the academic cultures of medical faculties. As a result the medical profession is struggling to accommodate social change while also seeking to preserve its professional privileges. The rise of courses on 'professionalism' in medical schools is an interesting development reflecting the decreased status of the medical profession and its urge to shore up professional autonomy for the future by explicitly inculcating particular attitudes among students (see Chapter 2 for further discussion on this).

Corrigan and Pinchen and Cockerham's chapters are included in Part III of the *Handbook*, examining medical education in national contexts.[1] One of our aims in this collection is to show how with globalization there are a number of common processes in the transformation of modern medical practice. Medicine played a core role in western colonialism and it has equally been caught up in struggles over neocolonialism. Western medical curricula and assessments were syndicated around the world without necessarily fitting the cultures in which they were implemented. The values inherent in these curricula have rarely been critically assessed by medical educators and hence further work is needed on postcolonial theory and medical education (Bleakley *et al.* 2008). A related issue is the current movement of international medical graduates from developing nations to high-income countries to fill physician shortages, partly brought about by the West's ageing population. Ivy Bourgeault and Jennifer Aylward (Chapter 16) analyse the ethical issues this migration raises, alongside the challenges to achieving medical workforce self-sufficiency in Canada. Barriers to training enough Canadian physicians include rising medical-school tuition fees, the increased length of and competition for medical training positions and a shortage of full-time medical faculty members.

In examining how globalization affects medical education, we need to keep in mind important differences between medical and educational systems, for instance between the United States and the United Kingdom. Cultural differences also play an important role. Fred Stevens (Chapter 17) considers why innovations in medical curricula have proliferated in some European countries (particularly the Netherlands) but not others, and contemplates the probable impact of the Bologna Declaration – stipulating the convergence of higher education systems across Europe – on medical schools. Stevens predicts that the competency-based medical education model will be conducive to European convergence and to the greater involvement of social sciences in medical curricula; however, it remains to be seen how such a development will interact with national cultures and systems of healthcare and educational governance. Global social changes will have varying effects on medical education, depending on national context.

Struggles over knowledge in medical curricula

A third focus of this collection is on the meaning of curricular change. In 1957 Merton listed a series of innovations in medical curricula that were instrumental in the rise of the sociology of medical education. The prevailing form of medical education worldwide at the time centred on the 'traditional curriculum', which, designed to further the biomedical sciences, consisted of a pre-clinical phase of two years of university-based training in the basic medical sciences (anatomy, physiology, biochemistry, pathology and so on), taught as separate disciplines and largely through didactic lectures, followed by two or three years of hospital-based clinical training in medical procedures, using bedside teaching techniques.

In the 1950s, in response to criticisms that the traditional curriculum involved too much emphasis on redundant science and failed to consider the social determinants of health, the first alternative medical-educational models began to emerge. *The Student-Physician* is based on studies of the innovative 'Comprehensive Care' programmes at Cornell, Colorado and Western Reserve universities in the United States, which integrated pre-clinical and clinical training, brought in the social sciences, and required students to follow the health needs of families within the community. While these particular programmes were short-lived, they marked the beginning of an era of medical curricular reform which has persisted ever since. As part of this movement of educational reform, most medical schools have moved to replace their traditional programmes with so-called 'innovative' or 'integrated' curricula which purport to overcome the pre-clinical/clinical divide, teaching science in the context of clinical problems and often involving some form of patient contact in the first two years. One of the most widespread innovations has been the introduction of problem-based learning (PBL), in which didactic teaching is replaced by self-directed learning; typically, small groups of students are presented with weekly paper-based patient cases from which they must derive their own learning objectives. The 1960s and 1970s also saw various non-biomedical disciplines find their way into medical curricula, notably the social and behavioural sciences along with bioethics.

Although reforms to the traditional curriculum have been taking place for half a century, they are not without controversy. There has been much recent publicity surrounding the phasing out of some traditional teaching methods, such as anatomical dissection, and there are widespread accusations over the supposed 'dumbing down' of curricula. Governmental and professional reforms continue to target both the form and content of medical education in the United Kingdom, United States, Canada, Australia and across Europe, yet there is little consensus concerning the direction which medical education should take. While many parties claim that medical education must be reformed in order to train practitioners who are able to respond to the healthcare needs of patients in the twenty-first century, others decry the changes which have already taken place, asserting that they are responsible for the erosion of medicine's knowledge base and professional autonomy. At the centre of these debates are questions about the character of knowledge as such: what type of knowledge distinguishes the medical profession from other groups? What sorts of knowledge are needed to produce a competent but caring doctor? These questions are being asked in an era when the status of medicine itself is contested, when interdisciplinary teaching and research is high on the policy agenda and when universities are increasingly forced to compete for research funding. The medical faculty with its traditional hierarchy of professors and specialists is confronted by a higher-education policy that has become more student-centred, again reflecting the democratization of knowledge in contemporary society.

Since Merton's time then, ongoing attempts at innovation in medical curricula have come to represent fundamental epistemological and social struggles. In Part II of the *Handbook*, four chapters examine the place of different types of knowledge within contemporary medical curricula. Samantha Regan de Bere and Alan Petersen question the state of anatomy teaching in the British system. As a traditional cornerstone of medical education, anatomy instruction has undergone some of the most profound reforms of all in recent decades. Regan de Bere and Petersen use an approach that is taken from the work of the French social philosopher Michel Foucault to unpack the rhetoric of 'crisis' and 'renaissance' which has accompanied these changes. While medical curricular reform has challenged the position of traditional disciplines such as anatomy, it has enabled new disciplines to flourish. In Chapter 11, Carla Keirns, Michael Fetters and Raymond De Vries outline the emergence of bioethics and discuss its current position in American medical schools, when and how bioethics is taught in medical curricula and what topics are covered (finding there is little consistency among schools). They then interpret these changes through a sociological lens, arguing that bioethics serves an effective legitimating rather than critical role in medical education at a time when medical practice appears increasingly to alienate rather than comfort patients.

Renée Fox (1997) notes that bioethics has recently overtaken social-science teaching in many medical schools. While bioethics is more closely aligned to medical professional interests, sociology has often been considered 'downright subversive' by the medical establishment (Stacey 1992: 112). In Chapter 12, Graham Scambler reflects on the past and present position of sociology in British medical education, through a case study of the London Hospital Medical Schools. He identifies four historic phases of 'innovation', 'consolidation', 'rationalization', and the current 'corporate' phase which have seen medical sociologists assimilated and thereby tamed within medical schools. Scambler interprets these shifts through the theories of Jürgen Habermas's system colonization of the life-world, George Ritzer's McDonaldization thesis, and postmodern theory. Essentially, Chapters 10 to 13 address one of the central questions for the sociology of medical education, namely what counts as legitimate knowledge within medical curricula? While this varies across time and place, forms of knowledge within medical curricula (and more generally) are typically framed as being either 'hard' or 'soft' and either 'scientific' or 'technical', with hard, scientific knowledge most often having the greater legitimacy. Margot Lyon (Chapter 13) puts forward a critique of these epistemological distinctions in medical education, while discussing an innovative course within a problem-based medical curriculum in Australia which strives to enable students to confront and question their assumptions about the epistemological basis of medicine. By encouraging students to reflect on the structure of knowledge systems, 'The Social Foundations of Medicine' course aims to make for better teaching of the science of medicine. Lyon's chapter provides at the same time a new critique of current medical education and PBL, an original set of curricular materials that attempts to address the problem within a PBL curricular structure and an explanation of why these materials are of use.

The continual evolution of medical curricula is a fruitful area for sociological analysis. Samuel Bloom concluded in 1988 that twentieth-century attempts to remedy the scientific reductionism of the traditional medical curriculum had amounted to 'reform without change'. The impact of medical curricular change is just one of many questions which it is time for sociologists to revisit. There are also many new questions to be asked. Our *Handbook* asks and answers some of them, but more importantly it attempts to reinvigorate the sociology of medical education and to provide the intellectual impetus for sustained theoretical and empirical engagement with the topic. The university medical faculty is a powerful and prestigious institution, providing training for students who will occupy not only a key position in the nation's income distribution, but who will become a significant social elite bound together and represented by respected professional associations. Medical science has been at the forefront of modern science as such and medical students can expect to share in that prestige. As a result medical faculties are resistant to social and educational change. It is our hope that this *Handbook* may make a modest contribution to the debate about the nature and function of medical education which in turn may contribute to the more effective care and treatment of patients.

Note

1 Note also that throughout the *Handbook* authors have used the terms appropriate to their own country, so that British and Australian authors refer to the highest stratum of practising doctors as 'consultants', while for North American authors they are 'attendings'. Medicine is a post-graduate degree in the United States and all doctors receive an MD as their basic medical qualification, whereas most British and Australian medical students are undergraduates who receive a Bachelor of Medicine and Bachelor of Surgery, with only a small number pursuing the post-graduate MD.

References

Albert, M., Hodges, B. and Regehr, G. (2007) 'Research in medical education: balancing service and science', *Advances in Health Sciences Education*, 12: 103–15.

Atkinson, P. (1981) *The Clinical Experience: the construction and reconstruction of medical reality*, Farnborough: Gower.

Becker, H., Geer, B., Hughes, E. and Strauss, A. (1961) *Boys in White: student culture in medical school*, Chicago, IL: University of Chicago Press.

Bleakley, A., Brice, J. and Bligh, J. (2008) 'Thinking the post-colonial in medical education', *Medical Education*, 42: 266–70.

Bloom, S. (1988) 'Structure and ideology in medical education: an analysis of resistance to change', *Journal of Health and Social Behavior*, 29: 294–306.

Colombotos, J. (ed.) (1988) 'Theme: continuities in the sociology of medical education', special issue of *Journal of Health and Social Behavior*, 29 (4).

Cribb, A. and Bignold, S. (1999) 'Towards the reflexive medical school: the hidden curriculum and medical education research', *Studies in Higher Education*, 24: 195–209.

Davis-Floyd, R. (1987) 'Obstetric training as a rite of passage', *Medical Anthropology*, 1: 288–318.

Dimitroff, A. and Davis, W. (1996) 'Content analysis of research in undergraduate medical education', *Academic Medicine*, 71: 60–7.

Flexner, A. (1910) *Medical Education in the United States and Canada: bulletin number four*, New York: Carnegie Foundation for the Advancement of Teaching.

Fox, R. (1979) *Essays in Medical Sociology: journeys into the field*, New York: John Wiley & Sons.

Freidson, E. (1970) *Professional Dominance: the social structure of medical care*, New York: Atherton Press.

—— (1972) *Profession of Medicine: a study of the sociology of applied knowledge*, New York: Dodd Mead.

General Medical Council (GMC) (1993) *Tomorrow's Doctors: recommendations on undergraduate medical education*, London: General Medical Council.

—— (2003) *Tomorrow's Doctors: recommendations on undergraduate medical education*, London: General Medical Council.

Hafferty, F. (1991) *Into the Valley: death and the socialization of medical students*, New Haven, CT: Yale University Press.

—— (2000) 'Reconfiguring the sociology of medical education: emerging topics and pressing issues', in C. Bird, P. Conrad and A. Fremont (eds) *Handbook of Medical Sociology*, 5th edn, London: Prentice Hall.

—— (2007) 'Medical school socialization', in G. Ritzer (ed.) *Blackwell Encyclopedia of Sociology*, Blackwell Reference Online, online at www.blackwellreference.com/subscriber/tocnode?id=g9781405124331_chunk_g978140512433119_ss1–74 (accessed October 2008).

Kapsalis, T. (2001) *Public Privates: performing gynecology from both ends of the speculum*, London: Duke University Press.

Light, D. (1980) *Becoming Psychiatrists: the professional transformation of self*, New York: W. W. Norton & Co.

McKinlay, J. and Marceau, L. (2002) 'The end of the golden age of doctoring', *International Journal of Health Services*, 32: 379–416.

Merton, R. (1957) 'Some preliminaries to a sociology of medical education', in R. Merton, G. Reader and P. Kendall (eds) *The Student-Physician: introductory studies in the sociology of medical education*, Cambridge, MA: Harvard University Press.

Merton, R., Reader, G. and Kendall, P. (eds) (1957) *The Student-Physician: introductory studies in the sociology of medical education*, Cambridge, MA: Harvard University Press.

Power, M. (1997) *The Audit Society: rituals of verification*, Oxford: Oxford University Press.

Schuwirth, L. and van der Vleuten, C. (2006) 'Challenges for educationalists', *British Medical Journal*, 333: 544–6.

Scully, D. (1980) *Men Who Control Women's Health: the miseducation of obstetrician-gynecologists*, Boston, MA: Houghton Mifflin Company.

Sinclair, S. (1997) *Making Doctors: an institutional apprenticeship*, Oxford: Berg.

Stacey, M. (1992) *Regulating British Medicine: the General Medical Council*, Chichester: Wiley.

Turner, B. (2004) *The New Medical Sociology: social forms of health and illness*, London: W. W. Norton & Co.

Part I
Theoretical perspectives

2 The hidden curriculum

A theory of medical education

Frederic W. Hafferty and Brian Castellani

Preface

It is 30 June and a new crop of interns has gathered to hear the Fish (Chief Resident and 'permanent Slurper'), Leggo (Chief of Medicine), the Pearl (an Attending), Dr Frank (the House psychiatrist), and other House representatives describe how things work (for example, parking, rounding schedules) and the values (for instance, covert autopsies) that govern the House of God. Amid this flurry of advice and information, the Fish and Dr Frank direct their trainees to seek their counsel if the demands of the House proved too formidable. However well intentioned, this edict contained several tacit messages: all problems are personal; organizational structures and practices are inviolate; trainees adapt and cope. In *The House of God* (Shem 1978) a book that is one of medicine's great primers on medical education's hidden curriculum (via Laws of the House of God, the Fat Man, and a montage of other emblematic characters and settings), this particular injunction slips by unnoticed – most certainly by the speakers (who are sincere if ritualized in what they say), but also by the interns who will not appreciate its normative undercurrents until long after the House began to exact its terrible toll. The hidden curriculum, after all, is most effective when it appears innocuous, innocent, and invisible.

Introduction

> ...the first wisdom of sociology is this: things are not what they seem.... Social reality turns out to have many layers of meaning. The discovery of each new layer changes the perception of the whole.
>
> (Berger 1963: 23)

In this chapter we examine the hidden curriculum as a theoretical construct using medical education as our template. To this end, we briefly introduce three natural histories, a case study and a futuristic scenario. The histories track the hidden curriculum as a theoretical construct within the literatures of education, medical education and sociology, in that order. In addition, and to better situate the hidden curriculum within the broader framework of sociology, we develop a conceptual map linking the hidden curriculum to a host of other sociological concepts that address issues of social relations, group dynamics and interpersonal change. The case study examines medicine's modern-day professionalism movement. The future scenario involves our attempt to link the hidden curriculum to systems theory and complexity science.

Critical to understanding the above materials is our distinction between the hidden curriculum as an overall theoretical framework (HC), and the hidden curriculum as one particular process of student learning (for example, the messages conveyed about core organizational values that are embedded within medical-school award ceremonies) that unfolds within the complex milieu of medical education. This distinction between theory and process is often obscured in the medical-education literature. Scholars frequently use the term 'hidden curriculum' to represent/symbolize one half of a dichotomy (the formal versus the hidden) in which lessons learned outside the formal stand in some opposition to what is being acquired within the curriculum-as-stated, or what Martin (1976) labels the 'curriculum proper'. While this framing of formal and hidden as polar opposites possesses a certain heuristic appeal, it also collapses a large number of heterogeneous types of learning processes into a single conceptual category, thus limiting our understandings of medical training as a complex social system. To move past this dichotomous roadblock, we employ the symbol 'HC' when talking about the theory as a whole and 'hc' when we explore one particular type or subset of learning that exists within that overall theoretical framework.

The HC and theories of education

> Hidden curriculum refers to messages communicated by the organization and operation of schooling apart from the official or public statements of school mission and subject area curriculum guidelines.... The messages of hidden curriculum usually deal with attitudes, values, beliefs and behavior.
>
> (Berger 1963)

The HC has its most extensive natural history within the education literature. As both a concept and theoretical framework, material on the HC routinely appears in education textbooks, encyclopaedias and journals. Historically, the HC traces its conceptual roots to Philip Jackson's 1968 volume *Life in Classrooms*. While this attribution is technically correct, it is somewhat misleading. Jackson did use the term in his study of student learning and did frame (à la Durkheim) school-based learning within an overall process of socialization. Nonetheless, the phrase appears only twice in this volume, once on pages 33–4 and once on the inside flap of the dust jacket. Instead, a more nuanced (if psychiatrically oriented) development of this concept would have to wait until Benson Snyder published his 1971 comparison of student life at MIT and Wellesley College. Snyder, a physician and psychotherapist, wanted to explore the dissonance students experienced as they negotiated the space between what each school formally required of its students versus the more tacit cues students picked up about what their school 'really' expected of them (something Snyder defined as the 'emotional and social surround of the formal curriculum' (p. 4)). Among other things, Snyder concluded that student success was determined less by academic prowess than by the ability of students to navigate the space between these two sets of expectations, and then to engage faculty in strategic gamesmanship based on these nuances. Moreover, the burden of having to negotiate this space also produced feelings of hypocrisy and cynicism in students. Snyder considered the ability to navigate these waters to be a skill and one not equally available across racial and ethnic lines. In a point we will revisit, Snyder drew upon the conceptual terminology of social ecology because he wanted to emphasize the interdependence of social actors and their surroundings, and thus the need (as we will argue) to address issues of the HC in terms of complexity and systems thinking.

Over time, the HC has undergone several waves of theoretical reframing within the education literature. Early treatments of the HC, focusing on K-12 education, adopted an uncritical functionalist perspective in noting how schools can operate as agents of social control via the teaching of 'virtues' such as patience, docility and respect for authority. Later writings were more Marxist in orientation with schools depicted as operating in the service of dominant sociopolitical and capitalist interests and by reproducing pre-existing relations of social class and power. Still later writings on the HC adopted more of a symbolic interactionist perspective by stressing the active participation of students in resisting dominant (if tacit) messages of social inequality and in creating countervailing forces such as student subcultures. Howard Becker and colleagues would employ this latter interpretive framework in their famous *Boys in White* study (Becker *et al.* 1961). Work on the HC peaked between the 1970s through the 1990s. While the concept remains widely used in the education literature, it has also been labelled a mythical social force and an irrelevant social construct (Lakomski 1988) – claims that have generated considerable debate within the education community (for instance, Eisner 1992).

Finally, and as a historical note, an awareness that learning involves more than formal pedagogy substantially predates Jackson and Snyder. Cotton Mather (1663–1728), for example, proposed a 'collegiate way of living' at Harvard as he advocated bridging the formal learning of the classroom with the more informal exchanges that emerge among students. Similarly, John Dewey's (1859–1952) concept of collateral learning, and William Heard Kilpatrick's (1871–1965) concepts of primary, associate and concomitant learning, depict teaching and learning as distinctive social phenomena.

The HC curriculum and medical education

If one wants to find out how a modern American city is governed, it is very easy to get the official information about this subject.... However, it would be an exceedingly naive person who would believe that this kind of information provides a rounded picture of the political reality of that community. The sociologist will want to know also the constituency of the 'informal

power structure'. When sociologists study power, they 'look behind' the
official mechanisms supposed to regulate power in the community.

(Berger 1963: 32)

Introduction

The HC is a relatively recent arrival in medical-education literature. Most contemporary publications in medical education date the HC to a 1994 article by
Hafferty and Franks. However, the concept was first applied to medical education more than a decade earlier by sociologists Jack Haas and William Shaffir in
their study of the new McMaster medical-school curriculum (Haas and Shaffir
1982). In this study, the authors employed a symbolic interactionist perspective
to examine student socialization and how students sought to create a 'cloak of
competence' via ritualized practices of impression management in their dealings
with faculty. Although Haas and Shaffir used the HC as an interpretive tool, they
did not extend or develop it as a theoretical construct – in spite of using the term
in their title.

Over the past 15 years, the hidden curriculum (HC) has become somewhat of
a buzzword within the medical literature. Both PubMed and ISI Web of Science
track articles using the HC as a keyword. Medical journals from education and
ethics to clinical orthopaedics, internal medicine, oncology and healthcare analysis, have highlighted the role of the HC in medical work and professional acculturation. The HC has also been featured in the nursing, physical therapy,
dentistry, emergency medicine and dietetics literatures, and across countries
such as the US, Canada, the UK, Australia and New Zealand. Special sessions
have been organized at national and international meetings, and efforts are
underway to measure its dimensions and impact (sponsored by organizations
such as the National Board of Medical Examiners (NBME) and the American
Board of Internal Medicine (ABIM)). Most recently, the Liaison Committee for
Medical Education (LCME) has used the concept (see below) to develop a new
medical-school accreditation standard. Within this broad and evolving set of
literature and educational practices, the HC is most often linked to issues of professionalization and professional socialization and to calls for a 'fundamental
change' or 'paradigm shift' in the organizational and occupational culture of
medical schools.

Over time, the HC has assumed a rather ubiquitous presence within the
medical-education literature. The Association of American Medical Colleges'
(AAMC) flagship journal *Academic Medicine* has published 73 articles employing this concept since 1994. A somewhat atypical and yet illustrative example is
a recent (November 2007) issue of *Academic Medicine* largely devoted to the
issue of professionalism. The issue includes a thematic overview by the editor,
three lead articles (the first by medical students on the disconnects in medical
training, the second by a leading physician–writer on medical professionalism,
and the third by the outgoing president of the AAMC), a research paper on peer
evaluation and professionalism, and case materials from nine medical schools.

All three lead articles and six (Vanderbilt, McGill, North Dakota, Mayo, Indiana, Chicago) of the nine school-specific articles draw upon the HC to advance their arguments. The three that did not (Pennsylvania, New York University and University of Washington) employed related concepts such as organizational culture, the informal curriculum and/or appreciative enquiry in their discussions on the creation of a new 'culture of professionalism'.

This growth notwithstanding, most authors who employ the HC use it as a sensitizing concept, making only minor attempts to develop it as a theoretical construct. When using the concept, most authors stress the theme of 'disconnects' – be that a disconnect between:

1   What is taught in the basic science versus clinical years.
2   What is taught in 'the classroom' versus 'the clinic'.
3   What role models preach and what they practice.
4   How formal organizational policies are transformed on the shop floor.

Overall, the HC is framed as having a negative impact on student learning – by promoting something bad (such as cynicism) or in preventing something good (such as professionalism). In association with, and in a partial outgrowth of, this literature, educators have begun to call for major changes in the structure, process and content of medical training (using terms like 'fundamental' or 'paradigm shift') in order to transform a faculty-centric emphasis on teaching to a student-centric emphasis on learning (see Hafferty and Watson 2006 for an examination linking the HC to learning communities).

In contrast to this thematic and reform-focused literature, there is a relatively small movement to assess the content, process and the products/outcomes of the HC. Notable efforts include work by Haidet and colleagues (Haidet *et al.* 2005), along with some preliminary efforts by the National Board of Medical Examiners (NBME) and the ABIM Foundation to measure the impact of the HC. Most striking (in terms of immediate impact) is the LCME's new (July 2008) accreditation standard (MS-31-A) that requires medical schools to 'ensure that the learning environment for medical students promotes the development of explicit and appropriate professional attributes (attitudes, behaviours, and identity) in their medical students'. This standard calls for medical schools to take responsibility for student learning – as opposed to faculty teaching – and is an obvious work in progress. How medical schools will attempt to meet this standard, including how the LCME responds to their efforts, will be grist for medical educators – and sociologists.

A shift in perspective: the popularization of the HC as an analytic tool

The fact that the HC fell on deaf ears within the medical-education community in the 1980s, yet attained cult-like status a decade later, invites an obvious question: 'What changed?' While singular answers are always suspect, one primary shift was organized medicine's discovery of its own 'crisis of professionalism'. Although medicine's status as a profession has been studied by sociologists since the late 1800s, and while sociology had been documenting medicine's loss of professional status since the late 1960s, organized medicine did not itself begin to acknowledge, and critically reflect on, its fall from professional grace until the early 1990s (Hafferty and Castellani 2008). The HC, in turn, became one tool by which medical educators sought to understand this fall.

Medicine's self-perceived crisis of professionalism represented a conundrum for medical educators. On the one hand (and according to the prevailing discourse of medical educators), medical schools were continuing to train 'excellent physicians'. On the other hand, evidence had begun to accumulate that the public-at-large no longer perceived medicine as having an unwavering commitment to public service. The rise of corporate medicine, the emergence of a medical marketplace (a relatively new term), Wall Street's discovery of healthcare as an object of capital investment, and even the growth of the academic health centre (AHC) as a research enterprise and the marginalization of the medical school's teaching mission in favour of emergent research and clinical enterprises, all helped to highlight medicine as an occupation that had 'lost its way'.

Medicine's acknowledgement of this crisis began to alter the way medical educators framed the nature of their work. It was not that educators had been altogether blind to the negative aspects of physician training. Studies documenting the loss of idealism and the rise of cynicism have long been a staple of medical-education research. So too are studies documenting a loss of moral reasoning and patient-centred skills by students during training. Other studies tracked the seemingly trenchant presence of medical-student abuse (termed 'bullying' in the UK medical-education literature). Persistent evidence of medicine's failure to recruit and train non-majority students only added to the picture of medical schools as negative and/or dysfunctional learning environments.

If evidence about medical training's dark side was nothing new, why are today's medical leaders calling for a shift in physician education at the level of organizational and institutional culture – something quite different from the decades of initiatives Bloom (1988) once characterized as 'reform without change'? What has shifted, we feel, is not the discovery of 'new' sins or even the accumulation of some critical mass of old transgressions, but rather a reframing of the meaning and import of long-accepted educational practices. Two factors have contributed to this conversion. First, new information technologies began to emerge to study healthcare quality – and thus new data sets from which to frame the consequences of medical-learning environments (be they school-based or the workplace). Second, and equally important, educators needed a new way of thinking about that training, something that held both face validity but would also be palatable (and thus reassuring) to those who were, after all, captains of the old (and sinking) ship. One such reframing was the HC. Thus, when researchers began to accumulate data in the 1990s documenting the widespread presence of health disparities in the diagnosis and treatment of disease, the fact that only 50 per cent of patients were likely to get recommended medical care, that medical errors were killing upwards of 100,000 patients per year in the US, and the presence of considerable conflicts-of-interest (COI) within medical practice and research ranks – and when medical education's long-standing defence ('yes-but-we-still-produce-the-best-doctors-in-the-world') began to crumble as the product of medical education came under increased scrutiny (and criticism) – the HC was there to fill the conceptual (and reassurance) void.

What turned out to be both conceptually assuaging and organizationally palatable for educators was a particular reading of the HC that emphasized that there was *another* curriculum at work – a 'hidden curriculum'. The problem (according to medical education's evolving discourse on the HC) was not the formal educational experience, but rather a subterrestrial set of factors that were hindering the formal curriculum from doing the job it was designed (by these very same medical educators) to do. The logic of the HC (again as constructed within medicine) was both reasonable and palatable – if ultimately self-serving.

If medical education was indeed buffeted by a self-defined crisis of identity and structure, and if indeed reform was needed at the level of culture, then the HC became the perfect oil to pour upon these troubled waters. There was, however, more than self-serving discourse at work. The slowly evolving realization that there was far more to medical education than the formal curriculum provided educators with an analytical framework from which to reconsider decades of data detailing the loss of student idealism, the rise of cynicism, the persistent (and troubling) presence of medical student abuse, the actual loss of moral reasoning skills and the failure of medical education to correct long-standing deficiencies in the recruitment and training of non-majority students. Some educators began to acknowledge that 'trying harder', admitting 'better' students, and/or adding more ethics courses to an already overburdened curriculum were not going to do the trick. Somehow the entire educational enterprise had to be reconceptualized. It is at this point of reconceptualization that we find medical education today.

Some issues of concern

There are some points of caution in this story of rediscovery and reclamation. For example, the LCME's new accreditation standard explicitly frames the HC (relabelled as 'learning environments') solely in terms of professionalism and this rather narrow focus limits the applicability of HC theory to broader issues of medical training. After all, the tacit lessons students learn during training are not limited to issues of ethics, patient communication or COI. For example, the science that faculty teach medical students is a fundamentally different science than what these same faculty teach to their graduate students. The difference is not a matter of amount (with medical students receiving 'the same but less'). Rather, medical students are taught a science of absolutes and certainties. Graduate students, meanwhile, are presented by these same faculty with a science grounded in uncertainties, ambiguities, probabilities and nuances. In short, while the HC is an important vehicle for teaching professionalism, it is also essential in conveying information to students about what it means to be a physician.

A second concern is how the LCME characterizes the HC. The LCME treats the HC as a dichotomous variable composed of a formal and 'informal' curriculum, the latter being shaped by 'informal lessons' that unfold as students interact with others. Within the HC literature, this distinction highlights that space between what the organization says is happening within its formal curriculum and the lessons students learn in the unscripted, idiosyncratic interactions that take place between students and faculty or students and their peers in the cafeteria, hallways, elevators, and/or on-call rooms (Hafferty 1998). One problem with this particular division is that it ignores the organization – and thus that space between what a medical school says it does (via its formal pronouncements, practices and policies) and how that school conducts 'business' on an everyday basis. In short, this new LCME standard ignores the hc and directs faculty (who are, after all responsible for meeting LCME accreditation standards) to focus on individuals (faculty and students) while ignoring the school as an operational force.

One possible downside of this marginalization is that medical educators (and administrators) may come to mimic a common medical-student coping device – and thus focus more on 'the test' than on what really needs to be accomplished. With schools being held responsible only for their formal and informal curriculum, medical educators may fail to examine (in terms of learning environments) the overall allocation of resources to the teaching, research and clinical service missions of the medical school, the actual formation of school COI policies versus their implementation and enforcement, or how the overall profile of medical-student or faculty awards sends messages to students and faculty about what is truly meritorious and 'award-worthy' within the organizational culture of a given school. Nor may schools be encouraged to imagine how the underlying value structure of the school itself, the overall structure of the curriculum (for example, patterns in the types of courses deemed required versus elective, or what courses or faculty get the prime times for class), or how a school's physical plant and architectural layout might contribute (in positive or negative ways) to student learning experiences. Nonetheless, the fact that medical educators will now be responsible (in ways yet to be determined) for more than what they teach is a notable step in making the HC more visible.

The HC as a dichotomous variable: extending the concept

The tendency of medical educators to frame the HC as a dichotomy (formal vs. informal) is more than limiting. It is also conceptually incorrect. The HC and the informal curriculum are not synonyms. While considerable student learning takes place within social networks, this is not the only 'alternative' site/source of learning. The education literature, for example, identifies a number of different ways to deconstruct student learning. Wilson and Wilson identify eight different types of curricula (overt, societal, hidden, null, phantom, concomitant, rhetorical and curriculum-in-use) (Wilson and Wilson 2007). Goodlad and colleagues identify five (ideal/ideological, formal, perceived, operational, experienced) (Goodlad *et al.* 1979), while Coles and Grant (1985) identify seven (using a Venn diagram of three overlapping circles). One notable example of an altern- ative curriculum is the null curriculum – or what gets learned when something is *not* mentioned (Eisner 1985). Our point here is neither to enumerate all possible learning modalities, nor to introduce new labels even for the sake of valid refine- ments, but rather to underscore that student learning is a multidimensional process – and one that is not well served by reducing complex social processes and a complex social system (medical education) to a dichotomy.

A related issue involves accessibility – this time the accessibility of the parti- cipants (faculty and students) to the learning processes taking place around them. Within the medical education literature, the hc has been linked to the concept of organizational socialization and organizational culture – the latter focusing on how new recruits 'learn the ropes' and come to understand 'the way things happen around here'. For example, Edgar Schein conceptualizes organizational culture as unfolding across three dimensions:

1 Artefacts.
2 Espoused values.
3 Basic assumptions and values.

(Schein 1992)

While artefacts (for example, dress, course syllabuses) are surface phenomena, quite visible yet difficult to interpret (their meaning to insiders may be quite dif- ferent from their meaning to outsiders), and while Schein's treatment of espoused values has important similarities to our formal curriculum, Schein con- siders the core of any culture to be represented by its basic or underlying values. Many of these values, however, reside at an unconscious or unexamined level, and thus are not readily available (if at all) to the immediate social actors. This unavailability represents a challenge to educators who call for change at the level of organizational culture. How exactly is this to take place? For students, medical training is fundamentally a process of identity change and personal transformation – something that unfolds, in many respects, at a subconscious or unreflexive level. While faculty and administrators may indeed have their fingers on the pulse of the formal curriculum, they too have only limited access to student subcultures, and to their own assumptions about how their medical school actually works – as opposed to how they feel it is (formally) supposed to work. In short, much of what goes on in a medical school is not readily accessi- ble to its inhabitants – unless promoted by direct (and often outside) questions and/or when 'jostled' by an unanticipated and unusual event. Nonetheless, medical educators continue to call for a 'culture change' and link this type/level of change to the HC.

Because the overall medical literature on the HC tends to bifurcate student learning into formal versus HC (thus lumping together the informal and HC), and because the LCME tends to focus on the formal versus the informal curriculum (leaving aside the hc), we find it helpful to:

1   Differentiate among *at least* three curricula (formal, informal and hidden).
2   Take particular care to differentiate between the informal and the hc.
3   Add other types of learning (for example, null) as needed for the deconstruction of student learning.

Second, we strongly suggest that the labels formal, informal, hidden and so on, not be unyieldingly linked to given settings, situations or roles. Although the medical literature frequently labels 'the classroom' as formal and 'the clinic' as informal, the classroom (as a physical place) can (and almost always does) contain all kinds of curricula (informal, hidden, null and so forth), just as the clinic can be a site of many important formal learning opportunities. Similarly, if the student handbook states, 'medical student well-being is our primary concern', then student well-being is a part of that school's formal curriculum. The HC, in turn, asks how this value statement is operationalized/manifested within school practices and policies. Conversely, while issues of 'lifestyle', 'balance' and 'student-centredness' currently have a high profile within medical education, what if a given student handbook fails to mention any of these themes? Perhaps what we have here is an instance of a null curriculum at work?

Role models are another example. Although role models have long functioned for students as an important source of tacit learning, the implicit nature of this learning changes if a given school:

1   Identifies 'role models' as a critical resource for student learning.
2   Establishes formal expectations for those faculty around this form of student learning.
3   Develops training modules to advance faculty skills in role modelling.
4   Employs assessment tools to monitor faculty performance as role models, then this school is treating role models as a part of their formal curriculum.

In fact, the recent move toward 'mentors' and mentoring programmes within medical education circles reflects a shift from something (role models) that has long functioned outside the formal curriculum to something (mentors) that fits more squarely within the formal curriculum. Role models, after all, need not even know they are considered as such by another. Mentors, however, cannot hide behind this form of social distance.

As our final example, while a medical school may announce, with great enthusiasm and sincerity, that it offers its students an 'integrated curriculum', it sends an altogether countervailing message when students are told to answer test questions based not on any sense of integration but rather on who wrote the question. In short, the potential to say one thing and do another is omnipresent within both organizational structures and social relations and thus it is a mistake to link particular settings or situations to particular types of curricula. The HC is about layers of learning and about systems of influence. A penchant for labelling X as 'formal' (in some overarching sense), Y as 'informal' and/or Z as 'hidden' often gets in the way of untangling medical student learning as a dynamic and integrated process.

The HC and sociological theory

The HC, as a formal construct, has virtually no presence within the sociological literature – and this despite the fact that many sociological concepts can be directly and indirectly tied to the HC. Even the presence of the HC within the general education literature matters little within sociology. The sociology of education is a well-established subdiscipline within sociology. Nonetheless, neither the *Sociology of Education* nor the *British Journal of Educational Studies*, both sociology of education journals, contain a single article whose primary focus is the HC – the *British Journal of Educational Studies*' primary contribution to this literature being a 2002 book review (50, 3: 393–5) of Eric Marolis's *The Hidden Curriculum in Higher Education*.

Nonetheless, and as captured in the quotes by Peter Berger that headline the previous two sections of this chapter, sociology is all about the HC. The distinction between formal and informal social norms or between official workplace rules and the more informal normative practices that govern work on the shop floor directly speak to the difference between the formal curriculum and other types (for instance, hidden, informal, null and so on) of learning. Also relevant are the sociological literatures on occupational culture, socialization and identity formation, the transformation from out-group to in-group status, interaction rituals and/or the differences that exist between surface (or manifest) social phenomena versus the 'deep structures', the 'underlying grammars', 'cultural codes', or the 'generative rules' that underscore social action. Finally, we note how everyday social action, because of its mundane and taken-for-granted nature, readily unfolds beneath the reflective radar of individuals and therefore exerts its influences at a pre-, sub-, or unconscious level. The great bulk of social life, after all, is rendered opaque by its very ubiquity.

One way to illustrate the centrality of the HC to sociological theory is to develop a conceptual map illustrating key links between sociology and the HC. Conceptual maps are useful visual tools for demonstrating the intellectual relationships among a given set of theoretical terms and/or ideas. In this respect, conceptual maps are encyclopaedias, not dictionaries. Instead of defining a term, they position each concept relative to other similar concepts. Conceptual maps are a type of network comprised of nodes (terms, theoretical ideas, concepts and so forth) and the links among them (direct ties, indirect ties, weak ties, strong ties), which, when positioned in two-dimensional Euclidian space, result in a measurable map that can be mined for important information.

To create our map, we first combed through several sociology dictionaries and encyclopaedias to create an exhaustive list of sociological terms we felt had something to do with either the spirit or specifics of the HC. For example, latent and manifest functions relate to the spirit of the HC, while secondary socialization relates to the HC's mechanics. Our final list contained N = 68 concepts (including the HC) which we grouped into six basic conceptual neighbourhoods:

1   Discourse (ideology, values and so forth).
2   Power relations (coercion, labelling, etc.).
3   Socialization (roles, front stage, etc.).
4   Formal organizations (organizational culture, informal structure, etc.).
5   Social institutions (latent and manifest functions, etc.).
6   Sociology of education (learning environment, student–teacher relations and so on).

Next, we took each concept and linked it to each of the other concepts associated with it. The HC, for example, was connected to every other concept with other concepts having a more limited set of links. Our process of linking all 68 concepts resulted in a database of 1,035 links. We entered this database of links into Pajek, a software program for the study of social networks. The result is Figure 2.1.

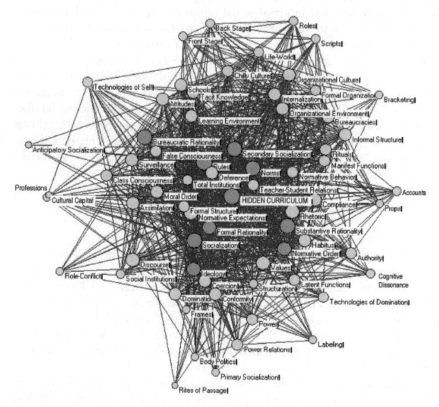

Figure 2.1 The Hidden Curriculum: a conceptual map.

Figure 2.1 is to be read as follows. The closer a node is to the centre of Figure 2.1 (where HC resides), the stronger its relationship to the HC. Similarly, the more proximal any two concepts, the more similar they are to each other. As a second-order association, the larger a given node, the more direct and indirect links that node has with the other 67 concepts. The largest nodes are referred to as hubs. Nodes that are both proximal and large have strong conceptual and relational links to HC and its associated 67 concepts.

A key to interpreting Figure 2.1 is to understand that it does not represent a definitive statement about the relationship of sociological theory to the HC. Rather, Figure 2.1 is a conceptual map depicting the relationship of these 68 concepts to the HC – *given their web of connections to each other*. Thus, Figure 2.1 does not depict how a given variable (for example, rituals) connects to the HC as an isolated entity. Rather, it captures how the term ritual links to the HC *given the relationship of ritual to all other concepts – and those concepts to each other*. Readers may select a different set of concepts and/or posit different connections. This would, in turn, produce a different map.

Figure 2.1, therefore, represents a particular window into the interconnections that exist between a theoretical framework (HC) that has largely been developed within one academic field (education) and the host of theoretical and conceptual traditions that have been developed within another academic domain (sociology). In all of these respects, we believe that Figure 2.1 represents an important first step toward exploring the place of the HC within the broader framework of sociological theory.

To illustrate how one might work with Figure 2.1, we offer two examples. First, we examined a particular sociological concept (socialization) along with its constituent parts (anticipatory, secondary and primary socialization) and watched how these various concepts emerged within the overall figure. Second, we selected one particular link (manifest and latent function – HC) to highlight and explore this particular relationship on a conceptual level. In the former instance (socialization) we sought to examine the map as a whole. In the latter instance (manifest and latent function) we wished to examine (conceptually) one particular connection.

Socialization

The link between socialization theory and the HC has considerable face validity. Within sociology, there is a long history identifying educational settings as sites of targeted learning and identity transformation, and much of the education literature on the HC speaks, both directly and indirectly, to issues of socialization, acculturation and to schools as sites of sociopolitical and economic reproduction. Thus, it is not altogether surprising to examine Figure 2.1 and find that socialization emerged as one of the ten nodal concepts within our web of 1,035 connections. Furthermore, the particular web of relationships captured in Figure 2.1 asks us to reconsider how different types of socialization (for example, anticipatory, secondary and primary) connect both to the master concept (socialization) as well as to each other. Figure 2.1, for example, suggests that primary and anticipatory socialization are more peripheral to issues of the HC than is secondary (adult) socialization. This makes perfect (conceptual) sense. We are, after all, dealing with the occupational training of quasi-adults (socially speaking). Figure 2.1 also suggests that anticipatory socialization and primary socialization reside within different conceptual constellations. Merging these two pieces of information suggests we might best consider the HC as operating more in the 'here and now' than in the past or the future – or at least consider time and place when exploring issues of the HC. On a more personal note, the conceptual constellation captured in Figure 2.1 also helped the authors identify a dimension of socialization we had neglected to include in our original database – namely the concept of 'resocialization'. We noticed this missing element when we explored the proximal relationship of 'total institutions' to the HC, and then recalled a small body of sociological work linking the socialization of physicians to this particular (and extreme) form of identity transformation (resocialization). Although we have not yet done so, the dynamic nature of the relationships that exist within Figure 2.1 also allows us to imagine a 'theory experiment' whereby we would insert resocialization into our underlying database, map its connections, and then see how Figure 2.1 re-calibrates. Such an experiment (along with others) would further enrich our understandings of the connections between the HC and sociological theory.

The HC and manifest/latent function

Robert Merton's concept of manifest and latent function (Merton 1957) is an excellent example of a prima facie link between the HC and sociological theory. Merton's distinction between the stated and/or recognized purpose(s) of a given social action or activity (to those participating) and the unstated or unrecognized purpose(s) of that action (latent function) has obvious parallels to the formal curriculum versus other forms of social learning. In developing his distinctions between manifest and latent functions, Merton drew attention to a number of different social properties and dynamics including:

1   The difference between insider accounts and observer/outsider accounts, thus legitimating the role of the social scientist as a valid source of interpretation.
2   Freud's distinction between conscious and unconscious motivations.
3   Durkheim's notion of social facts and the legitimacy of placing social situations and structure on the same playing field as psychological dispositions and biological tendencies in explaining human behaviour.
4   The ways in which culture and social structure might operate at cross purposes.
5   The paradoxical and counterintuitive aspects of social action.
6   The distinction between subjective disposition and objective consequences.
7   How irrational human behaviour may still be functional.

8   Links between manifest and latent functions and Merton's earlier work on unintended consequences.

Each of these themes has a parallel place within HC theory.

The HC and the symbolic interactionist (SI)/dramaturgical perspective

While there are a number of vantage points from which to explore the interface of HC and SI/dramaturgy, we will highlight Erving Goffman's (1959) work on how individuals engage in culturally and strategically managed interactions ('performances') as they seek to craft 'presentations of self' within strategies of 'impression management'. In developing his theoretical framework, Goffman utilized the metaphor of the theatre and of social life as a staged performance replete with props, sets, staging, scripts, costumes and an audience. One important parallel between HC theory and Goffman is Goffman's treatment of setting, particularly his distinction between front-stage (the performance as intended and viewed) and back-stage social action (not privy to the audience, but both accessible and necessary to the performers who share some social identity). For Goffman, the social action that takes place back stage can knowingly and intentionally contradict the formal presentation, with Goffman even characterizing back-stage renderings as being more 'truthful'.

The linking of social roles and dramaturgy also highlights the fact that individuals can give different performances to different audiences and that furthermore, what social actors present (in whatever setting) may not be what they think or believe. Goffman also differentiated between the expressions we give (intentional) and the expressions we give off – and thus (in part) the potential inconsistencies between what we say and what we actually do (both intentionally and not). Finally, Goffman's theoretical framework allows for a connection between his concept of situated identity and the HC's focus on situated learning.

The HC and professionalism: a case of pedagogical disruption

The rise of a modern-day professionalism movement within organized medicine (from the mid-1980s onward) has been detailed elsewhere (for example, Cohen *et al.* 2007; Hafferty and Castellani 2008). Here, we do not seek to decipher the forces underlying this movement, explicate its evolution or even explore its substantive implications for the future of medical practice. Rather we wish to highlight the HC and what happens when something that has traditionally functioned at a tacit and informal level (professionalism) becomes the object of formal pedagogy. Medicine's modern-day professionalism movement represents an excellent case study in this regard because of the way medicine has come to define the problem (the loss or lack of professionalism as a core occupational attribute); its principal solution (the 'rediscovery' of, or 'recommitment' to, that core); the principal locus of remediation (medical schools and medical training); and finally, the scope of that remedial effort (a change in the 'culture of medical education') (see Cohen *et al.* 2007). Stated differently, organized medicine has created a discourse of professionalism over the past 20 years where a focus on loss and reclamation has generated a cottage industry devoted to:

1   Establishing 'core definitions'.
2   Developing 'unambiguous assessment tools'.
3   Identifying professionalism as a 'core competency'.
4   Including professionalism within accreditation standards at the undergraduate and graduate medical education levels.
5   Creating formal statements of core organizational principles around issues of professionalism (for example, the *Physician Charter*).
6   Publishing special issues of journals, organizing special sessions at national meetings and special conferences sponsored by national medical organizations.
7   Creating national initiatives (for instance, conflict-of-interest policies within clinical and research settings).
8   Developing formal instruction in professionalism at medical schools across the UK and North America.

Taken as a whole, these initiatives and related discourses constitute a veritable 'professionalism project' within organized medicine.

Befitting medicine's framing of its professionalism problem (loss), its professionalism solution (rediscovery and recommitment), and its definition of the HC (as something that needs to be removed or neutralized in order for the formal curriculum to achieve its intended goals), it is not surprising to find medicine (as an occupation steeped in power and hierarchy) crafting highly traditional definitions which are then inserted into a top-down educational model (where faculty teach – and students learn). Furthermore, it is equally predictable that assessment tools have been designed to reassure faculty that students indeed are learning what they (faculty) teach and to buttress this newly formalized curriculum of professionalism. The fact that medical students may perceive professionalism differently from faculty, be resistant to faculty teachings, create subcultural or counter definitions of professionalism, or be cynical about their overall instruction generally are not part of this pedagogical picture – at least as constructed by faculty (Hafferty 2002). Nor should they be, at least from within medicine's discourse of professionalism. After all (and again according to this discourse), medical students are 'naturally' professional, and therefore faculty 'need only' flood the curriculum with formal instruction on core professional principles, all delivered by wise elder role models, in order to counter whatever problems may arise during an educational process that organized medicine itself acknowledges is a source of countervailing values.

If only educational reform was so simple.

In fact, the effort by medical educators to shift professionalism from the world of the tacit, informal and hidden to that of formal pedagogy is a study in organizational tension and irony – and one riddled with unintended consequences. Moreover, it is a lesson in the interconnected and symbiotic nature of medical-learning environments – and therefore, as we will discuss in just a moment, of the medical school as a complex social system. As students are introduced to formal definitions, and as they join faculty in formally structured discussions about these principles, students (unwittingly) are brought face-to-face – and inescapably so – with the presence of those inevitable disjunctures that exist between these principles and the values reflected in the actual work of medicine as it is carried out on the shop floor. For example, it is good to formally teach students that professionalism is steeped in altruism and the primacy of patient welfare (a 'nostalgic' view of professionalism – see Castellani and Hafferty 2006), but what values do students actually internalize when they find themselves in a variety of research and clinical-practice environments that are awash with normatively sanctioned and routinized conflicts of interests?

Furthermore, since faculty seek both to profess and evaluate, what lessons do students learn when students find that faculty seek only to evaluate students while exempting themselves from any similar set of standards? Even more disingenuous, what do students learn when some of these very same faculty are seen by students as being chronic violators of professional standards – and where such transgressions occur without rebuke or sanctions? One consequence, according to Brainard and Brislen (2007), is that students identify with learning environments where 'power and personality are more important than patients' and that the only way to 'navigate the minefield of an unprofessional medical school or hospital culture' is to become 'professional and ethical chameleons'. Although Brainard and Brislen do not reference the following, their arguments are reminiscent of Goffman's concepts of front stage–back stage as well as the impression management/cloak of competence language used by Haas and Shaffir in what was the very first article in medical education to use the HC as a conceptual tool.

While none of this collateral learning is a part of anyone's formal professionalism curriculum, this is what students are learning about professionalism – and inescapably so. Once again we find the HC at work, even as medical education launches a professional project built around the (flawed) premise that if medicine is to be saved, the principal method would be to bring the HC more under the control of formal pedagogy.

Conclusions: medical education as a complex system

In this last section we offer an alternative way to think about the HC based on the new science of complexity (for instance, Capra 2002). Complexity science is a far-reaching, interdisciplinary field of research devoted to the study of complex systems. Some of its more popular ideas include the small-world phenomenon, self-organization, emergence, fractals and agent-based modelling. The last concept is an umbrella term for the latest advances in computer-based modelling, ranging from neural networks to cellular automata to fuzzy logic (Gilbert and Troitzsch 2005).

One of the most popular areas of substantive inquiry in complexity science is the study of formal organizations – including businesses, educational institutions, non-profit companies and medical practices (see Anderson and McDaniel 2000 for an example of the latter). Across the managerial-sciences literature, the basic argument is that formal organizations are really complex social systems and therefore best studied and managed as such (Richardson and Cilliers 2001).

Our own research, for example, has explored the integration of complexity science and sociology (Hafferty and Castellani 2008), as well as the more focused question of multiple (and competing) types of medical professionalism (Castellani and Hafferty 2006).

Using this literature as a backdrop, our goal is to briefly sketch what the HC might look like from a complexity science perspective. A more formal review would be necessary to actually build a defendable model. In what follows, we will list our ideas as a series of numbered points.

The system of medical education

1   As argued in the body of this chapter, it is a mistake to imagine the formal curriculum as something educators construct 'ahead of time', deliver to students (as passive recipients), assess in terms of some point-in-time impact, and then make adjustments to (even if these adjustments are framed in terms of the HC). This model (develop, deliver, assess and remediate) is *relatively* hierarchical, static and unidirectional. Teachers still deliver pre-established blocks of material and students are still the objects of faculty pedagogical affections, all operating within one feedback loop. Transforming this model (which some might still characterize as 'progressive') to a systems perspective (where education is complex, emergent, self-organizing and so on) will require thinking about education in new and different ways. This will be the true 'culture change' called for (sometimes rhetorically) by medical educators.

2   Medical education is not something medical schools deliver. It is a system. It is a system formed by the intersection of several types of curriculum (formal, informal, hidden, null and so forth) – all of which function within a dynamic web of intersecting influences. The formal curriculum, while central to the educational enterprise, is not the only or 'most important' site of learning. Nor is the hc the only alternative learning process. The formal, informal, hidden and so on, are intersecting social practices – all of which create the system of medical education.

3   The term 'learning environment' is what medical education does. It is the system of medical education in practice. As practised (and as a system), learning environments are complex, emergent, self-organizing, evolving, adaptive systems where the whole is more than the sum of the parts (Capra 2002).

4 When we study (or attempt to reform) the system of medical education, we cannot do so by targeting one component or another in isolation. Instead, we work with and through the system to see how these segments form very specific, concrete instances of medical learning. Different schools will exhibit different learning configurations. Each overall learning environment for each and every medical school is a unique combination of the formal, informal and hidden curriculum. As such, each process of educational reform is unique. Nonetheless, educators still work with the same 'parts' (formal, informal, hidden), the same overall structure (network) and the same overall process (dynamic).

5 Because it is part of this overall system, the hc cannot be separated from the overall process of medical learning. Nor can it be removed or otherwise marginalized in terms of its impact. There is *always* a latent to every manifest, an informal to every formal, and/or a back stage to every front stage. One can shift (aspects of something) from the realm of tacit learning to the formal curriculum (such as role models to mentoring), but this does not minimize the effect of the HC. Nor does it make the HC less relevant as a theoretical framework. Rather, the system changes. Elements are rearranged and new processes emerge. However, the overall structure and dynamics remain. Change is ubiquitous, and it is the responsibility of educators to both anticipate change and respond to the system permutations (as best as possible).

6 The fact that there will always be hidden, informal, null and so forth, curricula operating alongside the formal curriculum does not relegate remedial efforts to the dustbin of wasteful or purposeless action. If for no other reason, educators have a moral responsibility to address those instances where students find themselves wallowing in learning environments awash with inconsistent or conflicting messages. In addition to these more reactive and instance-specific reclamations, medical educators are also beginning to explore proactive structural innovations that bear future scrutiny (from an HC perspective). One involves models of 'longitudinal and integrated training' – an example being Harvard's Cambridge Integrated Clerkship (Hirsh *et al.* 2007). There are great psychological and learning costs associated with medicine's traditional requirement that students and residents rotate through discrete clinical settings (for example, services, wards, departments), each with its own knowledge base, skill sets, cast of characters and 'ways of doing things'. Under such circumstances, students spend a prodigious amount of time and energy tacitly learning the ropes for each clerkship/rotation (particularly as they first enter these settings and situations) rather than focusing on the clinical skills that supposedly sit at the core of that learning environment's formal curriculum. Longitudinal learning experiences (for example, a single, integrated and continuous third-year clerkship), provide students with a more stable and focused – and certainly less disjointed and disruptive – opportunity to learn what the formal curriculum says it wants to impart. A similar movement involves efforts to

construct more vertically positioned learning structures, this time those that cut across the hierarchically ordered years of medical education (such as learning communities) and thus seek to link (and network) students at different levels of training. Other structural changes await our imagination.

References

Anderson, R. A. and McDaniel Jr, R. R. (2000) 'Managing health care organizations: where professionalism meets complexity science', *Health Care Management Review*, 25: 83–92.

Becker, H., Geer, B., Hughes, E. C. and Strauss, A. L. (1961) *Boys in White: student culture in medical school*, Chicago, IL: University of Chicago Press.

Berger, P. L. (1963) *Invitation to Sociology: a humanistic perspective*, New York: Anchor Books.

Bloom, S. W. (1988) 'Structure and ideology in medical education: an analysis of resistance to change', *Journal of Health and Social Behavior*, 29: 294–306.

Brainard, A. H. and Brislen, H. C. (2007) 'Viewpoint: Learning professionalism: a view from the trenches', *Academic Medicine*, 82: 1010–14.

Capra, F. (2002) *The Hidden Connections: integrating the biological, cognitive, and social dimensions of life into a science of sustainability*, Garden City, NY: Doubleday.

Castellani, B. and Hafferty, F. W. (2006) 'Professionalism and complexity science: a preliminary investigation', in D. Wear and J. M. Aultman (eds) *Medical Professionalism: a critical review*, New York: Springer.

Cohen, J. J., Cruess, S. and Davidson, C. (2007) 'Alliance between society and medicine: the public's stake in medical professionalism', *Journal of the American Medical Association*, 298: 670–3.

Coles, C. R. and Grant, J. G. (1985) 'Curriculum evaluation in medical and health-care education', *Medical Education*, 19: 405–22.

Cornbleth, C. (2003) 'Hidden curriculum', in J. W. Guthrie (ed.) *Encyclopedia of Education*, 2nd edn, New York: Macmillan Reference.

Eisner, E. W. (1985) *The Three Curricula That All Schools Teach: the educational imagination*, New York: Macmillan Publishing Company.

—— (1992) 'A reply to Gabriele Lakomski', *Curriculum Inquiry*, 22: 205–9.

Gilbert, N. and Troitzsch, K. G. (2005) *Simulation for the Social Scientist*, 2nd edn, Buckingham, PA: Open University Press.

Goffman, E. (1959) *The Presentation of Self in Everyday Life*, Garden City, NY: Doubleday.

Goodlad, J. I., Klein, M. F. and Tye, K. A. (1979) 'The domains of curriculum and their study', in J. I. Goodlad (ed.), *Curriculum Inquiry: the study of practice*, New York: McGraw-Hill.

Haas, J. and Shaffir, W. (1982) 'Ritual evaluation of competence: the hidden curriculum of professionalization in an innovative medical school program', *Work and Occupations*, 9: 131–54.

Hafferty, F. W. (1998) 'Beyond curriculum reform: confronting medicine's hidden curriculum', *Academic Medicine*, 73: 403–7.

—— (2002) 'What medical students know about professionalism', *Mt. Sinai Journal of Medicine*, 69: 385–97.

Hafferty, F. W. and Castellani, B. (2008) 'The two cultures of professionalism: sociology and medicine', in B. Pescosolido, J. Martin, J. McLeod and A. Rogers (eds) *The Handbook of Health, Illness & Healing: blueprint for the 21st century*, New York: Springer.

Hafferty, F. W. and Franks, R. (1994) 'The hidden curriculum, ethics teaching, and the structure of medical education', *Academic Medicine*, 69: 861–71.

Hafferty, F. W. and Watson, K. V. (2006) 'The rise of learning communities in medical education: a socio-structural analysis', *Journal of Cancer Education*, 22: 6–9.

Haidet, P., Kelly, P. A., Chou, C. and The Communication, Curriculum and Culture Study Group (2005) 'Characterizing the patient-centeredness of hidden curricula in medical schools: development and validation of a new measure', *Academic Medicine*, 80: 44–50.

Hirsh, D. A., Ogur, B., Thibault, G. E. and Cox, M. (2007) ' "Continuity" as an organizing principle for clinical education reform', *New England Journal of Medicine*, 356: 858–66.

Jackson, P. (1968) *Life in Classrooms*. New York: Holt, Rinehart & Winston.

Lakomski, G. (1988) 'Witches, weather gods, and phlogiston: the demise of the hidden curriculum', *Curriculum Inquiry*, 18: 451–63.

Martin, J. R. (1976) 'What do we do with a hidden curriculum when we find one?', *Curriculum Inquiry*, 6: 135–51.

Merton, R. K. (1957) *Social Theory and Social Structure*, Glencoe, IL: Free Press.

Richardson, K. and Cilliers, P. (2001) 'Special editors' introduction: what is complexity science? A view from different directions', *Emergence*, 3: 5–22.

Schein, E. H. (1992) *Organizational Culture and Leadership*, 2nd edn, San Francisco, CA: Jossey-Bass.

Shem, S. (1978) *The House of God*, New York: Dell.

Snyder, B. R. (1971) *The Hidden Curriculum*, New York: Alfred A. Knopf.

Wilson, L. and Wilson, O. (2007) *Wilson's Curriculum Pages*, online at www.uwsp.edu/Education/lwilson/curric/curtyp.htm#null (accessed 20 December 2007).

3   From classification to integration

Bernstein and the sociology of medical education

Paul Atkinson and Sara Delamont

Introduction

The recent history of medical education in the United Kingdom provides a perfect opportunity to exemplify and test a major theory in the sociology of education. While the sociology of education has been focused disproportionately on *schooling*, many of its key ideas derive from and apply to higher education. Indeed, it is important, analytically speaking, to ensure that the sociology of education encompasses higher and professional education. Professional education, and medical education within it, have been treated as specialist topics in their own right, but have been marginal to the mainstream sociology of education. Equally, although medical education has been the subject matter of several key sociological studies, and British medical education has given rise to a small number of monographs, the degree of engagement with current and recent issues in the sociology of medicine has been limited. This chapter is intended to be a contribution to a *rapprochement*.

Medical education in the United Kingdom has undergone a major change in recent years. The formal curricular arrangements for basic (undergraduate) training are laid out from time to time by the UK's General Medical Council (GMC). The GMC produced a set of recommendations and requirements that enshrined a major, even revolutionary, transformation in the organization and transmission of medical knowledge (GMC 1993, 2003). The underlying representation of medical knowledge and its realization into a model curriculum are the subject matter of this chapter, along with the analysis of curricular change and pedagogic message systems pioneered by Basil Bernstein. Before examining the transformations in medical education, therefore, we need to acquaint ourselves with the Bernsteinian model.

The classification and framing of educational knowledge

Basil Bernstein (1924–2000) was the most original and influential sociologist of education of his generation (Delamont and Atkinson 2007). He developed a sustained programme of sociological research on social reproduction and educational processes. His intellectual inspirations included the sociology of

Durkheim, viewed through a European lens, rather than the Anglo-American filter that portrayed Durkheim primarily in terms of a structural-functional meta-theory. Bernstein's sociology of education was, therefore, concerned primarily with the *forms* of social life in educational institutions, and other institutions of social reproduction, and the *forms* of knowledge reproduced in such settings. In a way that strikingly recalled the anthropological analysis of Durkheim and Mauss, Bernstein explored the formal homologies between the patterning of social organizations and the patterning of their distinctive cultural systems (Atkinson 1985). If one wishes to sense the overall flavour of Bernstein's sociology of knowledge, then a useful starting point would be Durkheim and Mauss on the structuring of Zuñi cosmology, or Mauss on the social and cultural universe of the Eskimo. These are classic accounts that propose distinctive affinities between the *ordering* of culture and key axes of *social organization*. Such accounts model cosmologies and social structure. They do so in ways that explore fundamental *principles* of ordering, not in terms of trivial, surface-level similarities.

There is therefore, a sense in which Bernstein was one of the heirs to a structuralist sociology/anthropology (Atkinson 1981). This was not a matter of slavishly adopting the fashionable theories of Parisian luminaries like Lévi-Strauss or Barthes, although there were parallels in the development of French structuralism and post-structuralism on the one hand, and Bernsteinian analysis of cultural reproduction on the other. Bernstein developed his own research out of a Durkheimian structuralism in a way that paralleled the work of Mary Douglas – another British social scientist who developed her own distinctive form of structuralist anthropology (for example, Douglas 1966).

Like Douglas – famous for her analysis of dirt and pollution – Bernstein is preoccupied with *boundaries*. Douglas's analysis of pollution, in terms of 'matter out of place', emphasizes the cultural significance of symbolic boundaries that define cultural categories, and so keep distinct the 'natural types' that constitute any given cosmology or cultural domain (Douglas 1966). In Mary Douglas's analysis, phenomena that appear to transgress such symbolic boundaries or are hybrid, ambiguous types, become treated as 'polluting' anomalies: such monstrous types in turn can be marked as especially dirty, or especially potent. Such categories and types thus become abhorrent forms. In an intellectually similar vein, Bernstein's sociology of the curriculum examines the principles whereby the contents of knowledge are made separate and distinct. In a thoroughly structuralist vein, Bernstein (1971) notes that any curriculum establishes two axes. It defines principles of *selection* and *combination*. Selection defines what contents (such as 'subjects' or 'topics') shall be identified from the universe of possible content. A curriculum, in other words, defines a number of knowledge domains and specialized contents. There are, therefore, boundaries that separate one subject or field or knowledge from another. There are also external boundaries that separate specialized, esoteric knowledge from everyday, mundane knowledge – which is normally excluded from formal curricula. (Changing definitions of what *counts* as esoteric or mundane can be of considerable moment, however.) In stressing these aspects of Bernstein's sustained theoretical and empirical research programme, we are guilty of perpetuating a one-sided and limited account of it. The ideas used in this paper are relatively early in his output. He went on to develop much more highly developed and complex models of pedagogic discourse and practice. We focus on some of his more fundamental ideas here not out of laziness, but because they correspond so closely to the current realities of curriculum and pedagogy in medical education. For accounts that stress the complexities of Bernstein's mature sociology see: Davies (1995); Morais *et al.* (2001); Muller *et al.* (2004); see also Bernstein (2000).

If any given curriculum defines the classification of contents, then it also prescribes how those contents can be *combined*. It may, for example, specify what contents must be taken together (as required, co-requirements), what may be taken in what temporal and developmental sequence (as in prerequisites). It will specify what contents must be studied (*compulsory*), what may be chosen (*optional*) and what may not be chosen (*prohibited*). Sequential and combinatorial principles thus define what is permitted and what is mandatory within any given curricular regime.

From this perspective, therefore, we can analyse any given curriculum in terms of its formal properties, more or less independently of its concrete subject matter. As we shall see, we can also use these basic analytic tools and elaborate on them further. It means, however, that following Bernstein we can make sense of a curriculum in classic semiotic terms. The analysis lends itself to a Saussurean understanding. The founder of general linguistics, Ferdinand de Saussure suggested that language could be analysed in terms of two axes: the *paradigmatic* and the *syntagmatic*. The paradigmatic axis defines what linguistic items (such as phonemes, morphemes or words) are selected, while the syntagmatic axis defines how those items are put together to form an utterance of message.

We can think of the selection of curricular knowledge as a set of paradigmatic knowledge relations, while the principle of combination corresponds to the syntagmatic axis. The semiotic 'message' so constructed will, therefore, consist of a culturally acceptable ('grammatical') array of disciplinary knowledge, constructed in accordance with cultural conventions governing what counts as acceptable combinatorial possibilities. Like any semiotic system, the classificatory boundaries and combinatorial options are 'arbitrary' in the sense that they are underdetermined by any inherent features of the natural and social world. (In common with many natural and cultural categories, however, they have referential value: 'arbitrary' in this context does not mean that categories are entirely whimsical, as it were.) Curricular knowledge, in other words, imposes categories and combinations on the world. Of course, cultural categories also help to *define* the world: cultural knowledge is thus naturalized. We do not normally perceive our worlds of knowledge as arbitrary constructs: we tend to see them as naturally given. Consequently, the cultural categories encoded in curricular arrangements can take on normative connotations: they define not merely how the world *is* but how it *ought* to be.

Bernstein, then, provides a suggestive framework for the analysis of curricular knowledge and its formal arrangements. In the earliest versions of his theories of curricular knowledge and pedagogical practice, he outlined some ideal-typical forms of curriculum – or, more precisely, of the ordering principles underlying curricula. These in turn related directly to Bernstein's yet more general theories concerning socialization and identity formation, some aspects of which we shall return to later in this chapter.

Bernstein contrasted two knowledge *codes*. These were derived from general observations concerning the organization of knowledge in schools – especially in English secondary schools – and, most crucially for this chapter, transformations in the organization of school knowledge. The first type of code Bernstein referred to as the *collection* type. (As we shall indicate, there are variants within this type.) The underlying ordering principle is one of strong boundaries between contents. The curriculum is, therefore, made up of a series of clearly defined, sharply differentiated knowledge-domains (such as academic subjects). The principle of ordering Bernstein refers to as classification, and the collection type is characterized by strong classification, in which the symbolic boundaries are relatively impermeable.

This collection code can operate within an equally strongly bounded domain. For instance, a curriculum could be put together prescribing, say, contents from physics, chemistry, biology and mathematics, in which they were treated as four relatively exclusive domains. Where these are – as in this case – all drawn from a broader, but equally bounded intellectual field ('science') then we can call this collection type a *pure* one. By contrast, it is possible to think of a collection type in which a student is required to learn from a more diverse range of academic contents, which still remain strongly bounded domains in their own right: hypothetically one might be required to take a science discipline, a humanities discipline, a modern language and a social science, where each of those categories is treated as more or less self-contained. This, therefore, remains a collection type, but the contents are drawn more promiscuously from more than one overarching domain. These are, as we have said, ideal types, but for ease of reference it may help to attach possible exemplars. The traditional single honours degree scheme in an English university (and we do mean English, as the Scots have a different tradition) corresponds to the pure collection type. The equivalent American undergraduate degree has normally been much more impure, given the normal 'general education' requirements that see humanities majors taking science courses or vice versa.

The contrast to the collection type is given by the *integrated* code. As Bernstein's term implies, this knowledge code is governed by a principle of weak symbolic boundaries. The underlying principle is, therefore, one of *synthesis* as opposed to the collection code's principle of separation. The fundamental organizing idea, therefore, would be 'science' – defined by the generic scientific method – and not (say) physics, chemistry, biology. Of course, there remain boundaries – for instance around 'science' – but even these may be weakened for, as we shall see, these differences in knowledge code reflect not merely different ways of organizing knowledge, but also different orientations to and evaluations of knowledge. At about the time that Bernstein himself was developing these ideas, forms of integration were prominent innovations in English schooling, reflected in the Nuffield Integrated Science or Integrated Humanities programmes, for instance.

In accordance with this model (a simplification of Bernstein's original formulation) a number of further contrasts can be drawn. In effect, they constitute predictions derived from the general theory of knowledge codes. When a curriculum is regulated by strongly classified subject boundaries, then the 'subject' is implicitly treated as the main *raison d'être* of instruction. The student embarks on a relatively lengthy and detailed study of (say) physics in order to learn physics, and even perhaps to become a physicist. It will be congruent with this implicit model of socialization that formal instruction will follow the development of the discipline itself, recapitulating classic experiments and demonstrations. The neophyte is thus drawn into a community of scholars who have all followed the same recapitulation of the discipline's collective identity. Formal socialization thus includes an extended period of apprenticeship. As with many extended initiations and ordeals, the initiate is admitted to the 'mystery of the craft' only as the culmination of this lengthy process. Strong identification and personal loyalty are implicitly encouraged and the 'subject' is a major source of personal identity for teachers and taught in equal measure.

The reverse, of course, is true of the integrated code. Specific subject matter is subordinated to general principles, such as 'the scientific method', 'individual and society', or 'language and culture' rather than individual disciplines. Rather than the essence of the disciplinary knowledge being a deferred revelation, it is the starting point for instruction. Consequently, rather than being *implicit* in the subject matter of the discipline, it is *explicated* in the general guiding principles. This contrast between implicit and explicit messages in curriculum codes is a key feature of Bernstein's general theory and it has considerable value for our discussion of medical education in the sections that follow.

The general model also predicts strong organizational boundaries that mirror strong cultural boundaries under a collection code. The socializing institution such as a school or university will be arranged primarily in terms of 'departments' or 'divisions'. There will be strong boundaries between them. Within them, there will be strong relations of subject-based identification and strong vertical (hierarchical) relations. This does not mean, incidentally, that everyone within an academic department has to like or get on with one another; clearly they do not in many cases. The implementation of an integrated code, on the other hand, calls for weaker, more permeable boundaries, and strong horizontal ties across anything like departmental boundaries. These are not necessarily static types. There is a dynamic implied in Bernstein's model. In particular, Bernstein himself was influenced by a pervasive movement apparently leading from collection code to integrated code, especially in English schooling. Clearly, it was a shift, at the level of knowledge, that was congruent with educational change associated with the more 'progressive' aspects of schooling.

These models are not merely ways of capturing contrasting types of curriculum; they also go beyond the description of educational change. They encapsulate and reflect significant shifts in underlying orientations towards knowledge, identity and reproduction. They are, in other words, ways of regulating cosmologies. As we shall see, the recent changes in medical education also embody major epistemic change, which will be outlined in the following sections.

Modelling medical education

The system of British medical education that we might consider 'traditional' was, in Bernstein's terms, strongly classified. It was built around a number of powerful symbolic boundaries. It represented a very clear exemplar of Bernstein's collection code. The divisions created by these boundaries were the main organizational, professional and epistemic building blocks of the undergraduate medical curriculum in the United Kingdom. The account that follows is, to some extent, ideal-typical itself. In the UK, medical schools over the past 30–40 years have been different. Some have been thoroughly 'traditional' while others have been modernizing institutions prior to the most recent interventions by the General Medical Council. The two major sociological/anthropological monographs on UK medical schools both describe 'traditional' arrangements, and they help to fix the social and intellectual style (Atkinson 1997; Sinclair 1997).

The traditional undergraduate curriculum was marked by one major boundary and the equally significant cleavage it gave rise to (Armstrong 1980). That was the distinction between the pre-clinical and clinical phases. The pre-clinical phase was devoted almost exclusively to the sciences, which were treated as prerequisites to clinical understanding and practice. Typically, the pre-clinical sciences would be based on anatomy, physiology and biochemistry. Other basic disciplines such as bacteriology or pathology might also be included. Each of these (and the precise mix always varied from medical school to medical school) was delivered by a separate academic department. As well as the major clinical/ pre-clinical divide, therefore, there were strongly classified, separated knowledge domains within the pre-clinical field. The same was true of the clinical phase of the curriculum. The subject divisions reflected the professional segmentation of medicine in terms of separate clinical specialities. The basics of clinical work would be instruction in medicine and surgery, each treated as a self-contained specialty (or collection of specialties). In subsequent phases of clinical work, finer discriminations and specializations were encountered, through such specialisms as obstetrics and gynaecology, haematology, neurology, ophthalmology and the like. Likewise, General Practice or public health were treated as specialisms in their own right. Just as in the pre-clinical phase, therefore, the clinical aspect of the undergraduate curriculum was comprised of strongly bounded domains, each with its distinctive content. Although the Todd Report on Medical Education in 1968 had proposed some radical changes in the content of medical education (including compulsory social science), it left intact the fundamental structures of strongly classified, bounded curricular domains and divisions, such as the pre-clinical/clinical divide and distinct academic/clinical departments (Royal Commission on Medical Education 1968).

The strongly classified contents and subjects, in both phases, reflected not merely complementary differences. In many cases each created a different scientific or medical reality. Each defined a distinctive thought style and mode of practice. There could be, for instance, differences in style between anatomy and physiology, even when similar topics were being taught. In the clinical phase, medicine and surgery introduced medical students to two different – sometimes starkly different – intellectual and practical domains (Atkinson 1977).

Within this strongly classified curriculum, therefore, it comes as no surprise – if we follow Bernstein's model – that the process of medical socialization was predicated on a lengthy apprenticeship, with major benchmarks and rites of passage along the way. It was a mode of socialization with multiple initiation ceremonies. In many ways, these processes of enculturation recapitulated key aspects of modern medicine, in ways that paralleled the 'classic' demonstrations of introductory laboratory sciences. The most vivid of these – simultaneously a *rite de passage* and a classic pedagogical recapitulation – was 'the anatomy lesson'. For many years the disciplines of gross anatomy were foundational in every sense. First-year medical students' first encounters with a cadaver in the Dissecting Room (DR) were the central feature of initiation into the world of medicine. It was widely regarded not merely as important in terms of learning topographical anatomy, but also in terms of instilling the right sort of attitudes and feelings (cf. Hafferty 1991). The DR, and the rigours of the pre-clinical curriculum more generally, were treated as mechanisms for testing whether students were the 'right stuff' to stand up to the demands of medical training and practice. More general rites of passage included major examinations that assessed voluminous amounts of factual knowledge. The rigours – emotional and cognitive, of a subject like gross anatomy – were used to test the mettle of young medical students; in the nineteenth century they had been used to test the commitment and capacities of female students and would-be female doctors.

The conclusion of the pre-clinical period of study was a major point of transition for the individual medical student. The university examinations at this stage represented a significant hurdle for students to overcome. Failure was not uncommon and students' medical studies could well be terminated at that point. By contrast, once students had successfully progressed to the clinical phase of the undergraduate degree, failure was much less likely. The transition from pre-clinical to clinical was a move from 'contest mobility' to 'sponsored mobility' (Turner 1964). Having been admitted to the clinical realities of medical training, students were treated more like 'junior colleagues' and less like 'students'.

The initiation of the first encounter with the cadaver was recapitulated in students' initial encounters with patients. The clinical settings in which early clinical work was done were predominately hospital wards, and students would learn basic clinical skills such as history-taking, auscultation or palpation, at the bedside of hospital in-patients, not in classrooms. As Atkinson's ethnography (1997) demonstrates, students would thus learn to perceive 'classic' clinical signs (skin colour, pulse, heart sounds, reflexes) and their pathognomic signifi-cance. Bedside instruction was therefore predicated on the professional and epis-temic centrality of 'the clinical gaze'. The twin epiphanies of encountering first the cadaver and then the patient were twin pillars on which rested students' emergent identity. They were among the key turning points in the medical stu-dent's moral career.

Medical students were, therefore, enculturated in a strongly bounded and seg-mented professional and intellectual domain (Atkinson 1977). The world of medicine was strongly demarcated from the profane world of everyday life; clin-ical practice was contained primarily within the hospital. The 'laboratory' and the 'clinic' defined the double gaze of the student, and hence the version(s) of medicine reproduced in the medical school.

This model of the 'traditional' medical-school curriculum is not intended to do justice to all the variations existing in the United Kingdom. There were many differences to be found, and many attempts to generate innovative arrangements. The latter were introduced independently of the General Medical Council's wide-ranging recommendations in *Tomorrow's Doctors*. As an ideal type, however, this outline services two purposes. It is in part an analyst's construct, used here in order to capture key aspects of the Bernsteinian theory. Equally, however, it was a model that was implicit in the world of medical education itself. The strongly classified and segmented divisions were widely recognized and were equally widely deprecated. There was, therefore, a constant pressure towards reform based on the progressive weakening of the classificatory bounda-ries. These were couched in terms of a movement towards both horizontal and vertical integration. Horizontal integration referred to the weakening of bounda-ries between subject domains and integration across the disciplines or special-isms at any given phase of the curriculum. Vertical integration referred to the weakening or even abolition of the clinical–pre-clinical divide.

Various forms of integrating curricula were thus introduced in UK medical schools. They were distinctive features of newly established medical schools in the 1970s. The 'old' centres of medical education such as London or Edinburgh tended to remain the most 'traditional' in style, while the newer and provincial medical schools (such as Leicester or Newcastle) were more innovative. Attempts at integration included the removal of the cleavage between pre-clinical and clinical work. Students did not have to assimilate the laboratory sci-ences before encountering their first patients. They did not have to cope with the Dissecting Room as a rite of passage before encountering the living (if sickly) bodies of patients. Moreover, the classificatory boundary encircling the medical school and its esoteric knowledge was weakened through the progressive incor-poration of community-based practice, family medicine and public health into the core curriculum. In at least one medical school, the pre-clinical–clinical divide was also transcended by the absence of a separate department of anatomy, and by having anatomy taught by surgeons (whose own occupational culture stressed that students forgot nearly all the anatomy they had been taught by the pre-clinical department and had to be taught it all over again in the context of clinical surgery). The weakening of boundaries and the promiscuous mixing of formerly separate categories has also been manifest in interprofessional instruction, whereby medical students have been taught together with students in other healthcare professions.

It would, therefore, be wrong to over-interpret our ideal–typical contrast. UK medical schools were not equally 'traditional' and there were many attempts at reform. It is clear, however, that the root-and-branch reforms of *Tomorrow's Doctors* were formulated against the backdrop of a curriculum and a mode of social organization that remained stubbornly classified and internally segmented. By contrast, *Tomorrow's Doctors* proposed a shift from a collection code to an integrated code. Indeed, the GMC might have read Bernstein and taken his theory as a blueprint in drawing up the report's major proposals. *Tomorrow's Doctors* projected into the future a very different model of social organization and knowledge reproduction in the UK's medical schools. Despite the fact that some of the GMC's written pronouncements are terse, they imply major changes in the underlying philosophy of medical education, certainly as traditionally implemented. For instance, the requirement that 'The clinical and basic sciences should be taught in an integrated way throughout the curriculum' (GMC 2003: 12) codifies a major shift in the discourse and practice of medical education. This was in turn part of a wider discursive shift. Changes in medicine were closely paralleled by curricular changes in other health professions, notably dentistry and pharmacy.

Tomorrow's Doctors

We now turn to examine just how the GMC attempted to transform the curricular code of undergraduate medical education. As we have already indicated, the innovations were driven by the search for integration and flexibility. They also sought to construct a different style of learning, and hence implied a different kind of medical student. Changes in curricular organization were mirrored by changes in pedagogy. The recommendations enshrined in the two versions of the GMC report (1993, 2003) are schematic in themselves. In describing the implications of the GMC's interventions, therefore, we draw not just on the text but also on the effect of GMC visitations to medical schools and the interpretation of the GMC requirements in practice. Again, we must stress that we construct an ideal type here: local implementations of the broad recommendations are variable across institutions. These shifts in emphasis are not confined to the GMC's requirements. In the UK system of higher education, all disciplines have 'benchmarks', compiled and published by the Quality Assurance Agency (QAA). The benchmarks for medicine affirm the principles of integration.

The de-classification of the traditional medical curriculum resulted in a re-classification, justified in terms of integration. (Of course, no curriculum can conceivably exist without some principles of selection, discrimination and combination.) Entirely in line with Bernstein's model, the curricular contents were reformulated in terms of broad organizing themes that transcended any disciplinary divisions, corresponding to the Bernsteinian integration type.

The curriculum is now predicated on generic *themes*, such as physical systems, health and society, or ethics and communication. A theme or strand that is based on a physical system – the gut and digestion, or the nervous system, for example – is intended to draw together physiology, anatomy, clinical practice, community and family issues. The separate disciplines or medical specialisms are thus subordinated to the organizing principle. Any given specialism could contribute teaching across several such superordinate themes. In contrast to the more traditional arrangements, there is no one-to-one correspondence between an academic department or clinical specialty and a segment of the curriculum. Indeed, this is a clear organizational difference between the two curriculum codes. Curriculum (or 'contact') hours are a major form of currency in higher education, being translated into fragments of 'full-time equivalent' (FTE) students, and hence into allocations of resources within the university. The arrangements of integrated, multidisciplinary curricula do not do away with such an institutional-cum-instructional calculus, but do render it more problematic. Under the new dispensation, groups of academic staff do not, in that sense, 'own' chunks of the academic programme. Separate departments equally do not own them. Major themes, which are intended to achieve horizontal and vertical integration, are managed by cross-disciplinary teams. Newer skills are introduced into the new curriculum content, such as IT and communication skills.

Tomorrow's Doctors also envisions a different approach to pedagogy and student learning. Reforms in medical education had long been predicated on several related problems. The curriculum itself was seen as unmanageably overloaded. As a consequence, students themselves faced overload, with little or no time for independent learning or reflection. It was also seen as damagingly based on the acquisition, retention and regurgitation of factual detail: students were felt to lack more generic skills of reasoning. These emphases were also reflected in dominant styles of assessment. The multiple-choice examination, focused on the accuracy of factual recall, and requiring (or indeed allowing) no reasoning from general principles, was the main technology of assessment. It is, incidentally, no accident that a substantial proportion of the published papers in journals devoted to research on medical education have been devoted to technical issues of setting and scoring multiple-choice question examinations. The pedagogy and assessment regimes were entirely congruent. As we have already seen, individualistic modes of work (which could readily become competitive) were replaced or at least supplemented with team-based, problem-solving modes of work.

This is a further feature of Bernstein's general model to which we have not yet referred. Bernstein's analysis of curricular classification is paralleled by an account of pedagogical *framing*. If classification refers to the organization of knowledge at the level of the formal curriculum, then framing refers to the management of knowledge in the pedagogical encounter (in the classroom, in the lecture theatre, at the bedside). While it is entirely conceivable to have mixed types, it is common to find strong framing with strong classification. When framing is strong, then the content and management of the teaching encounter are strongly controlled. The locus and justification of such control may come from multiple sources: from the requirements of national and professionally pre-scribed curricula, to institutionally imposed requirements, to the personal author-ity of the individual teacher. When framing is strong, then the content of any given encounter is closely regulated and controlled. So too is the *order* in which aspects of knowledge are introduced, and so is the *pacing* of pedagogy: that is, the tempo at which material is covered. These knowledge arrangements can be enshrined in documentary sources: textbooks (often with teacher's guides) can prescribe a course in such a way as to frame it strongly; assessment regimes may also frame the pedagogy, by prescribing the ordering of content, its pacing and indeed its form.

Of course, these features of pedagogy are not independent. They realize in practical terms the dominant assumptions and implicit models that inform and regulate any given system of instruction and learning. They therefore inscribe models of the student and of the teacher, and their respective positions. When framing is strong, then the respective positions of teacher and taught are them-selves circumscribed. They tend towards hierarchical relationships within a system of relatively fixed identities. When framing is weaker, then there is room for greater variation in the social relations of teachers and taught, and multiple ways of implementing pedagogical action.

Tomorrow's Doctors implied a shift in pedagogy, with a weakening in the framing. Medical students were to be more actively engaged in their own learn-ing, which was to be far less dependent on rote-learning and the assimilation of undigested facts. Instead, a far greater proportion of learning would be based on independent small-group and enquiry-led work, in which students learned to search for evidence, evaluate it, synthesize it and report it. To that extent, there-fore, students could exercise far greater control over their own direction and effort. (Sociological studies of medical education have in the past shown how students coped with factual overload: setting their own levels of effort and selec-tive negligence were methods of exercising some degree of control, but they were subversive strategies and not the overt aims of pedagogy.) There is, there-fore, a marked contrast with earlier approaches to pedagogy that stressed indi-vidual, competitive approaches to student learning, as well as the assimilation of large volumes of factual material. The model of socialization here aims to produce students and practitioners able to assess their own learning needs, to act as reflexive practitioners, and to ground their practice in the evidence base. It stresses collaboration and team-working in problem-solving.

The shift in pedagogy reflected an ideology of flexibility, and an implied repositioning of the medical student. The new emphasis on self-directed learning and the 'research' skills needed to seek out relevant information was linked to a wider attempt to re-fashion the epistemic basis of medicine itself. Recent and contemporary emphases on evidence-based medicine stress the value of gather-ing and assessing the available information, rather than a practice based on memorization and recipes for action. The ideology of medical education in con-temporary Britain thus presupposes a new and different relationship between students and medical knowledge. It also models a different kind of practitioner.

The principle of flexibility in the curriculum is carried through in defining a core curriculum and optional subject matter. In the 'traditional' arrangements, there really was no notion of optional subjects (although in practice there was always a hit-or-miss aspect to what students encountered and learned in the clinical years).

At the same time, previously strong symbolic boundaries are weakened. In the traditional, strongly classified and framed system of medical training, knowledge was imparted almost exclusively within the 'sacred' bounds of the hospital. The teaching hospital, site of modern medicine's most distinctive modes of knowing and perceiving (Foucault 1973), was the primary site of knowledge reproduction. Under the newer dispensation, medical students are required to learn, from the outset, in the more 'profane' environments of the community or the family. Educational opportunities '… might involve visiting families expecting a baby, visiting an elderly or disabled person, or taking part in community projects that are not necessarily medically related' (GMC 2003: 12).

The Bernsteinian model allows one to make some specific predictions, and they can be tested against *Tomorrow's Doctors*. In particular, the shift from a collection code to an integrated code presupposes a change in the basis of a student's educational identity. As we have seen already, traditional social and intellectual arrangements were predicated on the bounded academic discipline or specialty. In Bernstein's own terminology, identities were largely implicit in the structured divisions and positions of traditional forms. In integrated codes, on the other hand, two messages are rendered explicit. First, as we have seen, general principles and overarching themes are spelled out as organizing principles. Second, learners' identities and personal qualities themselves are made part of the pedagogical project itself. This is what has happened in the course of contemporary reform in UK medical education.

While the personal qualities of students were significant in the hidden curriculum of traditional medical education, the modern version places particular emphasis on them. This is entirely congruent with Bernstein's prediction that under an integrated, weakly framed curriculum, principles that were formerly treated as implicit will be rendered explicit. Consequently, we are not surprised to find that in *Tomorrow's Doctors* issues of attitude and behaviour are central to the formal curriculum. These include the establishment of successful relationships with patients and effective working with colleagues. Likewise, the notion of professionalism runs through the contemporary discourse on medical education. Whereas personal and professional values were implicitly inculcated in the course of prolonged exposure to the world of clinical medicine in the traditional mode, the newer curriculum and pedagogy treat them as topics for explicit socialization. Personal and professional qualities are, moreover, treated as contents susceptible to explicit evaluation and assessment. In the same way, 'ethics' and professional conduct more generally are treated as matters for explicit instruction and evaluation (Cribb and Bignold 1999). As a consequence, competencies that were formerly treated primarily as personal qualities have now become formal parts of the curriculum, subject to explicit instruction and

assessment. In curricular terms, these are subsumed under issues of communication, values and attitudes; 'attitudes and conduct' are subject to formal instruction, scrutiny and assessment. Personal, social and cultural aspects of medical
practice are explicitly part of curricular knowledge, and subject to formal assessment. This is entirely in keeping with the overall shift from collection to integrated code, where identities are increasingly rendered explicit, and integrated
within the message system of formal educational knowledge. In a similar way,
continuing professional development and a commitment to lifelong learning on
the part of the medical practitioner are among the goals of a reformed medical
training.

Discussion

As we witness major changes in the organization of the medical curriculum, we
seem to see the possibility of a major shift in knowledge, learning and the reproduction of a different form of medical knowledge itself. These fundamental
shifts redirect sociological attention towards some of the most important theorists of educational knowledge. As we (for example, Atkinson 1981) and a
number of other authors have suggested, Bernstein shares many interests with
French social thought, notably structuralist and post-structuralist in character.
Some comparisons with the work of both Bourdieu and Foucault are therefore
appropriate. Bourdieu and Bernstein are both concerned with principles of classification, and their mutual interest can be traced to common roots in the inspira-
tion of Durkheim and Mauss, most notably their work on systems of
classification (for example, Durkheim and Mauss 1963). Like Bernstein's,
Bourdieu's reflections on educational knowledge and its social formations are
concerned with symbolic boundaries. For both authors, the organization of cultural categories, including curricular knowledge and academic disciplines, is a
form of collective representation. It represents a system of discriminations
through which social differences are produced and reproduced. The order
imposed upon knowledge (such as curricular forms) inscribes a cultural and
moral order. Curriculum is not, therefore, a neutral medium for the representation of a natural or social order. It naturalizes essentially arbitrary distinctions
and boundaries to the extent that curricular knowledge seems to be a reflection
of how the world *ought* to be viewed. (As Davies (1995) points out, Bourdieu
himself managed to misrepresent Bernstein's ideas quite grotesquely, however,
and some degree of intellectual convergence should not be taken to imply perfect
congruence.)

   In key ways, therefore, this general mode of analysis has significant parallels
with that of Foucault. Like Bourdieu and like Bernstein, Foucault's general
approach emphasizes the relationships between forms of knowledge, social formations and social structure. Like Bernstein, Foucault asserts that regimes of
knowledge specify what is thinkable and what is not, what is permitted and what
is not. All three of these major theorists, in other words, draw attention to the
significance of symbolic boundaries within educational and other discursive

fields. Medicine has traditionally been a highly segmented field, and medical education equally so (Atkinson 1977). As we have seen, boundaries between phases of training and between different specialties have been among the most characteristic features of the medical school.

Within this highly segmented domain, distinctive identities have been fostered. Major specialisms such as medicine (including neurology and cardiology) and surgery (including obstetrics/gynaecology) have developed not merely specialized knowledge, but also distinctive social identities and epistemological styles (cf. Colditz and Sheehan 1982). These include characteristic attitudes and styles of language use (cf. Bourdieu and Wacquant 1992; Lingard 2007). Likewise, psychiatry has developed distinctive styles, and even more finely graded differentiations within it. The medical student and the junior, trainee doctor have traditionally circulated through a sequence of more or less discrete social worlds, each with its distinctive mode of understanding. The transformation of this segmented world in the translation of medical training into a system regulated by an integrated code represented a major transformation in the underlying principles of medical discourse. Such radical disjunctures in the discourse of medicine have the capacity to drive changes in medical knowledge and practice as much as any specific changes in biomedical technology. They deserve the close attention of sociologists – both of education and of medicine – working within the analytic tradition of Basil Bernstein and his collaborators.

References

Armstrong, D. (1980) 'Health care and the structure of medical education', in H. Noack (ed.) *Medical Education and Primary Health Care*, London: Croom Helm.

Atkinson, P. (1977) 'Professional segmentation and students' experience in a Scottish medical school', *Scottish Journal of Sociology*, 2, 1: 71–85.

—— (1981) 'Bernstein's structuralism', *Educational Analysis*, 3, 1: 85–95.

—— (1985) *Language, Structure and Reproduction: an introduction to the sociology of Basil Bernstein*, London: Methuen.

—— (1997) *The Clinical Experience: the construction and reconstruction of medical reality*, 2nd edn, Aldershot: Ashgate.

Bernstein, B. (1971) 'On the classification and framing of educational knowledge', in M. F. D. Yound (ed.) *Knowledge and Control*, London: Collier-Macmillan.

—— (2000) *Pedagogy, Symbolic Control and Identity: theory, research, critique*, rev. edn, London: Rowman and Littlefield.

Bourdieu, P. and Wacquant, L. (1992) *An Invitation to Reflexive Sociology*, Chicago, IL: University of Chicago Press.

Colditz, G. A. and Sheehan, M. (1982) 'The impact of instructional style on the development of professional characteristics', *Medical Education*, 16, 3: 127–32.

Cribb, A. and Bignold, S. (1999) 'Towards the reflexive medical school: the hidden curriculum and medical education research', *Studies in Higher Education*, 2, 2: 195–215.

Davies, B. (1995) 'Bernstein, Durkheim and the British sociology of education', in A. R. Sadovnik (ed.) *Knowledge and Pedagogy: the sociology of Basil Bernstein*, Norwood, NJ: Ablex.

Delamont, S. and Atkinson, P. (2007) 'Basil Bernstein', in J. Scott (ed.) *Fifty Key Sociologists*, London: Routledge.

Douglas, M. (1966) *Purity and Danger*, London: Routledge and Kegan Paul.

Durkheim, E. and Mauss, M. (1963) *Primitive Classification*, trans. R. Needham, London: Cohen and West.

Foucault, M. (1973) *The Birth of the Clinic: an archaeology of medical perception*, London: Tavistock.

General Medical Council (1993) *Tomorrow's Doctors: Recommendations on Undergraduate Medical Education*, London: GMC.

—— (2003) *Tomorrow's Doctors: Recommendations on Undergraduate Medical Education*, London: GMC.

Hafferty, F. W. (1991) *Into the Valley: death and the socialization of medical students*, New Haven, CT: Yale University Press.

Lingard, L. (2007) 'The rhetorical "turn" in medical education: what have we learned and where are we going?', *Advances in Health Sciences Education*, 12: 121–33.

Morais, S., Neves, I., Davies, B. and Daniels, H. (eds) (2001) *Towards a Sociology of Pedagogy: the Contribution of Basil Bernstein*, New York: Peter Lang.

Muller, J., Davies, B. and Morais, A. (eds) (2004) *Reading Bernstein, Researching Bernstein*, London: RoutledgeFalmer.

Royal Commission on Medical Education (1968) *Report of the Royal Commission on Medical Education* (The Todd Report), London: HMSO.

Sadovnik, A. (1995) 'Basil Bernstein's theory of pedagogic practice: a structuralist approach', in A. Sadovnik (ed.) *Knowledge and Pedagogy: the sociology of Basil Bernstein*, Norwood, NJ: Ablex.

Sinclair, S. (1997) *Making Doctors*, Oxford: Berg.

Turner, R. H. (1964) *The Social Context of Ambition*, San Francisco, CA: Chandler Press.

4 Pierre Bourdieu and the theory of medical education

Thinking 'relationally' about medical students and medical curricula

Caragh Brosnan

Sociologists have been studying medical education for more than 50 years. Rich empirical studies of life in medical schools and hospitals have been conducted by some of the most influential sociologists of the twentieth century. Nevertheless, sociology has yet to put forth a coherent and comprehensive theory of medical education. Fred Hafferty (2000: 241) has highlighted an analytical schism within the sociology of medical education between the majority of studies which focus on student socialization, and a less developed strand centring on organizational structure. In general, students' experiences have received ample scrutiny, while medical curricula, medical schools and the complex web of healthcare and higher-education institutions and policies impacting on medical education have received comparatively little attention. This divide is reflected in the use of theory within the sociology of medical education, which has tended to privilege agency over structure, and, less often, the reverse. As a consequence, sociology lacks a comprehensive theory accounting for both institutional arrangements and student practice in medical education, and the relationships between them.

This chapter offers one way of bridging this divide by drawing upon Pierre Bourdieu's theoretical framework in medical education. Bourdieu (1930–2002) was one of the most influential sociologists of his generation. Although relatively recently applied within the sociology of health and illness, Bourdieu's work has been profoundly influential in many other areas, particularly in the sociology of education, where his theories and empirical work have elucidated how the social order is reproduced through the educational choices and practices of individuals and institutions. Bourdieu seeks to overcome the theoretical opposition between structure and agency, urging us instead to 'think relationally' about social practices. This framework can potentially enrich a part of sociology which has tended to overemphasize either individual experience or institutional politics, thereby neglecting their interrelation.

The chapter begins by examining two key problems which sociologists have interpreted from a socialization and an organizational perspective respectively: the way medical students learn to value 'competence' over 'caring', and the lack of change brought about by medical-curriculum reform. It then explores how Bourdieu's central concepts of habitus and field could be used to reinterpret and reconcile existing interpretations, and to generate a comprehensive sociological theory of medical education.

Empirical and theoretical trends and gaps in the sociology of medical education

This section first discusses theories of medical-student socialization, focusing on studies of medical students' performance of 'competence'. It then examines the problem of 'reform without change' in medical curricula, which has been analysed from an organizational perspective.

Medical-student socialization: the production of 'competence'

How medical-student socialization takes place was the principal question in the first two major works in the sociology of medical education. Robert Merton and his associates produced the famous structural-functionalist study, *The Student-Physician* (1957), which analysed the 'professional socialization' of medical students. This was defined as:

> the processes through which he [sic] develops his professional self, with its characteristic values, attitudes, knowledge, and skills, fusing these into a more or less consistent set of dispositions which govern his behavior in a wide variety of professional (and extraprofessional) situations.
>
> (1957: 287)

The authors focused on the values, norms and roles of physicians and how the acquisition of this culture is central to becoming a member of the profession. Socialization is portrayed as a straightforward process, in which students are gradually assimilated into the medical profession. This process was uncontested and hence the outcomes were seen to be obvious and unproblematic.

In *Boys in White* (1961), Howard Becker and colleagues produced a study of Kansas medical students in which the experiences of medical students as social actors were privileged over the overt function of professional socialization. From within their symbolic interactional perspective, the authors discovered that part of the socialization process for students was learning how to survive the medical course itself. Becker's study identified a series of 'perspectives', each involving a different strategy that students engaged to organize their navigation through the course. For example, students learned how to impress the lecturers ('academic perspective') and to cooperate among themselves to decide how much work to do ('cooperation perspective'). While the Merton study assumed the consensual acquisition of norms, Becker's research drew attention to the competing versions of reality among staff and students and showed how students learned to manipulate the system.

These classic studies used competing theoretical perspectives, yet both were essentially concerned with students' experiences and they set the scene for later work. It is now generally acknowledged that both were correct (Light 1988: 313): medical students learn how to act like doctors through interaction with faculty members and with each other, but socialization does not always unambiguously reflect explicit institutional values. At the same time, both formulations left gaps; neither took account of the medical schools in which the students studied – their histories, their curricula, their faculties, and their prestige or power. Nor was there any consideration of the external social structures impacting on the culture or organization of medical education, or the perpetuation of social structure through medical education. Written during the 'golden age of doctoring', both studies ultimately valorized medicine as a profession (Cockerham elaborates further in Chapter 14 of this *Handbook*).

Though more critical, subsequent work has relied on similar conceptualizations of medical education as an interactional process, with the performative nature of medical-student socialization addressed in *Boys in White* providing the framework for a number of subsequent studies (for example, Atkinson 1997; Sinclair 1997). A common conclusion of these studies is that at the heart of student performance is a desire to appear 'competent'. Haas and Shaffir (1982) studied how students cope with the uncertainties of medicine and their novice status, concluding that they learn to adopt the 'cloak of competence'. That is, medical students work to give the appearance of knowledgeability and confidence whether or not this is well founded. A large part of their education involves learning to 'role play' in order to meet public expectations of professionalism.

Good and Good (1993) argue that medical-student socialization forces students to confront the 'dual discourse' of competence and caring. Students wish, and are expected, to master both aspects of being a doctor: competence (associated with scientific language, 'doing'/action and 'value-free' facts, knowledge and techniques) and caring (associated with values, relationships, attitudes, compassion and empathy) (p. 91). However, Good and Good argue that the structure of medical education has favoured the inculcation of competence at the cost of caring. Their and other studies have highlighted several factors which facilitate competence and discourage caring. Factual overload is often implicated – there are so many facts to be memorized in pre-clinical medicine that students only manage to learn selectively what they think is going to be examined, while the social and humanistic aspects of medicine receive the lowest priority (Becker *et al.* 1961; Sinclair 1997). Scientific language quickly becomes the norm at medical school (Good and Good 1993; Lief and Fox 1963; Sinclair 1997), but this discourse cannot express caring values and sentiments. Simultaneously, through undertaking anatomical dissection, students begin to conceive of human bodies as machines and to depersonalize patients (Good and Good 1993; Lief and Fox 1963; Sinclair 1997). Depersonalization is further encouraged by the emphasis clinical training places on technology rather than interactional care (Davis-Floyd 1987). Sociologists have found that ultimately cynicism and a loss of idealism result from the fundamental struggle students experience between their performance of competence for the benefit of the faculty and the concomitant need to quash their personal feelings and sense of idealism (Becker *et al.* 1961; Haas and Shaffir 1982; Sinclair 1997).

Studies concentrating on medical students' experiences have revealed problematic socialization patterns taking place which may have implications for the future treatment of patients. However, because virtually all studies have focused on interactions between students and staff in a single institution, they have left several questions unanswered: why are the same features of medical-student socialization, such as the emphasis on competence rather than caring, reproduced in different decades and in different places? Why are curricula dominated by bioscience in the first place? These questions point to the need for research on the organizational and structural aspects of medical education.

Organizational structure: curriculum 'reform without change'

Recognizing the narrowness of the socialization focus in the sociology of medical education, Donald Light commented in 1988 that:

> [I]n retrospect it seems remarkable that so many of us spent 20 years debating whether medical students were 'boys in white' or 'student-physicians'.... It is time to expand from this body of work, however insightful, to institutional and comparative analysis.
>
> (1988: 312–13)

Despite repeated calls for the sociology of medical education to move beyond its focus on student socialization, very few studies have examined medical education at a more macro or structural level. Almost all studies have been conducted within a single medical school, and have tended to take for granted the medical school itself as an institution, thereby ignoring medical schools' relationships to the healthcare system, the bioscientific research enterprise and the state. In short, there has been insufficient attention given to the whole national system of medical education, especially the competition between medical schools for students, funding, research grading and international prestige.

One issue which sociologists of medical education have tried to understand at an institutional level, at least theoretically, is curriculum reform. The traditional medical curriculum consists of two pre-clinical years focusing on basic sciences (such as anatomy, physiology and biochemistry), taught mainly by scientists in lectures and laboratories, and two or three clinical years, taught by doctors at the bedside. Curricular reforms since the 1950s have attempted to blend the scientific and clinical phases in order to reduce the factual overload and reductionistic focus noted above. These reforms also seek to address students' attitudes alongside knowledge and skills, in order to create medical practitioners with a more humanistic and holistic orientation to practice and patients. These changes are well documented elsewhere in our *Handbook*. However, research has repeatedly found that even in these so-called 'integrated' or 'innovative' curricula students continue to focus on 'competence' and learning 'facts' (Good and Good 1993;

Haas and Shaffir 1982; Knight and Mattick 2006). This outcome has led Bloom (1988: 294) to characterize medical-curriculum reform as 'reform without change'.

Sociologists have proffered various explanations as to why reform has been ineffective. Some argue that the reforms have not been implemented effectively. Hafferty (1998, 2000, and Chapter 2 of this *Handbook*) argues that reforms have targeted the formal curriculum, leaving intact the 'hidden curriculum' of medical education. The hidden curriculum is 'a set of influences that function at the level of organizational structure and culture' (Hafferty 1998: 403–4). Hidden curricular messages are encapsulated in organizational features such as: the allocation of resources; award ceremonies; staff appointments; the erection of new buildings; curriculum design; and the scheduling of some classes at 'prime time' while leaving others as electives (Hafferty 1998). One example is that, despite medical schools' public statements to the contrary, successful admission continues to depend mainly on students passing tests, rather than demonstrating qualities such as ethical awareness (Hafferty 2000: 249). Hafferty argues that this sends a clear message to students about what is truly valued by medical schools. The hidden curriculum is one of the few theories to attempt to connect student socialization to organizational structure. However, precisely how the hidden curriculum affects students' learning has not been empirically verified. Moreover, a curriculum-centred approach, while offering an explanation of why students' attitudes have not changed, cannot explain why particular values are reproduced at an organizational level, for example why students are judged on their test scores. Other theories point to major obstacles beyond the curriculum in the form of structural divisions within medical education.

Medical education is enmeshed in a complex structure of institutions, including hospitals, universities, the medical profession and the healthcare system, each of which have vested interests in the content of medical curricula. Bloom (1988) contends that the research focus of medical schools has prevented meaningful curriculum reform. He points out that the traditional curriculum was designed to incorporate and to further biomedical research. It resulted in powerful basic science departments being set up, each with their own agendas, and generated tension between the scientific and clinical faculties. As medical schools expanded into unwieldy bureaucracies over the twentieth century, they could no longer be supported by educational funds, and therefore came to depend on the resources generated through research (Bloom 1988). Research began to compete with and to be prioritized over teaching. Bloom (1988: 294) argues that research is now the main driver in medical schools and that 'medical education's manifest humanistic mission is little more than a screen for the research mission which is the major concern of the institution's social structure'. The development of these schools as centres of research prestige rather than teaching excellence is indicated spatially by the typical separation between medical faculties and the rest of the university.

Another competing factor is the clinical faculty's involvement in patient care. In the US, Ludmerer (1999: 372) suggests that through the expansion of faculty for-profit practice, a proprietary system is re-emerging: medical schools now rely on patient care to generate income, bringing hospitals back to the centre of medical education, as in the nineteenth century. Medical schools' link to the university has diminished as they have become 'enmeshed more firmly than ever in the health care delivery system' (Ludmerer 1999: 221). Many more clinical faculty members have been hired in order to bring in funds, but as Fox (1999: 14) points out, 'many of these clinician-nonteachers are faculty in name only' – their job is to see as many patients as possible. The resource-driven emphasis on both basic science research and clinical care in medical schools is supported by the traditional pre-clinical–clinical curricular divide, and therefore undermines attempts to instigate integrated medical curricula.

It has also been argued that curricular reform serves symbolic purposes. For example, Vinten-Johansen and Riska (1991: 82) posit that the American medical profession instigated reform from the 1960s as a strategy to maintain autonomy in the face of perceived threats of governmental intervention. The inclusion of social sciences in medical curricula may have served a symbolic function in expressing the medical profession's social commitment (Vinten-Johansen and Riska 1991).

While there are numerous theories of how structural and organizational factors impact on medical curricula, there has been little attempt to consider how they affect medical-student socialization. For example, what is the impact of structural features on the day-to-day experiences of medical students and what is learned both formally and informally via the hidden curriculum? In particular, there has been little theorization of the role of medical schools themselves, as the institutions which mediate between the demands of clinical care, bioscientific research and the education of students. The analytical schism between socialization and organizational perspectives in medical education must be repaired in order to begin to understand these issues. In the next section, Bourdieu's main concepts of capital, field and habitus are outlined, before examining how they may enable us to 'think relationally' to generate a more coherent understanding of medical education.

Bourdieu's theoretical framework

The most widely used concept within Bourdieu's repertoire is the idea of habitus, which is defined as:

> a system of lasting, transposable dispositions which, integrating past experiences, functions at every moment as a *matrix of perceptions, appreciations, and actions* and makes possible the achievement of infinitely diversified tasks, thanks to analogical transfers of schemes permitting the solution of similarly shaped problems.
>
> (Bourdieu 1977: 82–3, emphasis in original)

Habitus is essentially Bourdieu's theory of socialization. The dispositions which compose an individual habitus are disproportionately weighted by the early experiences of family life, through which all subsequent experience is perceived (Bourdieu 1977: 78). Familial habitus then underpins the structuring of school experiences, in turn changing the habitus and structuring future experiences (1977: 87). So, the habitus is structured by the past and structures the future. Crucially, the habitus generates action; it is 'this kind of practical sense for what is to be done in a given situation' (Bourdieu 1998: 25).

Consistent with Bourdieu's overall project, the function of the habitus concept is to overcome the dichotomy between perspectives which deny all individual agency and ascribe action to external forces, and those which posit that all action is the result of individual rational calculation (Bourdieu 1977). Bourdieu conceives habitus as being formed and operating within a social 'field'. A field is 'a network, or configuration, of objective relations between positions' (Bourdieu and Wacquant 1992: 97), functioning as an arena 'of production, circulation, and appropriation of goods, services, knowledge or status' (Swartz 1997: 117). Within the various fields, agents (individuals or institutions) occupy different relative positions of power, objectively defined according to how much of these resources, or capital, they possess (Bourdieu 1998: 5, 31–2; Bourdieu and Waquant 1992: 96–101). Bourdieu refers to capital not just in the economic sense, but as a term to describe any goods or characteristics which are valued and used to gain power and prestige in a given field. He discusses various types of capital – social, cultural, symbolic, academic and so on. Each field is characterized by a 'game' in which forms of capital are competed for, and in which the definition of legitimate capital is also struggled over. For example, in the scientific field the game involves the definition of legitimate science (what is 'good' science?), as well as competition over legitimated forms of scientific capital (Albert *et al.* 2007). It is the relative positioning of agents within a field which is of most significance to Bourdieu, for it is these relationships which determine what gets defined as legitimate in that field.

Fields overlap with each other but are also relatively autonomous (Bourdieu and Wacquant 1992: 98). However, the political and economic fields interact with all fields to some extent, and the degree to which fields are able to achieve autonomy – the ability to define the content of their own problems – varies along a continuum (Bourdieu 2000: 112; Maton 2005). In all fields there is a tension between their autonomous, inward-focused activities (associated with cultural capital) and their heteronomous orientation to political and economic success (or economic capital) (Maton 2005: 690).

Forms of capital interact and are often translatable; for example, having high cultural capital (the 'right' tastes) is likely to facilitate access to high social capital (the 'right' social connections). Judgements of what counts as legitimate capital are formed through the habitus, and agents compete strategically within fields to distinguish themselves from others through their capital. An individual's ability to accrue legitimate capital within a given field is determined by his/her habitus, thus the game played within a field is not a fair one: those whose prior experience has not imbued them with valued forms of capital will be relegated to the subordinate positions of the field, while those with legitimate habitus are able to ascend to dominant positions within the field and to gain more capital. It is in this way that the habitus reproduces the field, while the field simultaneously reproduces habitus. Both dominant and subordinate agents contribute to reproducing the field through their practices, because all agents in a field share the belief that the stakes they are struggling for are worthwhile, that the 'game' is worth playing: this is what Bourdieu defines as the *illusio* which unites any field and which makes social change so difficult to achieve (Bourdieu 2000: 11).

Bourdieu's theories were grounded in his wide-ranging empirical work and were always intended by him to be used as empirical tools (Wacquant 2005). Central to any Bourdieusian analysis is the need to 'think relationally' (Bourdieu 1992), to analyse the relationship between agents in a field, between field and habitus and between fields. As Bourdieu's colleague Wacquant (2005: 318) explains, 'a full analysis of practice thus requires a triple elucidation of the social genesis and structures of habitus and field, and of the dynamics of their "dialectical confrontation"'. I will now examine how Bourdieu's work has been and could be used to unpack the sociology of medical education, beginning by discussing the medical habitus.

The medical habitus

The concept of habitus has the potential to provide a more comprehensive theory of medical-student socialization than has been developed so far, and to move beyond the student-centred focus to examine how and why particular behaviours and attitudes are reproduced in medical education. Though he did not study medical education, Bourdieu has shown that education is central to the reproduction of habitus and the overall structure of fields. Elsewhere, medical education has often been described in terms that sound remarkably like the habitus. As cited earlier, Merton *et al.* (1957: 287) in their original description of medical-student socialization define it as the development of a 'more or less consistent set of dispositions which govern ... behavior in a wide variety of professional (and extraprofessional) situations'. Becker *et al.* (1961) also described the use of strategies in a field when they demonstrated that students focus on pleasing the faculty and working out 'what they want us to know', while Good's (1995) medical-student interviewees talked explicitly of learning to 'play the game' of medicine. Drawing from his own and others' observations of medical trainees' displays of 'competence', Light (1979: 313) concludes that 'Ironically, through this process of impression management, trainees get taken in by their own act until the self-conscious process of role simulation becomes the real thing', that is, strategies to succeed in the medical field become an unconscious practical sense. Therefore, medical education involves the development of lasting dispositions which imbue trainees with a practical sense of how to succeed in the field, and could potentially be seen as the production of a habitus.

Indeed, several empirical studies have found evidence for a distinct 'medical habitus' arising through medical training. Sinclair (1997) concludes from his ethnographic study of a London medical school that medical education involves the development of a set of dispositions which together form a medical habitus. Sinclair describes the way the world of medical students becomes 'scientific' and also how they embrace notions about 'pathology' in their new knowledge and the language accompanying it – this perspective becomes a way of seeing and interpreting the world and acting in it. Students also learn through their own bodies, for example by practising clinical skills on themselves. In this way, medical knowledge is embodied and generates a habitus; it involves a real cognitive and corporeal shift. Like Becker *et al.* (1961), Sinclair found that the medical habitus centres around producing competent practice, rather than caring dispositions, yet this clashes with the idealistic dispositions students have when they enter medicine, resulting in cynicism. Because it is part of their habitus, students are unable to reflect on their conflicting dispositions. Although students are aware that achieving competence is 'all a game' (Sinclair 1997: 303), they are otherwise largely unreflexive, tending to accept stress and other problems as linked to immediate experience rather than to broader social and political structures of training. The medical habitus is the source of, and helps sustain problematic dispositions within medicine.

Melia (1999) asserts that Sinclair's use of Bourdieu's concept of dispositions largely adds confusion to what is essentially an exact replication of Becker *et al.*'s study. Indeed, many of the 'dispositions' Sinclair derives are drawn directly from Becker *et al.* and actually sound more like forms of capital that might be struggled for in the field, for example the dispositions of 'status' and 'knowledge'. Sinclair's study was, nevertheless, the first sustained attempt to interpret medical education through Bourdieu's theory.

Haida Luke (2003) places the medical habitus at the centre of her analysis of junior-doctor training in her ethnographic study, *Medical Education and Sociology of Medical Habitus*. Luke's work explores the transition from undergraduate training to full professional status, as junior doctors go from being 'clinical doctors' (technically qualified) to 'social doctors' with a 'feel for the game' of medicine. Luke argues that in order to access valued forms of capital, such as a place in specialty training, junior doctors must develop a medical habitus – that is the set of dispositions needed to successfully practise, behave and look like 'a doctor'. Luke documents the way the junior doctors gradually learn to (in their own words) 'play the game' of medicine. For example, being at the bottom of the hierarchy, they had to 'suck up' to the right people, to be compliant and 'likeable'. They learned which consultants represented valuable social capital and how to use cultural capital to access it. Like Sinclair, Luke found that cynicism was an integral and inevitable part of the medical habitus.

Luke's study again highlights the embodied nature of the medical habitus. The junior doctors quickly began to dress conservatively and to mimic the posture and voice of the registrars. They learned where to stand and how to conduct themselves on ward rounds, until finally these behaviours had become natural for them. Thus, the habitus explains 'how professions succeed in reproducing themselves in the form of durable dispositions in people' (Luke 2003: 52).

Heidi Lempp's work (2003; and Chapter 5 in this *Handbook*) also draws on Bourdieu's metaphor of learning to play the game, and briefly touches on the medical habitus. Like Luke, Lempp contends that medical training can be conceptualized as learning to develop dispositions which facilitate access to the economic, social, cultural and symbolic capital held by members of the profession. Students in her study perceived that sanctioned dispositions included keeping quiet about their concerns or their academic problems, and, for some, refraining from showing emotion or 'being human'. In turn, they hoped to be rewarded through good marks and future job opportunities. The training process involves oppressive power dynamics; one of Lempp's major findings was that on the way to developing the correct habitus medical students were subjected to abuse and humiliation by senior doctors, which led to stress.

These studies of the medical habitus each identify the same two problems: medical students/junior doctors experience stress related to their professional role; and the medical habitus suppresses caring dispositions while producing competent practice. The performance of 'competence' is a social production defined by the field which becomes embodied through the habitus and structures medical students' perceptions of legitimate practice. This reconceptualization helps to move toward a more coherent and precise theory of how medical socialization works. However, there is a need for further investigation of the possibility of a medical habitus and how it functions.

The studies using habitus remain student-centred and therefore neglect to investigate the judgement of taste/practice. By only uncovering students' and trainees' perceptions, this research does not reveal how the dominant agents in the field, that is qualified doctors, distinguish 'good' from 'bad' practice. This may or may not be according to the same values as the students, who have yet to fully develop the medical habitus. It may also be revealing to examine the habitus which different medical students bring to the field. Bourdieu (1988: 56) in fact argues that the dispositions required for success within a professional group are 'learnt less by educational apprenticeship than by previous and external experiences'. Which sorts of habitus and capital facilitate access to medical school in the first place?

The possibility of a variety of different forms of habitus operating among medical students is yet to be explored. In his study of the academic field, *Homo Academicus*, Bourdieu (1988) identifies a schism within the medical faculty between the basic scientists and clinical practitioners, whose differing social backgrounds produce differing types of habitus and strategies within the academy. Sinclair (1997: 299) hypothesizes that medical students and junior doctors will develop a basic medical habitus by going through the same training, but will give it their own 'style' in terms of which specialty they choose. Do the social backgrounds of medical students influence their 'style' of medical habitus? Do students with the same backgrounds select the same institutions? Do some students have a habitus akin to the basic scientists and others to the clinicians? These are questions which Bourdieu's framework is primed to examine.

Finally, the use of the habitus concept alone cannot paint a full picture of the sociology of medical education. As explained above, Bourdieu's theoretical tools are designed to work together as a whole, with his central method being to think relationally about the positions of individuals and institutions within the field and the dynamic between the field and a given habitus. The previous studies of the medical habitus focus only on students' dispositions within single institutions, leaving the field of medical education, its history and objective structures (for example, the institutions in which education takes place) unexamined. Little explanation has been offered as to why similar medical habitus are developed across time and place. It is important, therefore, to analyse the 'field' of medical education, in which the medical habitus is forged.

Medical education as a field

The field can offer an integrative theory of the structure of medical education, incorporating existing perspectives which have pointed separately to the influences of research, clinical care and the symbolic value of reform. It is also a framework well suited to conducting the institutional and comparative analysis which has long been called for in studies of medical education. Bourdieu's compulsion to think relationally renders comparison a necessity in empirical work. The concept of field has not been used to study medical education, although the fields within higher education were among Bourdieu's central research sites. In *The State Nobility* (1996), Bourdieu examined the struggle for capital between elite French universities. He argued that the French higher-education field was structured by a double orientation towards autonomy and heteronomy:

> On the one side, we find establishments that, in their selection criteria, their faculty, and their curricula, as well as in the career prospects they open up, have close ties to industrial and commercial firms.... On the other side, we find establishments that stress strictly academic demands and ... are relatively independent of the demands of the economic system.
>
> (1996: 152–3)

At each university, applicants' dispositions, the curriculum content and the institution's ethos together comprised a 'marketable commodity' (Robbins 1993: 158), which attracted students who in turn added to that institution's capital and thereby reproduced the field structure. Drawing on Bourdieu's framework, Naidoo's (2004) study of the South African university field revealed three hierarchical tiers – the 'English' universities, the 'Afrikaans' universities and the 'black' universities – which differed according to research funding, the prestige of their qualifications, and their degree of independence from the state. Naidoo showed that the institutions' admissions policies were used strategically to maintain or gain capital in the field. Such work demonstrates the importance of inter-institutional comparison as a technique to study medical education, as medical schools' differing curricula and admissions practices, for instance, are revelatory of their relative positions within the field and therefore of what is at stake in the field at a given point in time. The values of the field in turn will shape the medical-student habitus.

Conceptualizing medical education as a field may shed light on the problem of 'reform without change'. While some commentators have pointed to the push for biomedical research as degrading teaching and impeding reform, others have implicated the demands of clinical work. Both theories suggest that a struggle is taking place in medical education to define the most legitimate forms of practice. As noted earlier, in *Homo Academicus* Bourdieu (1988) identified a dispositional opposition between scientists and clinicians in the medical faculty. The two groups struggled to distinguish themselves by legitimating different knowledge types:

> [T]he faculty of medicine alone duplicates, in a manner of speaking, the whole space of the faculties (and even the field of power) ... [T]he complex and multidimensional opposition between the clinical practitioners and the biologists in the medical faculties ... can be described as the opposition between an *art*, guided by the 'experience' culled from the example of their elders, and acquired over a period of time through attention to individual cases, and a *science*, which is not satisfied with the external appearances which prompt diagnosis, but seeks to grasp the underlying causes.
>
> (1988: 59, emphasis in original)

These faculty members had different agendas within the academic field – while the clinicians followed heteronomous strategies, seeking economic and political capital, the medical scientists conducted pure research as much as possible in order to remain autonomous (Bourdieu 1988: 60). Although Bourdieu's study was conducted in France in the 1960s, a struggle between scientists and clinicians in medical education has been documented since the earliest days of curriculum reform in both the US and UK (see for example, Bonner 1995), suggesting that this 'game' is characteristic of the medical-education field. This may mean that, while there are structural demands on medical schools both to conduct biomedical research and focus on clinical care, it is also the case that these practices take priority over teaching because they enable scientific and clinical faculty members to gain sought-after forms of capital and to distinguish themselves from each other. Simultaneously, these practices would maintain the different habitus of scientists and clinicians and their dispositions towards legitimate medical knowledge (science versus art). Hence, curricular reforms which attempt to blend science and clinical work would not fit with the central game of the field and would be discounted by both scientists and clinicians.

It has been argued that medical-curriculum reform serves symbolic purposes rather than effecting real change. Bourdieu's framework can help extend and test this theory by examining precisely which forms of symbolic capital are struggled for in the medical-education field, by whom, and what other forms of capital they are translated into. In *Homo Academicus*, by turning his analysis on the academic field itself, Bourdieu (1988: 123) demonstrated that all scholarship is political: 'declarations in the domain of theory, method, technique or even style are always social strategies in which powers are affirmed and claimed'. In Bourdieu's terms, medical-curriculum reform can be seen as a strategy to either gain legitimate forms of capital or to subvert the field by asserting the value of a new type of education. The strategy followed depends on the position within the field of the institution or agent instigating the reform. As suggested by Bourdieu's (1996) analysis of French universities, differences between medical schools' curricula may be particularly demonstrative of social strategies to gain or retain power, and of the relative positioning of medical schools in the field. In the UK, for example, the medical schools with the highest research profiles have tended to retain largely traditional medical curricula, while the newest medical schools, which generally have lower research income and prestige, typically claim to have 'innovative' curricula which integrate science with clinical practice. This may represent attempts on the part of the new schools to symbolically differentiate themselves from the dominant players in the field, rather than to attempt to compete on the same terms. A study of the symbolic purposes of curriculum reform would again need to centre on an analysis of the objective positions of institutions within the field and their relation to one another.

The field theory can help to consolidate the different explanations sociologists have proffered for why curriculum reform does not result in change. It can be seen that those theories which place an emphasis on the content of the curriculum itself, implicitly conceptualize medical education as autonomously orientated – as deciding internally what is to be valued. The theorists who point to the competing interests of research and patient care, on the other hand, are emphasizing the heteronomy of medical education – its reliance on capital from outside the field. Bourdieu shows that in fact all fields are structured by both autonomous and heteronomous principles. The field concept can help to unpack the relationship between the internal and external factors influencing curriculum reform. The 'hidden curriculum' theory comes close to a Bourdieusian conceptualization of the field when Hafferty points to features of organizational structure and culture, such as corporately sponsored buildings, as influencing students' perceptions. However, a Bourdieusian study would look empirically at *which* schools have carried out *which* practices, such as redesigning their curriculum or employing large research faculties, how this affects their status relative to other schools and, in turn, how this affects which students attend which schools. Finally, the argument that curriculum reform is some sort of symbolic gesture serving the purposes either of medical schools or the medical profession, can be reconceptualized in Bourdieusian terms as a struggle by competing agents to attain symbolic capital in the field, which is translatable into other forms of power.

As a tool for empirical research, the field concept can take account of the multiple influences of biomedical research, patient care, government and public pressure and higher-educational politics on medical education, and how these are played out within specific institutions. Importantly, the theory of the field also provides a framework for understanding students' experiences and attitudes. The formation of a medical habitus will always take place within the medical education field and reflect and reinforce the values of the field. The dynamics of the interaction of habitus and field in the context of medical education requires sustained empirical investigation. The significance of medical schools themselves as institutions which mediate this interaction is also an important question. Those studies which have described a 'medical habitus' assume the cross-institutional homogeneity of medical students' experiences. Indeed, Bourdieu (1996) does show that students of the same discipline tend to share many dispositions, because of that discipline's place in the field. However, he also demonstrates in *The State Nobility* that students with similar backgrounds, dispositions and stances tend to select the same universities. That is, universities 'draw and honor mainly those students who are most strongly attracted to them in the first place because their dispositions are living embodiments of the kind of capital these schools demand and valorize' (Wacquant 1996: xii). At the same time, educational institutions work to perpetuate the perception among their students that that institution confers the most legitimate form of capital. This is partly accomplished through the curriculum and its delivery. Thus, in order to understand the development of medical students' attitudes and preferences for practice, it is necessary to pinpoint their particular medical school's position in the field.

There is already some evidence that the reproduction of institutions' ethos through the dispositions of their students takes place in the medical-education field. Roath *et al.*'s (1977) UK study showed that medical students at Cardiff and Sheffield were more favourable towards the traditional curriculum and more concerned with prestige than students at Dundee or Southampton, where students were more likely to value early patient contact. Students' preferences reflected their school's practices. The Cardiff and Sheffield students also tended to agree with each other on a number of other issues, as did the Dundee and Southampton students, demonstrating a social grouping of medical schools in the UK. Maheux *et al.* (1989) produced similar results in a survey of three Michigan medical schools: a very 'traditional' school which placed an emphasis on science and high admission grades; another 'conventional' school with a strong reputation for clinical practice; and an 'innovative' school which emphasized social and behavioural sciences and community-based practice. The students at each school tended to cite, respectively, the 'biomedical research', 'clinical medicine' or 'human and social' orientation of their school as being most valuable. Students' backgrounds differed by school: the 'innovative' school students were, in short, older, and more likely to come from minority and lower socioeconomic backgrounds than the other two groups. Other US studies have shown an association between medical-school type and primary-care specialization: public medical schools with low research profiles tend towards the production of primary-care doctors (Bland *et al.* 1995: 624). Though not referring to Bourdieu, these studies document a relationship between medical schools, medical students' profiles, the curriculum and students' preferences, which resembles the interaction of a field and agents' habitus. This illustrates how Bourdieu's central concepts of habitus and field may be used together to examine the dynamic between the organizational features of medical education and the socialization of medical students, with medical schools at the centre of their interrelationality.

Conclusion: thinking relationally about medical education

Sociological studies of medical education have uncovered problems with both the socialization of medical students and the reform of medical curricula. Medical students learn to perform 'competently', narrowly defined within medical culture as the acquisition of 'hard' knowledge and the exclusion of caring behaviour. Medical-curricular reform has not significantly altered this fundamental value system. The interrelation of these two problems has never been fully explored, because of a lack of application of a comprehensive theoretical framework within this area of sociology. Rather, the two issues have been treated as separate phenomena, reflecting the analytical separation of studies of students' experiences and theories of the organizational structure of medical education. Bourdieu's theoretical bastion of 'thinking relationally', along with his key concepts of habitus, field and capital, can be used to unpack the mutual constitution of medical students' perceptions of legitimate practice and the structure of medical curricula.

The traditional medical curriculum, with its distinction between scientific and clinical education, reflects the oppositional relationship between the scientific and clinical faculty members in medical education – each with their own definitions of what counts as legitimate knowledge and practice. This relationship reproduces the structure of the curriculum, while the curriculum simultaneously maintains the oppositional relationship between these groups. The struggle by these different faculty members to gain power and distinction in the field is played out in their pursuit of different forms of capital, such as the income generated through clinical care and biomedical research. In turn, this struggle determines what counts as legitimate within the medical education field, meaning that scientific and clinical forms of knowledge and practice take precedence over social or humanistic forms. Curricular reform which attempts to integrate science and clinical work and to promote the social within medical education is anathema to the very game which unites the field and thus has little success.

Rather than being a separate problem located at an individual level, the socialization of medical students takes place within this same field, and therefore reflects these same values. Studies which have drawn on habitus to conceptualize medical-student socialization show that students' performance of scientific or clinical competence is used to access valued forms of capital, while caring is rarely seen as a legitimate or valued practice. The relationship between field and habitus is not unidirectional, however: at the same time as students' dispositions are shaped by the field, students perpetuate the field struggle through their habitus, by playing the game of medical education themselves in their struggle to be seen as 'competent'. A further example of students' reproduction of the field is through their choice of medical school; for example, in the UK students with the best secondary school results tend to choose the most traditional (and most prestigious) medical schools, thereby lending legitimacy to the traditional curriculum. Rather than simply having institutional values imposed on them, students are drawn towards institutions which share their values. Thus, medical students' dispositions both shape and are shaped by the field, as are medical curricula. Curricular 'reform without change' and students' perception that competence has greater value than caring are not two different issues; instead, each is sustained by and reproduces the other, both being underpinned by the *illusio* of the field.

By privileging the relationships between institutions and agents and between field and habitus, a Bourdieusian analysis opens up a new and more coherent way of understanding how medical education works. It helps to reconceptualize some prior theories of medical education. For example, the concept of agents strategically competing for capital in a defined field enables a more nuanced analysis than Bloom's (1988) contention that reform is a 'screen' for medical schools' research mission. In addition, the idea of a habitus which shapes students' preferences for medical schools and their judgements of legitimate knowledge, helps to explain how the 'hidden curriculum' hypothesized by Hafferty works in practice. Bourdieu's work has the potential to move the sociology of medical education beyond the false division between student experiences and organizational structures that has plagued it so far. Ultimately, Bourdieu's concepts are tools for research, and their use in empirical studies would better elucidate the social processes of medical education while at the same time enabling a fuller assessment of their strengths and weaknesses through their application to a new empirical area. Future research might usefully draw on Bourdieu to take account of the relationships between medical students, faculty members and medical schools, and what counts as legitimate knowledge and practice in the field of medical education.

References

Albert, M., Hodges, B. and Regehr, G. (2007) 'Research in medical education: balancing service and science', *Advances in Health Sciences Education*, 12: 103–15.

Atkinson, P. (1997) *The Clinical Experience: the construction and reconstruction of medical reality*, 2nd edn, Aldershot: Ashgate.

Becker, H., Geer, B., Hughes, E. and Strauss, A. (1961) *Boys in White: student culture in medical school*, Chicago, IL: University of Chicago Press.

Bland, C., Meurer, L. and Maldonado, G. (1995) 'Determinants of primary care specialty choice: a non-statistical meta-analysis of the literature', *Academic Medicine*, 70: 620–41.

Bloom, S. (1988) 'Structure and ideology in medical education: an analysis of resistance to change', *Journal of Health and Social Behavior*, 29: 294–306.

Bonner, T. (1995) *Becoming a Physician: medical education in Britain, France, Germany and the United States, 1750–1945*, Oxford: Oxford University Press.

Bourdieu, P. (1977) *Outline of a Theory of Practice*, Cambridge: Cambridge University Press.

—— (1988) *Homo Academicus*, Cambridge: Polity Press.

—— (1992) 'The practice of reflexive sociology (the Paris workshop)', in P. Bourdieu and L. Wacquant (eds) *An Invitation to Reflexive Sociology*, Cambridge: Polity Press.

—— (1996) *The State Nobility: elite schools in the field of power*, Cambridge: Polity Press.

—— (1998) *Practical Reason: on the theory of action*, Cambridge: Polity Press.

—— (2000) *Pascalian Meditations*, Cambridge: Polity Press.

Davis-Floyd, R. (1987) 'Obstetric training as a rite of passage', *Medical Anthropology*, 1: 288–318.

Fox, R. (1999) 'Is medical education asking too much of bioethics?', *Daedalus*, 128: 1–25.

Good, B. and Good, M. (1993) '"Learning medicine": the constructing of medical knowledge at Harvard Medical School', in S. Lindenbaum and M. Lock (eds) *Knowledge, Power and Practice: the anthropology of medicine and everyday life*, London: University of California Press.

Good, M. (1995) *American Medicine: the quest for competence*, London: University of California Press.

Haas, J. and Shaffir, W. (1982) 'Ritual evaluation of competence: the hidden curriculum of professionalization in an innovative medical school program', *Work and Occupations*, 9: 131–54.

Hafferty, F. W. (1998) 'Beyond curriculum reform: confronting medicine's hidden curriculum', *Academic Medicine*, 73: 403–7.

—— (2000) 'Reconfiguring the sociology of medical education: emerging topics and pressing issues', in C. Bird, P. Conrad and A. Fremont (eds) *Handbook of Medical Sociology*, 5th edn, London: Prentice Hall.

Knight, L. and Mattick, K. (2006) '"When I first came here, I thought medicine was black and white": making sense of medical students' ways of knowing', *Social Science & Medicine*, 63: 1084–96.

Lempp, H. (2003) 'Undergraduate medical education: a transition from medical student to pre-registration doctor', unpublished thesis, Goldsmiths College, University of London.

Lief, H. and Fox, R. (1963) 'Training for "detached concern" in medical students', in H. Lief, V. Lief and N. Lief (eds) *The Psychological Basis of Medical Practice*, New York: Harper & Row.

Light, D. (1979) 'Uncertainty and control in professional training', *Journal of Health and Social Behavior*, 20: 310–22.

—— (1988) 'Towards a new sociology of medical education', *Journal of Health and Social Behavior*, 29: 307–22.

Ludmerer, K. (1999) *Time to Heal: American medical education from the turn of the century to the era of managed care*, Oxford: Oxford University Press.

Luke, H. (2003) *Medical Education and Sociology of Medical Habitus: 'It's not about the stethoscope!'*, Dordrecht: Kluwer Academic Publishers.

Maheux, B., Beland, F., Pineault, R., Rivest, P. and Valois, L. (1989) 'Do conventional and innovative medical schools recruit different students?', *Medical Education*, 23: 30–8.

Maton, K. (2005) 'A question of autonomy: Bourdieu's field approach and higher education policy', *Journal of Education Policy*, 20: 687–704.

Melia, K. (1999) 'Review of S. Sinclair, *Making Doctors: an institutional apprenticeship*', *Sociology of Health and Illness*, 21: 126–7.

Merton, R., Reader, G. and Kendall, P. (eds) (1957) *The Student-Physician: introductory studies in the sociology of medical education*, Cambridge, MA: Harvard University Press.

Naidoo, R. (2004) 'Fields and institutional strategy: Bourdieu on the relationship between higher education, inequality and society', *British Journal of Sociology of Education*, 25: 457–71.

Roath, S., Miller, E., Kilpatrick, G., Hudson, G., Dallas-Ross, P. and Biran, L. (1977) 'Factors influencing students' choice of medical school', *Medical Education*, 11: 319–23.

Robbins, D. (1993) 'The practical importance of Bourdieu's analyses of higher education', *Studies in Higher Education*, 18: 151–63.

Sinclair, S. (1997) *Making Doctors: an institutional apprenticeship*, Oxford: Berg.

Swartz, D. (1997) *Culture and Power: the sociology of Pierre Bourdieu*, London: University of Chicago Press.

Vinten-Johansen, P. and Riska, E. (1991) 'New Oslerians and real Flexnerians: the response to threatened professional autonomy', *International Journal of Health Services*, 21: 75–108.

Wacquant, L. (1996) 'Foreword', in P. Bourdieu, *The State Nobility: elite schools in the field of power*, Cambridge: Polity Press.

—— (2005) 'Habitus', in J. Beckert and M. Zafirovski (eds) *International Encyclopedia of Economic Sociology*, London: Routledge.

Part II
Key issues

Medical students and medical knowledge

5 Medical-school culture

Heidi Lempp

Introduction

The structure of western medical education over the last 150 years has been remarkably unchanged (Sinclair 1997: 11) and largely unaffected by the wider world despite the many intellectual and social transformations in society and its health. In parallel fashion, the continuity and homogeneity of medical-school culture appear surprisingly unaltered. How has such stability been maintained?

This chapter will start with a description of the role of medical schools and will provide a definition of medical-school culture. Attention will be paid to a number of influential internal and external issues that have shaped the medical-school climate in recent decades. Underpinned by findings of a recent study conducted in a UK medical school, this discussion provides further evidence about the insulated life of a medical school, thereby illustrating the saying that 'there is more to see than what meets the eye'. The integration of three sociological theoretical models – Bourdieu's concept of 'playing the game' (Bourdieu 1994), Goffman's notions of 'the presentation of self in everyday life' (Goffman 1971) and 'total institutions' (Goffman 1961) – add an important theoretical relevance to the results of the recent UK study.

Aspects of medical-school culture

The function of a medical school as a social organization has been characterized as follows:

> It is their function to transmit a culture of medicine and to advance that. It is their task to shape the novice into the effective practitioner of medicine, to give him [sic] the best available knowledge and skills to provide him with a professional identity so that he comes to think, act and feel like a physician.
>
> (Merton *et al.* 1957: 7)

Jefferys and Elston (1989) have stated that the medical school is charged with two fundamental functions, which Sinclair (1997) claimed are implicit in the very term 'medical student'. These are to become a competent doctor *and* to become a member of the medical profession.

In official medico-historical accounts, medical education, like medicine itself, has often been represented as a story of continuous and sometimes heroic progress, in which medical students' lives and experiences have received little attention. Instead, students have been portrayed as voiceless and passive participants in an impersonal, yet important process. Historically, the reasons for change in medical education have to be understood within a context of social, industrial, political, economic and educational transformations between the Enlightenment and the Second World War (Bonner 1995). A number of social changes had major implications for health, especially the rapid growth of the population and an increase in the size of cities during the Industrial Revolution in the eighteenth and nineteenth centuries. The newly emerging economy triggered a widespread change of secondary and higher education in the nineteenth century. This in turn stimulated progress in the explanatory power of observational and experimental sciences. In this context of transformation, the Medical (Registration) Act approved by Parliament in 1858, is generally regarded as a major landmark for the medical profession in its accumulation of power in the UK. First, it provided the backbone for professional autonomy. Second, it set out in statute the medical profession's right to self-regulate. Third, the unification of three, previously competing, professional groups (physicians, surgeons and apothecaries) was a good example of the use of professionalism as an ideological strategy to gain upward mobility and to demarcate legitimate doctors from other competing occupations. Fourth, this merger facilitated the standardization of medical education and the establishment of the General Medical Council (GMC). Finally, the standardization of medical knowledge led to the agreement of the state and the general public that the medical commodity was 'superior' to other services. There is little doubt that medical education is intimately linked with the profession of medicine itself. Indeed what students learn and how they learn medicine are closely embedded within each historical and social context (Bonner 1995).

The notion of medical-school culture can be defined as the customs, ideas and social behaviour of teaching staff and undergraduate medical students within a medical-school. Those dimensions are influential for students during their undergraduate training and beyond, mainly within the context of the hidden curriculum (Hafferty 1998) that is described in detail in Chapter 2 of this book. Against a background of the dual function of medical schools and the definition of medical-school culture, a number of important aspects that students tend to passively absorb as an integral part of the institutional climate are, I shall argue, strongly related to the hidden curriculum. The concept was first highlighted within the context of medical education by Becker and Geer (1958). This notion draws attention to processes, pressures and constraints which fall outside of, or are embedded within, the formal curriculum (Cribb and Bignold 1999). The various learning processes (Lempp and Seale 2004) of the hidden curriculum, for example, emotional neutralization, ritualized professional identity and acceptance of hierarchy, appear instrumental in the enculturation of students as they develop into both medical practitioners and members of the medical profession. The long overdue modification of medical-school culture, I argue, needs to be brought about by the same fundamental changes to the hidden curriculum as the formal curriculum has undergone in recent years in the UK.

Four in-depth studies of undergraduate medical-school culture – two early American ones (Becker *et al.* 1961; Merton *et al.* 1957) and two later conducted in the UK (Atkinson 1981; Sinclair 1997) – highlighted a number of important issues: the role of medical schools as powerful institutions; the socialization process that medical students undergo during their period in training; and that medical education appears to take place in an 'unreal world'. Sinclair achieved significant progress through his representation of medical-school culture within Goffman's encompassing conceptual framework on the 'presentation of self in everyday life', enabling deeper insight into the official and unofficial front and back stage of medical education, and their relationship to each other, rather than partial perspectives on medical education (Merton and Atkinson focused on the official 'front stage' and Becker concentrated on the official 'back stage').

Notably, all four studies paid no or very little attention to the experiences of female or black and ethnic-minority students. The medical-student population has undergone unparalleled sociodemographic diversification in the last four decades in the UK in terms of gender and ethnicity (Goldacre *et al.* 2004), but less so in relation to social class (Sinclair 1997), having traditionally been dominated by students from mainly middle- and upper-class backgrounds.

Apart from the socialization process and diversification of the medical-student population, the concept of medical-school culture also needs to be understood against a background of unprecedented sociopolitical changes in medical education and in the National Health Service (NHS) in the UK. Growing disillusion among medical students about the overwhelming burden of factual overload culminated in the General Medical Council document *Tomorrow's Doctors* (1993), which acted as a major catalyst in altering medical education in the UK. Major structural transformations within the NHS subjected the healthcare system both to a state of continuous flux and to enormous pressures, some of which were in response to widely publicized medical scandals. Such pressures to some extent undermined public trust, which the profession had consistently claimed for itself for so long. Doctors, for example, perceive increasing political interference by the government through target-setting, as weakening professionalism. The wider society and its changing healthcare needs have raised expectations, including demands to establish an equal relationship between patients and medical professionals. These forces have dominated the medical-political landscape in recent years. Concurrently the medical-education system has faced unparalleled monitoring. There has been a political imperative to improve the quality of outcomes in relation to the auditing of the undergraduate curriculum.

In the next section, a study carried out in one UK medical school between 2000 and 2002 will illustrate clearly how medical-school culture continues to impact both positively and problematically on individual medical students on their way to becoming doctors.

Medical students' perception of medical-school culture

The focus of the study was the students' individual experiences in years one to five of their undergraduate course and their professional socialization, during their transition from student to junior doctors. This work took place at a time when the medical-student population was becoming more socially diverse. The point of the discussion is to contribute to a more differentiated picture of contemporary medical-school life than that described in previous sociological studies, and to address whether students recognize that their ethnicity and gender could constitute barriers against their success in the medical profession.

In this prospective qualitative study four key questions were originally investigated. Two questions that are discussed here have particular connotations for medical-school culture (two other questions focusing on gender and the hidden curriculum are discussed in this *Handbook* in Chapters 2 and 6 respectively):

1   How does the power of senior medical-school and hospital staff (as perceived by students) influence the experiences of their training?
2   How does ethnicity emerge as an influence on the experiences of students undergoing undergraduate medical training?

Thirty-six undergraduate medical students from one British medical school were interviewed, complemented by formal and incidental non-participatory observations of various teaching sessions, for example, dissection, outpatient-teaching, ward-teaching and clinical skills-teaching over an 18-month period. The participants were selected at random by quota sampling, across all the five years of training and stratified by gender and ethnicity, using the entire medical-school population as a sampling frame. As an 'insider' the researcher had access to students and teaching situations and could directly communicate the results and implications of the study to the senior people of the medical school concerned.

From the interview and observational data, the results conveyed how the transition from entry to the medical school to the final examinations mirrored a passage through time where the students progressed towards the final goal of graduation, with a complex mixture of personal rewards and costs.

The emergent analytical framework consisted of vertical and horizontal strands. The vertical strands reflected three critical transitional phases through which the students moved in their training, namely:

Phase 1: entry from school (or university or employment) into the first years (pre-clinical) of medical training (Years 1 and 2).
Phase 2: students move across from the two pre-clinical to the next two years of clinical training (Years 3 and 4).
Phase 3: the last year of clinical teaching (Year 5).

Each transitional phase presents specific challenges and experiences for the students, which can be represented in four horizontal strands:

1 Receiving ambivalent messages: throughout their training, as a fundamental character of the medical culture. These double messages related mostly to students' status and role inside the medical school, and outside as seen by friends, family and the public.

2 Loss of identity: through unpredictable rewards and punishments, which are closely accompanied by attempts to achieve a balance between holding on to the 'old self' and at the same time acquiring a new professional identity.

3 Sense of fragmentation: personally, through an increasingly deconstructed identity, and educationally through disjointed curriculum content and unpredictable teaching, delivered to a vast number of students and across a geographically dispersed university campus.

4 Survival strategies: used as a means to an end to get through the disjointed training, mostly driven by intrinsic and external motivation.

The findings of the study are summarized, starting by describing the three transitional phases students need to go through to reach their final destination of graduation. Finally, the results are presented and interpreted within the context of the two research questions on which this qualitative work was based. As will be shown, students' accounts reflect the extent to which the medical-school culture plays an important part in undergraduate medical education today, despite recent formal medical-curriculum reforms.

Phases of transition in medical education

Traditionally, the first two years of medical training can be summarized as a time of rigid pre-clinical structure of lectures and laboratory work, which existed within a 'cocoon' (in comparison to the second and third transitional phase). During this phase, students at the school studied are introduced to the basic sciences that underpin medical practice and have limited opportunities to 'play doctor'. Direct contact with people takes place in the form of the dissection of cadavers, during which they learn about the internal and external aspects of the human body in practical weekly sessions in the medical school (and by observations of operations when patients are anaesthetized), or with live patients, where the focus is on the manifestations of health and disease.

At this stage, students' knowledge of people's experience of health and disease is largely focused upon somewhat disembodied, abstract concepts as taught within sociology, psychology and ethics. In addition to the academic demands upon them in terms of 'frontloading' (before students start their clinical part of their training in the hospital and community) and 'overloading' the students with factual medical knowledge, many became involved in the social life of the university and this often included the challenge of finding their own independence.

Students entered medical school as outsiders who came from the 'real world' and who went into an 'unreal world', still with a largely integrated sense of self. For the majority of newcomers, this integrated identity arrived from being successful in their application to study medicine, following on from very good high-school results, and for some after a successful previous degree or professional career. Furthermore, this sense of a largely coherent inner self can be traced back to a number of other influences, such as a combination of strongly held personal motives to become a doctor, support from family members and teachers in their pursuit of a medical career, and the high social status of medicine, combined with an expected ethos of hard work. To the disappointment of some, such positive attributions were echoed less within the medical school itself where students found themselves to have the very lowest status within the institution, mostly segregated from the hospital activities, the medical profession and from friends and family. These mixed signals puzzled the students. Many adjusted to the fact that hard work is an expected minimum for them, and that they start out right at the bottom of a long and steep hierarchy. At this stage, many students were also looking forward to a secure career as doctors, a varied and interesting job for life.

> I've had a serious low confidence problem recently – in a way that was quite difficult. Because I took a year off, and that really bolstered my confidence – [working with adolescents in America with behaviour difficulties] and now I come here and it's ... there are aspects like I went to a state school, and I only know about three other people on my course that went to a state school! ... that kind of shocked me quite a lot – like the amount of times I was asked where I went to school.
>
> (Student Year 1)

> When I established I wanted to do medicine ... I think it was appealing because there's a career at the end of it; you qualify and then you get a job, which is quite nice.
>
> (Student Year 3)

The start of the clinical teaching phase in Year 3 of undergraduate training presented an important symbolic passage and watershed where students moved on from having been mostly passive recipients of theoretical knowledge to becoming active, clinically involved apprentices. The previous highly structured timetable was now replaced by less well-organized outpatient clinics or bedside-teaching situations within the context of a teaching-ward round, across a number of teaching hospitals or district general hospitals, local primary-care settings, centrally organized campus teaching, brief placements abroad for a few selected students and self-directed studies. The whole year group underwent substantial reconfiguration: firstly, about 50 per cent of previous second-year students rejoined the 'new' third year following completion of an intercalated BSc and at the same time 50 per cent of second-year students left their familiar year group to embark on optional BSc one-year courses. In addition, a small number of students who commenced their pre-clinical years in other universities joined the third-year student group. Finally, the newly constituted third-year students were split up into so-called 'firms', usually six to ten students, which are named after the clinical consultant they were grouped under. This could be a 'make-or-break' stage for some students.

This organizational upheaval of the year group, where again students are mostly strangers to each other, was paralleled by a division of the curriculum content – essentially a splitting-up of the physical body – the focus of their undergraduate medical education – into manageable educational units, similar to the theoretical lectures and dissection sessions of the first two years. Students had to get used to a different educational style and also begin to establish professional relationships with patients, senior medical and multidisciplinary ward, hospital and primary-care staff, learn how to care for and manage sick individuals and perform practical procedures under clinical supervision. This phase can be characterized as a further deeper immersion 'into' the world of medicine. Many perceived themselves in various degrees as unwelcome 'outsiders from within'.

> Umm, I feel like I'm at the bottom of the heap recently! You know, you feel you are right at the bottom – the nurses are at the bottom, and we are way below that! We're way down there – you kind of get lower and lower!
>
> (Student Year 3)

The transition to the clinical years is eased by an introductory course to prepare the students for their practice of medicine in the hospital and community and so alleviate their anxiety. This 'rite of passage' is signified by wearing the white coat (provided by the medical school), which symbolizes a dress code of a professional nature, a stethoscope around their necks, and a copy of the British National Formulary (prescription guide) in the outside pocket of the white coat. The apprehension of becoming a clinical student is usually accompanied by high expectations and excitement.

> We are now *real* medical students and no longer only *any other* medical students.
>
> (Student Year 3)

The final phase of the undergraduate training until graduation could be characterized as a period where students look forward to entering the 'real world of medicine' and the prospect of an end to being kept in suspense. They also have to pass their final examinations. In this last year students are expected to consolidate and bring together all the different strands of the manifest curriculum, which need now to be integrated and strengthened during this final stage. Moreover, if students can financially afford it, they have the opportunity to work abroad during the so-called 'elective period'. The status of the elective appears to be of similar significance to the dissection in Years 1 and 2, where the pre-clinical students enthusiastically applied their theoretical knowledge within a practical context for the first time.

> I think, you know, by the time you're coming to your final year, you actu-ally do have that sense of a realization, because you can get through finals knowing, you know, very basic medicine. And it just comes off, you know, on the fact that you have a responsibility now.
>
> (Student Year 5)

Given these three transitional phases with their various educational focuses on the one hand, other – covert – learning processes also left their mark on students' undergraduate medical-school experiences.

Power of medical staff over medical students' experiences

Historically the medical profession has enjoyed a powerful and privileged status since the time of the Industrial Revolution (Bonner 1995). Numerous efforts by the medical profession to actively exclude female and black and ethnic commun-ity doctors from its most senior ranks have combined to produce an image of medicine as a white, male-exclusive club. The results of this study suggest that one of the mechanisms the profession has used to maintain these forms of pro-fessional power has been to convey understandings of who can join 'the magic circle' via the hidden curriculum. The established rules are therefore communi-cated early to successive generations of doctors and are not openly challengea-ble. Traditionally, the culture of medicine has developed and prevailed within closed institutions (Goffman 1961), where hidden practices often survived unquestioned, either by those within or outside the profession. The students were acculturated to the realization that their future career prospects depended in important respects upon their ability to tolerate and excuse humiliation and dis-respect and being ignored with little evidence of overt complaint, and especially without their questioning the underlying power relations and rules of engage-ment whereby they quietly learn how to behave as doctors.

Such self-restraint was evident in many ways within students' accounts. For example, several female students reported feeling vulnerable during their psy-chiatry rotations, but they felt inhibited and were unable to articulate their concerns.

> I didn't like psychiatry, I was just really scared being with mad patients. It sounds really bad, but I just didn't like it at all. I couldn't relate to the patients, we didn't have very good teaching and I just found it really scary.
>
> (Student Year 4)

Furthermore, most students, whatever their gender or ethnicity (apart from mature students), preferred not to admit any academic problems to medical-school staff, as they assumed that this would be judged as weakness. A few students, throughout all three transitional stages, picked up a clear message that 'being human' or showing any emotional or physical weakness does not fit in with some aspects of medicine. Consequently, the net effect of the impact of these experiences of disempowerment was a form of self-censorship by students. In effect, students appeared to choose silence for their own good.

> I just don't think there's an appreciation of being who you are, being a woman, being a man, just being a *human being.* And I think there is this sort of: you must be a super human, steel person that is slightly … that can cope with everything – and as a junior doctor, you *will* have to cope with everything!
>
> (Student Year 5)

Such learned behaviour is closely related to Pierre Bourdieu's concept of 'playing the game' (Bourdieu 1994), as students assumed such conduct would help them to progress in their training and help them to pass their examinations, although such messages were nowhere to be found in the manifest curriculum. The implication was that as long as they went along with what the teachers wanted from them, rightly or wrongly, without challenge, such behaviour would keep them in good stead with their seniors and help them to reach their goal of qualification and entering the powerhouse of medicine.

In these ways students learned through experiences and observations of other medical staff a form of 'habitus', which Bourdieu described as 'a set of dispositions', which assisted them to develop a 'second sense', to adhere to the established and often traditional unwritten rules and regulations of the cultural group, in this instance the medical profession with its own rituals and rites. Therefore, educational settings can be viewed as establishments that sow seeds that shape and form their students in their own interests. The qualified doctors' concern is to gain and exercise control and power through the accumulation of economic, social and cultural capital over the novices. Only once the newcomers have complied with all the unwritten rules and practices, in other words completed their rites of passage, will they be rewarded by being accepted 'into the magic circle' of the medical profession and obtain their legitimate professional identity and privileges.

A further manifestation of the effect of medical power during undergraduate training was the choice of role models by students. Having knowledge or expertise was the attribute most highly ranked by students when selecting them. One result of this study, that students attached high importance to academic status, is only partially supported by previous work.

> The [male] professor was calm, knowledgeable, powerful, enjoyed teaching.
>
> (Student Year 4)

The study of Wright *et al.* (1998) found that academic standing was not highly rated, while Sinclair (1997) did discover that students were drawn towards doctors with status and responsibility and less so towards staff who showed interest in social attributes, such as integrity, or a patient-centred approach.

This attraction of students to powerful medical figures was both striking and suffused with ambivalence as these individuals had the power both 'to make and break' the careers of their protégés. What the students' accounts exemplified with their selection of role models, however, was that in medicine, (male) gender, being 'white' and having knowledge and therefore power was very closely interlinked. Some evidence that female doctors were also motivational for students emerged although the attributes they valued were less likely to include scientific knowledge.

> Enthusiastic about her discipline, involved students actively in the work, excellent knowledge and practical skills, nice to patients, staff and students.
>
> (Student Year 5)

The ripple effect of this power of medical staff also became apparent in that male doctors carried out almost all the teaching considered to be humiliating. Students' encounters with this special and often influential subgroup of medical teachers were commonly referred to as the 'old boys' network'.

> I came out of theatre and he was going on about something, he was ranting, 'oh you are a stupid slug anyway'. I think I fainted or something and I came out. And he came and said in front of everyone: 'oh you can't cope with the blood' and then he said 'you are a stupid slug anyway, I don't know why you bother'.
>
> (Student Year 3)

The reality of teaching by humiliation (verbal) was that it was applied almost exclusively by senior male doctors towards both male and female students. In a curious variant, there was also evidence of female nurses, midwives, patients and junior staff treating many medical students disrespectfully during their training in a way that could indicate professional rivalry.

> Some of the nurses actually try and give you a hard time; the midwives especially.... They'll fob you off ... most male medical students, you know, when they do obstetrics and gynaecology, they will have this totally biased opinion of midwives – they are the women from hell.
>
> (Student Year 5)

These forms of humiliation can perhaps best be understood as expressions of the inconvenience that medical students cause to nurses' work, and the blurred roles such students occupy, needing supervision without clearly sharing the workload, as nursing students do. Furthermore, Sinclair (1997) speculated that the increasing number of female medical students has effected a transformation in the previously stable and established relationship between nurses (female) and medical students (male) – changes that may suggest implicit jealousies. Furthermore, nurses are witness to the humiliation of students by consultants, and might therefore see such behaviour as legitimate.

A further indicator of the power of the medical staff was the haphazard nature of teaching, particularly by clinical staff. This disregard to the overt timetable resulted in frequent unintentional time-wasting and profound demotivation in students.

> I mean we've had so many days where we've had, sort of, five different sessions scheduled – and no one turns up! You just think, you know, why bother coming in? So that's irritating. It does happen a lot to everyone, I think. I mean, obviously the people who are teaching have another job – it's not their only job to teach you – but it's when you turn up and they don't get somebody else to do it, or they don't even let you know that they haven't turned up.
>
> (Student Year 3)

All students tended to excuse both teaching by humiliation and the perceived lack of commitment to teaching by remarking how the busy clinical work of doctors took priority over teaching.

All of these processes appear to have acted as accumulating signals to the students about who and what is important and powerful in the medical school as an institution.

The density of these components and the fact that hardly any of these issues were openly discussed with their teachers, but rather in most cases 'taken as a fact of medical life', suggested that they could be expected to persist in the foreseeable future. In the ways described above, the 'senior' culture of the medical profession is reflected by the 'junior' medical student culture from the very beginning in ways that mimic and appear to revere that of its 'elders'. This subtlety in the transmission of power within the medical profession appears to be illustrated by and imitated within the hidden curriculum.

Apart from Bourdieu's notion of 'playing the game', the findings also point closely to Goffman's ideas concerning the presentation of self in social situations (1971). What has become apparent from these accounts is that the medical students clearly recognized that they are in a weak power position in relation to the teaching staff and that their career prospects will be improved by controlling their behaviour to closely conform to the expectations of their seniors.

How can this role performance be understood? In the case of medical students, the need to perform to an audience applied to their everyday lives in the medical school, as they underwent continuous assessment of their clinical and professional work. Goffman (1971) analysed such complex social encounters from the perspective of the dramatic performance. This metaphor of the theatre, which he divided between the 'front' and 'back stage', and where an audience is essential, was easily translatable to the hospital situation (Sinclair 1997). Throughout undergraduate training, students took on different roles on the 'front stage' (where they are observable by patients appearing as the audience). On the 'back stages', however, which included the library, the bar, the sports fields and the halls of residence, students played different roles. On each 'stage', students have various audiences, which they try to impress. Increasingly through the clinical-training years, the only meaningful audience for the students' perform-ances are the teaching consultants who will rate and rank them. Students learn that they must carefully manage what they say to whom to elicit approval from seniors. Revealed gaps in their knowledge may lower their endorsement ratings, while successfully 'staged' contributions, for example, during a ward round, could increase their credibility. One consequence of this 'staging of self' might be that 'successful' students include those who could mask any incompetence, and do so in a way that complied with unwritten professional rules, such as accepting without complaint verbal abuse by a consultant, or exhibiting competitiveness.

Undergraduate medical training therefore can be interpreted within this theatri-cal metaphor as moving from a period of rehearsal or learning 'the play' in front of a powerful audience of senior colleagues to 'going live' in public after graduation. This series of staged transitions in their formal training status was mirrored by a series of inner transitions in which students' 'old selves' (established prior to enter-ing medical school) were rearranged before culminating in a degree of 'reintegra-tion of themselves' at the end of the training, during which time they gradually appeared to assume the professional identity as emerging doctors-to-be.

How do 'race' and ethnicity influence medical students' experiences?

The number of black and ethnic-community students in medical schools nation-ally has risen substantially in recent years. In all the transitional phases and in several of the key strands, important variations and distinctions surfaced among student groups, either between some of the 'ethnic' groups themselves, or between the 'ethnic' and 'white' students.

Almost half of the study cohort identified themselves as 'non-white' and described themselves as Indian/Asian, Pakistani and Bangladeshi, African, African-Asian, Chinese, Iranian and Arab. Most of these students were UK-born and therefore second-generation UK citizens. Several key aspects challenged Asian students in particular, there was parental pressure to study medicine as it was seen to be linked with high status and good career prospects. In some Asian cultures this is a second-generation phenomenon. Furthermore, becoming inde-pendent from parents was more difficult for both female and male Asian students and for the African-Asian student than for many 'white' students. These two cul-tural aspects were particularly pertinent during the first transitional phase.

> I'm a Muslim and, you know, I wasn't allowed to grow up until really, really late – my parents would flip if I wasn't home by midnight if I hadn't

called. Umm, so it was quite ... it wasn't tightly controlled – as Asian parents my parents are very liberal – but you know, living in a western society, it was still quite tight. But it's completely different to now, where I have complete freedom over what I do: I'm freely mixing with, like, girls – because my parents were not happy with me mixing with girls that much. Sometimes I feel that, you know, they wouldn't recognize that I am an adult until I was married.

(Bangladeshi male Student Year 1)

Other ethnicity-related issues also emerged. The perceived absence of 'ethnic' role models among senior medical staff (only two out of 46 were identified in positions of authority in all three transitional phases) was significant and illuminating. 'Ethnic' students primarily identified this discrepancy when considering the composition of the medical-student intake and when looking towards their future career prospects.

There is something about doctors and position of power, and the fact that it's just so ... *obvious* that it's just ... consultants are all Caucasian; and registrars are mostly all Asian – it's an amazing clear-cut line, that you can actually *see* it! So it's not like they're sort of spread out; I mean, you can actually, literally, notice the difference between the two.

(Iranian female Student Year 4)

Aspirations of becoming powerful and in control were particularly important for male 'ethnic' students and to a lesser extent for 'white' and 'ethnic' females. Once again, these features fell entirely under the rubric of the hidden curriculum in relation to a perceived ethnic 'glass ceiling'. What students seemed to have understood and which has been confirmed in the relevant literature (although this appeared not to be discussed within the manifest curriculum), is that ethnic-minority medical students, despite their increasing representation in UK medical schools over the last 25 years, had made relatively little inroads into the higher echelons of the professional hierarchy, especially at the prestigious teaching hospitals.

Further important themes also arose from the data analysis in relation to religious observation. For example, considerations about students' religious beliefs and practices, such as Islamic rules that a male doctor should not be alone with a female Muslim student, or that a female student should not be alone with a male patient, might be in conflict with conventional medical practice. Female 'ethnic' students' accounts implied that such salient issues for the ethnic-community students were not always openly discussed with teachers.

Religion may have a big role to play in medicine, because I am a Muslim and I do know that some female students who are Muslim found it difficult with the clinical placements, because I think there are some rules along the line, they shouldn't be left alone in the room with a guy. I know this female medical student who went for work experience and she was placed with a male General Practitioner and she said to him that she wouldn't … couldn't talk to his patients … with the doors closed and this would be ladened [laden] by her religious beliefs [which would deem this encounter to be unacceptable].

(African-Asian female Student Year 1)

Some experiences were common to all ethnic-community students while others were subgroup specific. The lack of culturally consonant role models was reported to be an important barrier for Asian, African-Asian and African students. In contradistinction, a very important issue arose. Black (African) female students reported that they at times felt the need to justify their very existence as medical students. In other words, their experience suggested the possibility that the wider 'white' culture may have accepted Asians as legitimate medical students, but regarded black (African) medical students as somehow problematic.

I do find [I'm] having to sort of defend myself all the time and justify the fact that I *did* get into medical school, you know it wasn't that I just *got in*! I got in because I *did* work hard and I got in because I am capable of doing it. People sort of say, 'Oh my daughter tried to get into medical school and she *didn't*', and it is kind of you know, I do feel that I do have to sort of justify my intelligence all the time. I suppose because, okay, I'm black, I'm female – and also, I suppose, I don't particularly look kind of studious or whatever. People just do not think I fit the image. And I do find myself trying to conform, and be a different person sort of in hospital, so I *look* like a medical student.

(African female Student Year 4)

Related to the issue of legitimacy as medical students, it was striking that when teachers failed to attend their timetabled teaching sessions 'white' students commonly criticized such behaviour, while the 'ethnic' students passed comments less often, particularly in the second transitional phase. The 'ethnic' students' behaviour might suggest a desire to fit in to the medical system, to raise no ripples, and certainly not to 'rock the boat'.

Furthermore, some evidence surfaced relating to important interactions between ethnicity and gender. For some, being 'Asian' and female was understood among some female 'white' and 'ethnic' students as being more likely to receive verbal abuse from 'white', male consultants and some 'ethnic' female students were more often ignored by consultants during teaching-ward rounds than were 'ethnic' male students or 'white' students. Conversely, more female 'ethnic' students in the second and third transitional phases in particular pointed out that the teachers who they identified as positive role models were those who treated them with respect, gave them confidence and did not humiliate them.

These close interpersonal dynamics identified by 'ethnic' female students in relation to teaching situations and nominated role models are significant as they suggested two opposing perceptions. First, that to some degree ethnicity might be a disadvantage in some parts of the training, and second, that recognition and respect can sometimes be shown to students as people regardless of ethnicity.

Interestingly, some students also identified the diversity of medical students as an advantage that allowed them to become more open-minded. It was revealing that they perceived the different ethnic backgrounds of students constructively rather than as a barrier. Some students reported that this allowed a widening of their horizons, particularly for those who came from close (d) families and communities, so that they learned from meeting colleagues and patients who were ethnically, socioeconomically and religiously diverse.

> Coming to the medical school was a real eye opener for me. It is the Year 2000 and I have never spoken to an Asian or black person before I came here.
>
> (White British female Student Year 2)

Several of the differences experienced by 'ethnic' students can be understood as being overdetermined by their power status within medicine. Despite an increasing number of 'ethnic' students and doctors, they tend to occupy positions of inferior status within the profession, similar to that of women. Such manifestations of power within medicine are essentially aspects of a covert reality. These results are somewhat consistent with the conclusions of Hafferty and Franks (1994) who pointed out that 'neophyte medical students – particularly those from diverse backgrounds – are more sensitive to the presence of the hidden curriculum'.

While all these processes are contained within the hidden curriculum, this in no way reduces their impact upon the experience of 'ethnic' students. A few reported that their ethnicity had at times an importance for their own treatment as students and for their future career prospects. However, they mostly described their ethnic status in terms of barriers and said that their ethnicity conferred no advantage.

Just as the increase in numbers of women might contribute to changes in aspects of medical practice, the ethnic diversification of the medical-student population might also make a gradual mark, for example, greater tolerance towards 'the other'. This may lead in turn to positive changes in the culture of medicine. However, the results of this study are consistent with the findings of previous work in illustrating a certain reluctance and/or slow progress by the medical profession to accept 'the others' as equals following qualification, to which some students in this study bore eloquent witness.

These accounts of the students are reminiscent of the all-embracing demands of total institutions. According to Goffman, these institutions are:

> purportedly established the better to pursue some work-like task and justifying themselves only on these instrumental grounds: army barracks, ships, boarding schools, work camps, colonial compounds and

large mansions from the point of view of those who live in the servants' quarters.

(1961: 16)

Because of the inward orientation of such institutions, these organizations often fail to keep pace with changes in the outside world. This is relevant here in relation to the experiences reported by 'ethnic' students. A hierarchy exists which dictates the system and distributes privileges and punishments, some of which can be described as humiliating, among the 'inmates'. The close resemblance between Goffman's characterization of a 'total institution' and students' reports on medical-school life in relation to their social identities are revealing and the degree of separation from the outside world can be seen to contribute to the permeation, unchecked by external constraints, of the hidden curriculum.

To some extent, the attempts by medical schools in general, and the school under study in particular, to become more inclusive by increasing the number of female and 'ethnic' students and students from lower socioeconomic backgrounds can be understood as a gradual refinement of Goffman's theory. One could argue that the diversification of the student population at the admission stage of medical training is a first step to greater openness (of the institution).

Taking a wider view in relation to these findings, two important sociological and methodological aspects need to be taken into consideration, to reach a balanced view. First, the majority of the study cohort and the generality of medical students come from socioeconomically privileged backgrounds, and can rely on a great deal of financial and emotional support from their families. Therefore it is reasonable to conclude that although in the short term many students did have a clear sense that at various stages in their training they were having a 'rough ride', nevertheless they also clearly realized that in the long term they would make considerable social and financial gains.

Summary

A key adage – 'there is more to see here than meets the eye' – emerged as a powerful image in this study of medical-school culture. The recognition of the existence and importance of unwritten rules may contribute to the processes of professional and emotional socialization. The hidden curriculum has emerged in this chapter as the most powerful overall overarching theme. It runs through elements of the students' accounts to explain why their behaviour in many ways is shaped and guided not only by what they are formally taught, but also by their shared understanding of what it means to be seen as a successful medical student. Such knowledge is transferred to them in ways that become more persuasive during the later clinical years, and which reward conformity to the model of professional behaviour they observe in their seniors.

Conclusion

To achieve fundamental changes in undergraduate medical education and medical-school culture, recognition and reform of the hidden curriculum are required. This means not only paying attention to the formal curriculum but also to the way in which students are enculturated into the medical profession. Such changes can be achieved in a variety of ways that focus on the behaviour and attitudes of students and teachers rather than the acquisition of medical knowledge and skills. Professional development modules focusing on self-reflection, multidisciplinary teamwork, personal-mentor schemes, learning about health in community-based teaching, health promotion and ethics teaching could be starting points, as well as ensuring that medical teachers are accountable for their behaviour. Apart from alterations to the medical curriculum, Cribb and Bignold (1999) also suggest that reflexive medical-education research might contribute to greater openness and self-understanding that can spill over and become integrated into the curriculum of medical schools.

References

Atkinson, P. (1981) *The Clinical Experience: the construction and reconstruction of medical reality*, Farnborough: Gower.

Becker, H. S. and Geer, B. (1958) 'The fate of idealism in medical school', *American Sociological Review*, 23: 50–6.

Becker, H., Geer, B., Hughes, E. and Strauss, A. (1961) *Boys in White: student culture in medical school*, Chicago, IL: University of Chicago Press.

Bonner, T. (1995) *Becoming a Physician: medical education in Britain, France, Germany and the United States, 1750–1945*, Oxford: Oxford University Press.

Bourdieu, P. (1994) *In Other Words: essays towards a reflexive sociology*, Cambridge: Polity Press.

Cribb, A. and Bignold, S. (1999) 'Towards the reflexive medical school: the hidden curriculum and medical education research', *Studies in Higher Education*, 24: 195–209.

General Medical Council (1993) *Tomorrow's Doctors: Recommendations on Undergraduate Medical Education*, London: GMC.

Goffman, E. (1961) *Asylums: essays on the social situation of mental patients and other inmates*, Harmondsworth: Penguin.

—— (1971) *The Presentation of Self in Everyday Life*, Harmondsworth: Penguin.

Goldacre, M. J., Davison, J. M. and Lambert, T. W. (2004) 'Country of training and ethnic origin of UK doctors: database and survey studies', *British Medical Journal*, 329: 597–600.

Hafferty, F. W. (1998) 'Beyond curriculum reform: confronting medicine's hidden curriculum', *Academic Medicine*, 73: 403–7.

Hafferty, F. W. and Franks, R. (1994) 'The hidden curriculum, ethics teaching, and the structure of medical education', *Academic Medicine*, 69: 861–71.

Jefferys, M. and Elston, M. A. (1989) 'The medical school as a social organization', *Medical Education*, 23: 242–51.

Lempp, H. and Seale, C. (2004) 'The hidden curriculum in undergraduate medical education: qualitative study of medical students' perception of teaching', *British Medical Journal*, 329: 770–3.

Merton, R., Reader, G. and Kendall, P. (eds) (1957) *The Student-Physician: introductory studies in the sociology of medical education*, Cambridge, MA: Harvard University Press.

Sinclair, S. (1997) *Making Doctors: an institutional apprenticeship*, Oxford: Berg.

Wright, S., Kern, D. E., Kolodner, K., Howard, D. E. and Brancati, F. L. (1998) 'Attributes of excellent attending-physician role models', *New England Journal of Medicine*, 339: 1986–93.

6 Gender and medical education

Elianne Riska

Introduction

In the early sociological literature on professions, the medical profession came to be viewed as a prototype of expert knowledge and of the expert–client relationship that emerged in the process of modernization. It was Talcott Parsons (1951) who outlined the sociological approach to describe and explain physicians' professional behaviour and attitudes. For Parsons, those in the role of physicians adopted other values and expectations than those in the private sphere of the family. According to this view, gender pertained only to the relations of the family and the sex roles acquired through primary socialization. By contrast, professional behaviour was formed by another type of socialization which emphasized the values of achievement, universalism, functional specificity, affective neutrality and collectivity orientation (Parsons 1951: 454). The assumption is that a man or a woman is above all a physician at work, and the achieved status and the professional orientation and behaviour will guide the individual's interaction and that of colleagues and patients (Parsons 1949: 197).

Early studies on the medical profession set out to explore the way in which professional behaviour and attitudes were socially acquired and the professional role institutionalized. Two classic works on medical education set the stage for the ensuing theoretical debate and research. The first, headed by Robert Merton, was *The Student-Physician*, a study of students at three US medical schools (Merton *et al.* 1957). Known as the Columbia University study, it examined how students learned the norms of the medical profession. The second study, *Boys in White*, known as the Chicago School study, was done at the University of Kansas Medical School and led by Howard Becker (Becker *et al.* 1961). The theoretical approach was symbolic-interactionist, in contrast to the structural-functionalist of the former. Becker's study interpreted the medical students' response to problematic situations as a form of situational adjustment and the outcome as 'pragmatic idealism'.

Both these studies portrayed the professional education of doctors as mainly an enterprise of training (white) men and thereby made gender, race and ethnicity invisible (Lorber 1975: 85). Merton's study presents medical students in gender-neutral or in masculine terms and does not mention women as medical students. For example, the medical school is said 'to shape the novice into the effective practitioner of medicine, to give him the best available knowledge and skills, and to provide him with a professional identity so that he comes to think, act and feel like a physician' (Merton 1957: 7) and in the next sentence the physician is called a 'medical man'. Only once are women mentioned – in a footnote commenting on the results of students' career decisions. The footnote suggests that 'because well over 90 per cent of medical students observed are males, the interpretations given here may be more adequate in describing the career decisions of young men than of young women' (Rogoff 1957: 120).

Becker's study omitted the data on the handful of women in each class by using as rationale existing gender discrimination: the authors argued that because of the overwhelmingly male composition of the medical profession, 'we shall talk mainly of boys becoming medical men' (Becker *et al.* 1961: 3).

The next sociological studies on medical education were published almost a decade later. Stephen Miller's *Prescription for Leadership* (1970) does not even consider women as medical students as a viable option. Miller (1970: 18) states that his research problem 'was to discover the patterned relationships by observing what actually did happen to young men during a year at Boston City Hospital'. The study refers only to 'men' and 'fellows' and there is no entry for 'women' in the index (Lorber 1975: 86). By contrast, Emily Mumford's *Interns: from students to physicians* (1970) not only includes women but also explores the tracking by gender in the selection of internship. Hence, this study opens up two questions that later studies have explored when women began to enter medicine in increasing numbers: why do female students choose different specialties to male students, and why are there so few women in academic positions in charge of teaching and research? The former question relates to the horizontal gender segregation of medical practice, while the latter question is connected to the vertical gender segregation – that is, the scarcity of women at top positions in healthcare and in academic medicine. In gender politics, these two issues capture the demands for gender equality and gender equity in medical education and in healthcare.

This chapter will review three topics related to gender and medical education. The first topic is the enrolment of a growing number of women in medical schools worldwide. This trend will result in an increasing number of women among physicians in the future. The numerical shift in the gender composition of medical-school classes and of the profession of medicine is often portrayed as the 'feminization of medicine', a term that will be further examined.

The second topic concerns medical knowledge and its gendered content and the way in which gender-bias is being reproduced in the medical curriculum.

The third topic addresses the choice of specialty during medical training: how do medical students end up in different specialties and on different levels in the academic and healthcare system on the basis of gender? Three major explanations for the impact of gender on the choices of medical specialty will be reviewed.

Throughout this chapter gender will be used in a narrow sense and imply differences between men and women. Although there is increasing research about the treatment of gay, lesbian and bisexual (GLB) patients in the healthcare system, there is still little knowledge and research about this group among medical students and doctors. The few existing studies point to the difficulties that the group has during the early stages of medical training, but a disclosure of sexual orientation seems to become easier at the time of residency selection (Burke and White 2001; Merchant *et al.* 2005; Risdon *et al.* 2000). In order to address the situation of GLB medical students and doctors, the term hegemonic masculinity will be used to indicate not only the homogeneous male culture of medicine but also the hierarchy of gender in that system.

Enrolment in medical schools: a sign of a future 'feminization' of medicine?

In the early 1970s, a new trend in the enrolment in medical schools could be discerned in most western countries: a shift from first-year medical-school classes being predominantly male to a composition featuring an increasing number of women. It is worth remembering that this trend is not unique to medical education, but has been part of a larger development in higher education. Women have entered university education in growing numbers, becoming a majority in many western countries. But this trend has evoked a reaction particularly in medicine. This section will look at how the demand for gender equality before 1970 led to the metaphor of 'feminization of medicine' in the 2000s. The new discourse on the 'feminization of medicine' addresses the assumed impact that female medical students are going to have on the way that medicine is practised when there is an increased proportion of women doctors.

When women tried to gain access to university education in the nineteenth century, medical education became a litmus test of their acceptance in the system of higher education. Both the United States and Russia were pioneers in offering medical education to women in the mid-nineteenth century, although often by means of special tracks or special medical schools for women (Riska 2001). The North European system of an integrated medical education for both men and women resulted in a later entry for women but allowing them to gain the same degree and qualifications to practise medicine as men. By the early twentieth century, the formal barriers for women's entry to medical education had been abolished in most western countries. However, progress was slow and it was not until the early 1970s that the current trend of women's rapid numerical increase among first-year medical students became evident. Today women constitute from 40–70 per cent of first-year medical students in most western countries.

The new situation of a female majority among first-year medical students has resulted in three discourses – the research discourse, the medical discourse, and the public discourse – whose actors speak about the 'feminization of medicine'. The research discourse has been put forward by sociologists to illuminate the changes in medical work as the number of women has increased. The medical discourse is represented by editorials in medical journals while the public discourse appears in news media (Riska 2008).

The discourses contain basic assumptions about the relationship between the gender composition of medicine and the character, but above all the quality, of medical work. There are two visions in both the research and medical discourse: an optimistic and a pessimistic. The optimistic vision sees women physicians as a vanguard of holistic medicine. It is argued that women will bring into medicine humanistic values, a new empathic approach and a concern for women's health issues. Women physicians are, according to such a view, to bring back the golden age of doctoring when the family doctor was familiar with the social context and the complexity of ordinary diseases. This view has not only been heralded by women's health advocates but has more recently also found its way into editorials in major medical journals. This vision holds an essentialist view of women's gender-related skills. It homogenizes women physicians as a group but it also sets unrealistic expectations about the substantial changes that a group which in the past has lacked major influence in medicine would be able to bring about.

The pessimistic vision is that female medical students, and hence women physicians-to-be, constitute a threat to the autonomy and quality of work of the medical profession as it has been known. The scenarios and arguments come in different versions, and the two views presented here are but simplified versions of more complex portrayals. The first pessimistic view presents a prophecy about the future re-segregation of the medical profession: from having been a male-dominated one – both in a cultural and numerical sense – it is becoming female-dominated. Re-segregation is not hailed as a victory for gender equality (that is, women gaining entry to and constituting a majority in a high-status and high-income occupation) but is rather interpreted as turning a high-status profession into 'merely' women's work. It is envisioned that the increase of female medical students will scare off future qualified males from applying to medical school and thus further escalate the 'feminization of medicine' and turn medicine into a low-status, female health profession (Riska 2008).

The second pessimistic view contains the same broad scenario as this but in addition presents more detailed accounts of the kinds of threats that the influx of female medical students is going to have on medical practice. The predictions concern the availability of doctors in various specialties and regions. It has been supposed, for example, that some primary-care specialties will be the main choice of female medical students, while other areas, such as surgery, will not attract women. The assumption is that the different career choices women will make, if women become a majority of medical students, result in a scarcity of qualified candidates in certain fields – for example, surgery and research. Another assumption has been that more doctors will have to be trained in the future because women doctors work shorter hours than their male colleagues, take long child-care leaves, and are unwilling to be on duty or to practise in rural areas. But while some North American and European research has documented this trend, the career choices and practice patterns of women physicians might be found to be related to their previous minority status in the profession rather than a permanent pattern when the medical profession becomes gender balanced and different practice styles become more prevalent.

While medical educators have recently called for a wider social diversity among medical students, such concerns have mainly included a quest for a wider diversity in social class, race and ethnicity in order to address the needs of different patient categories (for example, Whitcomb 2006). In such calls, gender is seldom included, which may mean that medicine is either perceived as already gender-balanced (or even dominated by women) or that it is unmarked by gender. Some medical educators and representatives of medicine are concerned that women are going to radically change medicine, but little research has addressed what male medical students are doing and how their careers are changing (for example, Kilminster *et al.* 2007: 45).

Gendered medical knowledge and medical skills in medical education

Researchers who have examined the character of gender hidden in medical knowledge have been surprised to find that little of the feminist concerns and of the factual knowledge of female sexuality represented by sexologists has filtered down to the level of medical training. Even after 30 years of feminist research on women's bodies and of women's health advocates' promotion of women's health issues, knowledge about gender differences in health and illness has not been fully integrated in medical curricula (Verdonck *et al.* 2006). A recent Canadian study suggested that the ideal of impartiality and neutral – colour-blind, class-blind and sex-blind – medical knowledge in medical education conceals the constructed and socially and culturally located character of such knowledge. The study concluded: 'Claims of universality construct as normal and neutral what is actually the knowledge of socially dominant groups' (Beagan 2000: 1262).

When the feminist movement in the 1970s turned its gaze on medicine, gender-biased medical knowledge became a crucial indicator of the way that medicine misrepresented factual knowledge about the female body. Medical textbooks offered evidence of the way in which knowledge of women's physiology was either absent or overtly gender-biased. The texts were also seen as a crucial tool for how this knowledge was reproduced through the medical curriculum. Most studies on this topic have been American and they have documented the gender-biased portrayal of female sexual organs and female sexuality in medical texts. A classic in this genre of research is Scully and Bart's (1973) study of the contents of general gynaecology texts written during 1943 to 1972, which showed that the material contained sexist stereotypes of female sexuality. Later studies have examined the history of the portrayal of female anatomy in nineteenth- and twentieth-century anatomy textbooks (Laqueur 1990; Lawrence and Bendixen 1992; Moore and Clarke 1995; Petersen 1998). For example, Moore and Clarke (1995) examined how female genitalia were portrayed in the anatomical drawings and in the accompanying text in major anatomy texts used at American medical schools from 1900 to 1991. Four different periods were identified. The first period (1900–1952) showed the male and female sexual organs as homologous – that is, having a corresponding structure. The second period (1953–1971) showed a surprising absence of female sexual organs in general although the era witnessed some of the classic studies on human sexuality that also documented the features of female sexuality. The third period (1971–1981) gave rise to a 'feminist imaging' of the female genitalia and a new awareness and openness about female sexuality. The fourth period (1981–1991) is characterized as the 'clitoral backlash' because of the reintroduction of narratives of heterosexuality based on evolutionary theories of male primacy. This last period showed how anatomical representations are part of a narrative that constructs a discourse of difference based on a naturalization and normalization of such differences. Moore and Clarke (1995: 255) conclude that anatomy is a key site for the production and maintenance of sex and gender as binary categories. The visual representation of the female sexual organ in anatomy illustrations and texts constructs, portrays and preserves the 'naturalness' of the female body. Hence, the anatomical pictures visualize a specific aspect of biological sex as the definitive marker of that sex. This cultural production of the natural can also be described as the construction of the 'essentials of essentialism' (Moore and Clarke 1995: 258).

Another contemporary American study also confirmed a gender bias in medical textbooks (Mendelsohn *et al.* 1994). It included five anatomy and five physical-diagnosis texts and two atlases used in five medical schools in the Philadelphia area in the early 1990s. The results showed an almost equal distribution of women and men in the texts on diagnosis, but gender distribution was more unequal in the anatomy texts. For example, women appeared on average in 21 per cent of the illustrations about reproduction, compared to 44 per cent for portrayals of men, and 34 per cent for neutral portrayals. The most overt imbalance appeared in normal non-reproductive anatomy: women appeared in 11 per cent and men in 43 per cent of the portrayals.

Alan Petersen (1998) convincingly argues that anatomy has played a key role in shaping cultural understandings of the body and in the production of cultural images of the 'sexes' as embodied dualities. His study of 38 editions of Gray's *Anatomy*, a major anatomy textbook, from 1858 on, examines the way that sex differences have been constructed in portrayals of sex organs, pelvises and skulls. He shows that the text and illustrations reflect an assumed two-sex model, with the male body as the universal standard. In this way 'anatomy texts are a key means of conveying cultural knowledge about "sex" and "sex differences" to generations of students and practising physicians' (Petersen 1998: 14).

The gender biases implicit in the production of scientific knowledge of sex differences continues today, but the teaching device is different. Today there is an increasing use of simulators as stand-ins for patients in medical education. Such simulators are tools both for medical students and for instructors in the teaching of medical skills. Two types of computerized simulators of patients are used:

1   Mannequin-based simulators with sensors that represent a human patient's body are used in teaching physical skills.
2   Virtual-reality surgical simulators are used for teaching minimally invasive surgery (MIS) procedures.

The surgical MIS simulator teaches the skills in minimally invasive surgery, a procedure taking place on a screen. These simulators constitute a simulated 'patient-on-demand' and solve many practical and ethical problems in gaining access to 'teaching material' in learning technical skills in medicine.

In two respects, however, the simulators continue the traditions of reductionism in anatomical teaching. The first tradition is the reproduction of the 'unrealistic realism' of past anatomical sketches which offer clearly delineated pictures of organs and tissues. As Michel Foucault (1975: 9) has suggested, the anatomical atlas spatializes diseases, which then become apparent in the body. The medical gaze enables the physician to see the interior of the body and to locate the organs and their pathology, and medical students have to be initiated into such readings of the body. Nevertheless, the 'real' body is a messy mixture of tissues, vessels and organs. The visually constructed anatomical body enables the student to see its material representation in the patient's body. For example, the 'hands on' skills of the surgeon are gradually acquired as a result of an ability to create a visual anatomical model in the patient's body, an act of 'mutual articulation' where the physician's gaze and the patient's body come into being together through practice (Prentice 2005: 841).

The second tradition is the tacit construction of gender, because simulators continue to represent the notion of a 'one-sex body'. In medical discourse the 'standardized patient' is based on a notion of the 'standard human' constructed through the model of an adult male body (Epstein 2007: 277). As a Swedish study shows, the digital full-patient mannequin used in anaesthesiology training in a Swedish university hospital was modelled on a generic full-grown male body. This teaching device contained a hierarchical notion of gender: the male body represented the generic human body and the norm and the female body was only used when it differed from the male (Johnson 2005: 151). The mannequin had a removable insert which could be used to change the genital region from male to female (Johnson 2005: 143).

The same Swedish study also examined the use of a special pelvic simulator which is a model of the female reproductive organs. This simulator allows students to learn the technical skills of doing a pelvic examination without risking the discomfort of a live patient (for example, the sensors indicate whether the examiner has pushed too hard on organs). Although students learn the technical skills with the aid of such a pelvic simulator, the simulator not only neglects variations in the nature of the body but also dematerializes it. The female patient is detached from the medical procedure, and the culture of interaction is sanitized by the computerized method. So far, the simulator's repertoire of built-in learning devices does not include any means of acquiring social-interaction skills or of observing cultural values and practices during the examination of the genital area (Johnson 2005: 149).

The use of simulators as teaching devices will probably therefore allow the gendered practices of anatomical teaching and the character of the informal socialization to continue in this area of medicine. For example, studies on cadaver stories circulated among medical students have pointed to the sexist character of such stories and how their sexist content confirms traditional gender-based power relations in medicine (Hafferty 1988).

In some countries the integration of gender-sensitive aspects of health and illnesses into the medical curriculum has been a way of addressing the gender-neutral or gender-biased content of the medical curriculum of the past. For example, in Sweden and the Netherlands, medical schools have taken initiatives to include gender-related medical knowledge in the medical curriculum (Hammarström 2003; Verdonck et al. 2005, 2006, 2008). The Dutch approach has been to introduce gender-specific topics to the curriculum. This approach is defined as bringing into medical education the knowledge of the meaning of sex and gender for health and illness and its application to practice (Verdonck et al. 2006: 402). Such gender-specific topics include gender differences in coronary heart disease (CHD), sexual violence, falling accidents in old female patients, men's health risks and infertility in highly educated women.

A survey of US medical schools in 2004 found that a core curriculum on women's health topics (courses or clerkships) related to gender differences in health and illness and women's health issues were not fully integrated into the curriculum. A surprisingly uneven development in this area has prevailed at US medical schools (Henrich and Viscoli 2006). The results showed that only nine schools (of a total of 126) offered a women's health course. Another set of schools (23) listed sessions with a non-reproductive women's health focus, and some (13) listed courses with a gender-specific focus. In general there was little gender-specific information about many conditions that cause the greatest morbidity and mortality in women (Henrich and Viscoli 2006: 481). A noteworthy finding was that the presence of a female medical-school dean was positively associated with the range of topics taught on gender. This confirms how important it is to have women in top positions in academic medicine if the culture and attitudes to gender in medical education are to change.

In American medical education the establishment of a specialty area in women's health and more recently in andrology (a male-focused specialty) reinforces an understanding of gender-related health needs and illnesses as merely matters of biology. Some scholars have been critical of a sex-based biology approach to gender differences in health. The argument has been that the sex-based biology approach to gender and health confirms essentialist notions about medical differences between men and women and diverts attention away from the social and economic structures underlying gender inequalities in health (Epstein 2007: 281).

The term 'hidden curriculum' has been used to indicate the processes and constraints outside the formal curriculum and tending to remain unarticulated or as hidden structures (Hafferty 2000; Lempp and Seale 2004). An exploration of the hidden curriculum at one UK medical school showed the presence of four such mechanisms with a negative impact on learning: the role of mainly male role models; the low priority of teaching, especially among clinical staff; degrading mechanisms of reproducing existing hierarchies in medicine; and the competitive character of medical education (Lempp and Seale 2004).

Medical practice: selection of specialty

The classic studies of medical education showed how medical schools socialize students to professional behaviour and attitudes. The pressure for homogeneity creates a culture characterized by time pressure and conformity. The norm of the 'impartial knower' – the ideal of impartiality and colour-, class- and sex-neutral medical knowledge – guides the teaching of professional knowledge and skills (Beagan 2000: 1262).

In consideration of such pressure for conformity, students make surprisingly diverse decisions in their choice of specialty on the basis of gender. As studies in many countries have shown, first-year female and male medical students express nearly the same level of interest in a career in surgery, paediatrics, obstetrics and gynaecology or academia, but the gender gap tends to have widened considerably among third-year students and residents. The different career choices are reflected in the current profile of medical specialization by gender. In healthcare systems where statistics by gender are available, a marked gender segregation of medical specialization tends to prevail, regardless of the increasing proportion of women among practising doctors. In 2004, although 70 per cent of the physicians in Lithuania were women, only 11 per cent of the surgeons but 76 per cent of the obstetricians/gynaecologists and 93 per cent of the paediatricians were women (Riska and Novelskaite 2008: 220). There are comparable figures for the Nordic countries, which have had a high representation of women among physicians during the past three decades. Women constituted 52 per cent of the practising physicians in Finland in 2008, but only 20 per cent of the surgeons, compared to 63 per cent of the paediatricians and 70 per cent of the obstetricians/gynaecologists (FMA 2008). The figures for Sweden show a similar pattern: in 2008, although 46 per cent of the practising physicians were women, only 18 per cent of the surgeons, but 62 per cent of the obstetricians/gynaecologists were women (SMA 2008). Female students now tend to be in the majority in training for obstetrics and gynaecology in the UK and male medical students' interest in a career in obstetrics and gynaecology is falling (Higham and Steer 2004).

With female students constituting a growing proportion of the first-year students and residents, researchers have noted that gender equity has improved for women, while new forms of gender inequities have emerged for men. For example, there was an increase in female residents in surgery – from 13 per cent in 1988 to 21 per cent in 1999 – in the US. This contrasts with the UK, where men's choice of and preference for surgery as their area of specialization has remained almost unchanged (Bickel 2001: 264; Drinkwater *et al.* 2008; Fysh *et al.* 2007). Furthermore, American women who choose surgery are very satisfied with their work as surgeons and find it a rewarding career (Bickel 2001: 267).

Female medical students report difficulties in finding a mentor, and there is a lack of support in choosing surgery. For example, a survey of an American surgery faculty showed that 71 per cent of the men but only 14 per cent of the women agreed that there were good role models within the department (Bickel 2001: 265). This has been known for some time but a new form of gender discrimination has begun to appear in obstetrics and gynaecology residencies. Male students tend to face problems in gaining adequate clinical experience in obstetrics and gynaecology training, in contrast to women. British male medical students tend to get less clinical exposure than female students, and the feeling of being excluded from clinical opportunities is further reported to be influenced by midwives who are less helpful to male than they are to female students. The result is that women do better in assessments of clinical examinations. The phenomenon is already called the 'anti-male environment in obstetrics and gynaecology' (Higham and Steer 2004: 143). This new gender-biased culture in obstetrics and gynaecology has also been confirmed in a recent qualitative study on the hidden curriculum of the UK undergraduate medical curriculum. The study found that nurses and midwives tend in general to treat medical students disrespectfully, especially male students. Male students tend to be resentful of midwives and characterize them in degrading terms during obstetrics and gynaecology training at teaching hospitals (Lempp and Seale 2004: 772). A similar situation has developed in US medical education (Krueger 1998). While women constituted 15 per cent of the residents in obstetrics and gynaecology in US medical schools in 1975, they constituted 70 per cent in 2000, and they are expected to amount to 60 per cent of the obstetrics and gynaecology practitioners in 2020 (Emmons *et al.* 2004: 331). The American findings also show that male students in obstetrics and gynaecology report gender discrimination more often than female students (Emmons *et al.* 2004; Nora *et al.* 2002: 1230). A basic reason for this is that female patients prefer female students to do pelvic examinations, and so male students perform fewer clinical procedures than do female students, who have a greater chance to gain a better clinical experience (Emmons *et al.* 2004: 329). A reverse finding has been reported for American students in family practice. The results show that male and female students seem to get different clinical-skills experience and female students were exposed to fewer clinical experiences in family practice than were male students (Kilminster *et al.* 2007: 42).

What kind of explanations can be given for the gendered choices and final distribution of doctors by gender in medical practice? There are three major sociological explanations: gender socialization, structural barriers and embedded values in medicine and healthcare. The first explanation is that gender socialization continues to influence the choices that students make in medical school. Expectations concerning gendered skills and expected gender-related behaviour influence, if not overtly then at least tacitly, students' choice of residency and medical careers. Expectations of work–life balance and regular working hours have been rated as more important among female medical students than among male ones in North American and European studies. These aspects of the character of medical work and practice tend to influence students' later career decisions as well. This explanation has been given different names: some call it the sex-role theory, others the human-capital theory or more recently preference theory (Riska 2008). The common denominator of these theories is the assumption that individuals make their choices on the basis of their individual life situation. The aggregated outcome of the individual career choices is a certain pattern of medical specialization by gender.

The second explanation is critical of the voluntaristic explanation of the gender-socialization theory and considers it too narrow. The argument is that gender-socialization theory does not take into account the structural and cultural barriers preventing women from gaining entry as equals with men into male-dominated specialties and practice settings. One such barrier is the lack of mentors: women are not encouraged and cannot find a mentor who provides the kind of informal socialization that is a crucial part of a career in medicine. Surgery is often mentioned as a case of the existence of hidden barriers or even explicit discouragement of women from entering into training. Both autobiographical reports (Conley 1998) and ethnographic studies (Cassell 2000; Katz 1999) point to the male ethos of surgery. Surgery is characterized by a dominant masculine culture, and women find it difficult to fit in or to even be invited to join surgical internships. The male ethos is characterized by an emphasis on such personal (male) qualities as aggressive, competitive behaviour and physical strength as prerequisites for becoming and being a good surgeon (Bickel 2001).

Yet surgery is changing: much surgery today is minimally invasive and done by a laparoscopic procedure which can be followed on a computer screen. This kind of surgery demands different kinds of skills (precision, diligence) and team-work rather than the quick decisions and physical strength required for long operations mainly performed by the lone, heroic (male) surgeon. The new work arrangements in most routine surgery have therefore been thought to change the previous masculine culture and to give physical and cultural space for women to practise in surgery (Zetka 2003).

This kind of cultural turn in the definition of professional skills required for work in a specialty has already taken place in pathology, where the old-fashioned dissection of cadavers is today a minor part of pathologists' work. Instead, the analysis of autopsies by means of microscopy and the identification and diagnosis of pathology in tissues taken from live patients is a major part of the pathologists' work profile. A Finnish study showed that visualization skills and an exceptional sense for details and a capacity for memorizing were mentioned by both male and female pathologists as the necessary gender-neutral skills for doing the work (Riska 2001, 2004). Women pathologists still felt that the master status of the specialty was defined in male terms. As a strategy of inclusion, the female pathologists defined their skill in microscopy as female-gendered because microscopy requires precision work, which the women pathologists perceived as the essential skill for today's pathologist. In their view, women pathologists' gender-specific skills better matched the professional qualities needed for good work. In the accounts of the male pathologists, gendered qualities for professional work in the specialty were not mentioned because for them the specialty was unmarked by gender (Riska 2004).

The third explanation for the gendered career choices in medicine is the embedded feature of gender in complex organizations like medicine. It has been argued that organizations (Acker 1990; Britton 2000) and professions (Davies 1996; Witz 1992) are inherently male-gendered: the workings of these institutions valorize the masculine and features associated with masculinity (for example, scientific objectivity, efficiency, hierarchical structures, autonomy of the professions). In today's terminology, hegemonic masculinity as a culture and social structure shapes the values and social structure of medicine. It has therefore been suggested that even if women enter medical schools and the profession in increasing numbers, the values in medical education and the organization of medicine will remain male-gendered, because men control the knowledge and power of the profession. More recently the term 'inequality regimes' (Acker 2006) has been introduced as a way to understand the production of gender, race and class in organizations and to shed light on why so many organizational-equality projects have failed or have had minor impact.

The embedded character of gender has been used as an explanation of why there is still both horizontal and vertical gender segregation in medicine. 'Vertical gender segregation is a term used to describe the concentration of men in top positions and the difficulties women have in reaching top positions in a profession and its organization of work. In medical education, the scarcity of women as professors of medicine and as medical-school deans has been used as proof of the existence of a 'glass ceiling' in medicine. The latter term has been used as an analytical tool to illustrate the invisible barriers that seem to hinder women in advancing to top positions. For example, in 2005, women constituted merely 10 per cent of the professors of medicine in the UK, although women have constituted over 40 per cent of the students over the past 20 years and now compose 60 per cent of them. Furthermore, women constituted 21 per cent of the clinical academics and, in fact, six UK medical schools had not a single female professor of medicine (Sandu et al. 2007). In the US, women constituted 15 per cent of full professors in medicine in 2005 (Hamel et al. 2006) while 45 per cent of entering students in 2004 were women (Emmons et al. 2004). Statistical figures for EU countries show that women composed the following proportion of the equivalent of professors in medicine in 2004: 22 per cent in Finland, 17 per cent in Norway, 15 per cent in Denmark, Sweden and France, 11 per cent in Italy and 6 per cent in Germany and the Netherlands (EC 2006: 60).

Gender discrimination and sexual harassment has been found to be a problem for female medical students in US and UK medical schools (Emmons et al. 2004; Higham and Steer 2004; Nora et al. 2002). A survey conducted in 1997 of senior medical students at 14 US medical schools examined the prevalence of gender discrimination and sexual harassment (GD/SH). There were only minor gender differences in answers about whether the respondent had heard about or observed gender discrimination or sexual harassment. By contrast, 83 per cent of the women but 41 per cent of the men had themselves experienced gender discrimination and sexual harassment in academic or non-academic contexts (Nora *et al.* 2002). The experiences of discrimination reported by both male and female students were greatest outside the medical training environment. Both male and female students perceived significantly higher rates of GD/SH in general surgery and obstetrics and gynaecology than in the other specialties. In the academic setting, discrimination and harassment was most prevalent in core clerkships, where 63 per cent of women compared to 30 per cent of men reported GD/SH. Such experiences tend to also affect choice of specialty. Female students, who had reported exposure to GD/SH, indicated significantly more often than men that this experience had influenced their specialty choice and residency ranking (Stratton *et al.* 2005).

There seems to be one exception in exposure to GD/SH: Dutch medical schools have been found to have an exceptionally low rate of sexual harassment of medical students. One in three to five female Dutch medical students had experienced unwelcome sexual attention from patients, colleagues or supervisors (Rademakers *et al.* 2008).

Conclusion

This chapter has reviewed three topics pertaining to gender and medical education: the increasing enrolment of women in medical schools; the new forms of reproduction of gendered medical knowledge in medical teaching; and the gendered career choices that result in a horizontal and vertical gender segregation of medical practice.

The topic of gender in medical education was indirectly addressed in the early research on medical education because the classic literature focused on how male medical students were socialized to professional conduct and attitudes. During the past 30 years 'gender' in medical education has meant the status of women and gender equality and equity in medical training and careers for women. The early 2000s witnessed a backlash because various 'problems' in medicine were interpreted as the result of the growing proportion of women among medical students and practising physicians. As suggested in this chapter, the use of the term 'feminization of medicine' is part of a discourse about the impact of female students and physicians on medicine as a profession and practice. The thesis about the feminization of medicine assumes that male medical students and men doctors are continuing their education and practice in the way that they have done in the past and it is only female medical students and doctors who cause the changes. Such assumptions are homogenizing both groups and creating essentialist notions about the attitudes and behaviours of male and female medical students and doctors.

Medicine as a science and technology is undergoing dramatic changes, and neoliberal policies in the area of healthcare policy are changing the way that medicine is organized and delivered. Hence, female medical students or doctors are not the sole or main agents of the structural changes in medicine. Instead, broader economic and cultural changes in healthcare and medical technology have challenged the autonomy and practices of the medical profession. Medical education has been a way that the profession has consolidated its position in the past but reforms in medical education have also been able to integrate changes that could alter future professional behaviour. The feminization debate has therefore raised an important concern: there are different styles of doctoring and there is a need for new approaches in medicine. The task ahead is to de-gender the different styles of doctoring and to teach these styles early in medical education. For example, emotion-skills training has been integrated into the medical curriculum and these skills seem to be acquired in the same way as physical-examination skills (Satterfield and Hughes 2007). A systematic review of the evaluation of the impact of communication-skills courses (with controlled trials) showed all positive outcomes (Smith *et al.* 2007).

The foregoing review brought up the persistent gendered character of medical knowledge and gender segregation of medical practice. Although a slow change in the most marked gender segregation of medical specialties – for example, surgery – can be witnessed, an awareness of the gender dimensions of medical knowledge needs to be addressed in medical education. Further research – for example, in science and technology studies – will generate more information in this area. Meanwhile, current knowledge about gender and health and illnesses should be more visibly integrated into the medical curriculum in order to address gender aspects of medical practice.

References

Acker, J. (1990) 'Hierarchies, jobs, bodies: a theory of gendered organizations', *Gender and Society*, 4: 139–58.

—— (2006) 'Inequality regimes: gender, class, and race in organizations', *Gender and Society*, 20: 441–64.

Beagan, B. L. (2000) 'Neutralizing differences: producing neutral doctors for (almost) neutral patients', *Social Science and Medicine*, 51: 1253–65.

Becker, H. S., Geer, B., Hughes, E. C. and Strauss, A. L. (1961) *Boys in White: student culture in medical school*, Chicago, IL: University of Chicago Press.

Bickel, J. (2001) 'Gender equity in undergraduate medical education: a status report', *Journal of Women's Health and Gender-Based Medicine*, 10: 261–70.

Britton, D. M. (2000) 'The epistemology of the gendered organization', *Gender and Society*, 14: 418–34.

Burke, B. P. and White, J. C. (2001) 'Wellbeing of gay, lesbian and bisexual doctors', *British Medical Journal*, 322: 422–4.

Cassell, J. (2000) *The Woman in the Surgeon's Body*, Cambridge, MA: Harvard University Press.

Conley, F. K. (1998) *Walking Out on the Boys*, New York: Farrar, Straus and Giroux.

Davies, C. (1996) 'The sociology of professions and the profession of gender', *Sociology*, 30: 661–78.

Drinkwater, J., Tully, M. P. and Dornan, T. (2008) 'The effect of gender on medical students' aspirations: a qualitative study', *Medical Education*, 42: 420–6.

Emmons, S. L., Adams, K. E., Nichols, M. and Cain, J. (2004) 'The impact of perceived gender bias on obstetrics and gynecology skills acquisition by third-year medical students', *Academic Medicine*, 79: 326–32.

Epstein, S. (2007) *Inclusion: the politics of difference in medical research*, Chicago, IL: University of Chicago Press.

European Commission (EC), Directorate-General for Research (2006) *She Figures 2006: women and science: statistics and indicators*, Luxembourg: Office for Official Publications of the European Communities.

Finnish Medical Association (FMA) (2008) *Lääkärit 2008*, online at (www.laakariliitto.fi/tilastot/laakaritilastot/taskutilasto.html) (accessed 17 June 2008).

Foucault, M. (1975) *The Birth of the Clinic: an archaeology of medical perception*, New York: Vintage Books.

Fysh, T. H., Thomas, G. and Ellis, H. (2007) 'Who wants to be a surgeon? A study of 300 first year medical students', *Biomed Central Medical Education*, 7, 2, online at http://www.biomedcentral.com/1472–6920/7/2 (accessed 7 November 2007).

Hafferty, F. W. (1988) 'Cadaver stories and the emotional socialization of medical students', *Journal of Health and Social Behavior*, 29: 344–56.

—— (2000) 'Reconfiguring the sociology of medical education: emerging topics and pressing issues', in C. E. Bird, P. Conrad and A. M. Fremont (eds) *Handbook of Medical Sociology*, 5th edn, Upper Saddle River, NJ: Prentice Hall.

Hamel, M. B., Ingelfinger, J. R., Phimister, E. and Solomon, C. G. (2006) 'Women in academic medicine – progress and challenges', *New England Journal of Medicine*, 355: 310–12.

Hammarström, A. (2003) 'The integration of gender in medical research and education: obstacles and possibilities from a Nordic perspective', *Women and Health*, 37: 121–33.

Henrich, J. B. and Viscoli, C. M. (2006) 'What do medical schools teach about women's health and gender differences?', *Academic Medicine*, 81: 476–82.

Higham, J. and Steer, P. J. (2004) 'Gender gap in undergraduate experience and performance in obstetrics and gynaecology: analysis of clinical experience logs', *British Medical Journal*, 328: 142–3.

Johnson, E. (2005) 'The ghost of anatomies past: simulating the one-sex body in modern medical training', *Feminist Theory*, 6: 141–59.

Katz, P. (1999) *The Scalpel's Edge: the culture of surgeons*, Boston, MA: Allyn and Bacon.

Kilminster, S., Downes, J., Gough, B., Murdoch-Eaton, D. and Roberts, T. (2007) 'Women in medicine – is there a problem? a literature review of the changing gender composition, structures and occupational cultures in medicine', *Medical Education*, 41: 39–49.

Krueger, P. M. (1998) 'Do women medical students outperform men in obstetrics and gynecology?', *Academic Medicine*, 73: 101–2.

Laqueur, T. (1990) *Making Sex: body and gender from the Greeks to Freud*, London: Harvard University Press.

Lawrence, S. C. and Bendixen, K. (1992) 'His and hers: male and female anatomy texts for US medical students, 1890–1989', *Social Science and Medicine*, 35: 925–34.

Lempp, H. and Seale, C. (2004) 'The hidden curriculum in undergraduate medical education: qualitative study of medical students' perceptions of teaching', *British Medical Journal*, 329: 770–3.

Lorber, J. (1975) 'Women and medical sociology: invisible professionals and ubiquitous patients', in M. Millman and R. Moss Kanter (eds) *Another Voice: feminist perspectives on social life and social science*, Garden City, NY: Anchor Press/Doubleday.

Mendelsohn, K. D., Nieman, L. Z., Isaacs, K., Lee, S. and Levison, S. P. (1994) 'Sex and gender bias in anatomy and physical diagnosis text illustrations', *Journal of the American Medical Association*, 272: 1267–70.

Merchant, R. C., Jongco, A. M. and Woodward, L. (2005) 'Disclosure of sexual orientation by medical students and residency applicants', *Academic Medicine*, 80: 786.

Merton, R. K. (1957) 'Some preliminaries to a sociology of medical education', in R. K. Merton, G. Reader and P. Kendall (eds) *The Student-Physician: introductory studies in the sociology of medical education*, Cambridge, MA: Harvard University Press.

Merton, R. K., Reader, G. G. and Kendall, P. L. (eds) (1957) *The Student-Physician: introductory studies in the sociology of medical education*, Cambridge, MA: Harvard University Press.

Miller, S. (1970) *Prescription for Leadership: training for the medical elite*, Chicago, IL: Aldine Publishing Company.

Moore, L. J. and Clarke, A. (1995) 'Clitoral conventions and transgressions: graphic representations in anatomy texts, c.1900–1991', *Feminist Studies*, 21: 255–301.

Mumford, E. (1970) *Interns: from students to physicians*, Cambridge, MA: Harvard University Press.

Nora, L. M., McLaughlin, M. A., Fosson, S. E., Stratton, T. D., Murphy-Spencer, A., Fincher, R.-M. E., German, D. C., Seiden, D. and Witzke, D. B. (2002) 'Gender discrimination and sexual harassment in medical education: perspectives gained by a 14-school study', *Academic Medicine*, 77: 1226–34.

Parsons, T. (1949) 'Professions and social structure', in *Essays in Sociological Theory: pure and applied*, Glencoe, IL: Free Press.

—— (1951) *The Social System*, New York: Free Press.

Petersen, A. (1998) 'Sexing the body: representations of sex differences in Gray's *Anatomy*, 1858 to the present', *Body and Society*, 4: 1–15.

Prentice, R. (2005) 'The anatomy of a surgical simulation: the mutual articulation of bodies in and through the machine', *Social Studies of Science*, 35: 837–66.

Rademakers, J. J. D. J. M., van den Muijsenbergh, M. E. T. C., Slappendel, G., Lagro-Janssen, T. L. M. and Borleffs, J. C. C. (2008) 'Sexual harassment during clinical clerkships in Dutch medical schools', *Medical Education*, 42: 452–8.

Risdon, C., Cook, D. and Willms, D. (2000) 'Gay and lesbian physicians in training: a qualitative study', *Canadian Medical Association Journal*, 162: 331–4.

Riska, E. (2001) *Medical Careers and Feminist Agendas: American, Scandinavian and Russian women physicians*, New York: Aldine de Gruyter.

—— (2004) 'The work of pathologists: visualisation of disease and control of uncertainty', in I. Shaw and K. Kauppinen (eds) *Constructions of Health and Illness: a European perspective*, Aldershot: Ashgate.

—— (2008) 'The feminization thesis: discourses on gender and medicine', *NORA: Nordic Journal of Feminist and Gender Research*, 2008: 3–18.

Riska, E. and Novelskaite, A. (2008) 'Professionals in transition: physicians' careers, migration and gender in Lithuania', in E. Kuhlmann and M. Saks (eds) *Rethinking Professional Governance: international directions in healthcare*, Bristol: Policy Press.

Rogoff, N. (1957) 'The decision to study medicine', in R. K. Merton, G. Reader and P. Kendall (eds) *The Student-Physician: introductory studies in the sociology of medical education*, Cambridge, MA: Harvard University Press.

Sandu, B., Margerison, C. and Holdcroft, A. (2007) 'Women in the UK academic medicine workforce', *Medical Education*, 41: 909–14.

Satterfield, J. M. and Hughes, E. (2007) 'Emotion skills training for medical students: a systematic review', *Medical Education*, 41: 935–41.

Scully, D. and Bart, P. (1973) 'A funny thing happened on the way to the orifice: women in gynecology textbooks', *American Journal of Sociology*, 78: 1045–50.

Smith, S., Hanson, J. L., Tewksbury, L. R., Christy, C., Talib, N., Harris, M. A., Beck, G. L. and Wolf, F. M. (2007) 'Teaching patient communication skills to medical students', *Evaluation and the Health Professions*, 30: 3–21.

Stratton, T. D., McLaughlin, M. A., Witte, F. M., Fosson, S. E. and Nora, L. M. (2005) 'Does students' exposure to gender discrimination and sexual harassment in medical school affect specialty choice and residency program selection?', *Academic Medicine*, 80: 400–8.

Swedish Medical Association (SMA) (2008) *Läkarfakta 2008*, online at www.lakarforbundet.se/upload/lakarforbundet/trycksaker/PDFer/Arbetsmarknad/L%C%karfakta-2008.pdf (accessed 17 June 2008).

Verdonck, P., Mans, L. J. L. and Lagro-Janssen, T. L. M. (2005) 'Integrating gender into a basic medical curriculum', *Medical Education*, 39: 1118–25.

Verdonck, P., Mans, L. J. L. and Lagro-Janssen, T. L. M. (2006) 'How is gender integrated in curricula of Dutch medical schools? A quick-scan on gender issues as an instrument for change', *Gender and Education*, 18: 399–412.

Verdonck, P., Benschop, Y. W. M., de Haes, H. C. J. and Lagro-Janssen, T. L. M. (2008) 'From gender bias to gender awareness in medical education', *Advances in Health Sciences Education*, online at www.springerlink.com/content/77770050012xjk81/fulltext.pdf (accessed 17 June 2008).

Whitcomb, M. E. (2006) 'Who will study medicine in the future?', *Academic Medicine*, 81: 205–6.

Witz, A. (1992) *Professions and Patriarchy*, London: Routledge.

Zetka Jr, J. R. (2003) *Surgeons and the Scope*, Ithaca, NY: Cornell University Press.

7 The inclusion of disabled people in medical education

Gary L. Albrecht[1]

Disability is an integral part of the personal and work lives of health professionals yet is most often neither well understood nor adequately conceptualized. On
a population level, the recent *World Report on Disability and Rehabilitation* co-
sponsored by the World Health Organization and World Bank estimates that the
prevalence rate for moderate or severe disability in the world is 15.3 per cent or
over one billion of the global population (Albrecht *et al.* in press). While disability prevalence rates vary according to the income level of the country (ranging
from 16.9 per cent for low-income countries to 14.2 per cent for high-income
countries), percentage of citizens living in poverty (25.4 per cent in the poorest
quintile of wealth to 10.4 per cent in the richest quintile), stage in the life course
(children and the elderly experience more disability), sex (12.9 per cent male;
21.6 per cent female) and exposures to risks causing eye diseases, hearing loss,
depression, unintentional injuries, drug and alcohol dependency, and chronic
conditions such as heart and pulmonary diseases, disability is clearly a universal
experience in every nation in the world.

On a personal level, most individuals are likely to experience disability personally in their lifetimes and almost certainly to have members of their immediate family, friends and co-workers who are disabled. These personal disability
experiences may be of limited duration where an individual is temporarily
restricted in function, activity and participation following an injury, heart attack
or bout of depression or persistent as with Alzheimer's, arthritis, asthma, HIV/
AIDS, spinal-cord injury and Parkinson's disease. Among family, friends and
co-workers, disability requires adjustment and accommodation on a personal
level and to their environments. A worldwide phenomenon is that people are
living longer with chronic diseases and disabilities. Consequently, families,
particularly children, need to care for their disabled and dying parents and in due
course manage their own disabilities. In all these circumstances, individuals and
their families face living with disability and managing their care, finances and
lives around the disability experience.

On a professional level, healthcare and social-service workers discover that
the people they see often have conditions with apparent or subtle disability consequences. Managing acute episodes or only a part of a set of co-morbid conditions avoids disability considerations in the short term but postpones the

inevitable with costly consequences in terms of function, activity levels and finances for individuals and their families. To deal effectively with these issues, it is imperative that healthcare professionals incorporate disability into their lives as an integral part of their educational and socialization experience.

If physicians and healthcare professionals are to be comfortable with and knowledgeable about disabled people, they have to include them in their professional and social networks. Consequently, this chapter takes a social-network approach to including disabled people in medical education. First, I outline how social-network theory provides a framework for thinking about medical education. Second, I show how a social-network approach to medical education addresses and incorporates the sound advice of disability advocates and activists, 'Nothing about us, without us'. Third, I suggest that the inclusion of disabled people in medical education helps to redirect physicians' thinking from episodic and problem-specific care to a holistic and lifespan view of the patient. Fourth, I point out that familiarity with disabled people will focus physicians' attention on broad-based patient outcomes. Fifth, I indicate that understanding disabled people and their health conditions will reinforce a team approach and emphasize continuity of care. I conclude by pointing out that healthcare disparities result in disability disparities and that physicians and public-health professionals can improve life chances and quality of life for disabled people, provide better care and reduce the expense of healthcare by addressing these disparities.

Social-network theory

People tend to think and behave like the people around them and usually share their values. Homogeneity of experience and context is either actively sought out because it is comfortable to be surrounded with like-minded people, or individuals with a difference are pressured to conform and adapt to the norms and expectations of the groups in which they find themselves. In either instance, diversity is often avoided, feared and controlled. The 'other' is someone different, not well known or understood and is often stereotyped to compensate for this lack of knowledge and contact with 'strangers'. If families do have someone different like a disabled relative in their midst, they often hide or gloss over the disability markers of this person. As a result, few people are knowledgeable about or comfortable with disabled people. Unfortunately, this is true of physicians and healthcare workers as well as the general public.

Social-network theory provides the theoretical basis for understanding how individuals relate to and influence one another and how disabled people fit into their families, friendships and work groups (Latour 2007). Network analysis helps us discover how disabled people become informed about their health problems, seek and utilize care and develop social-support groups to help them manage their disabilities. In network theory, the emphasis is on describing and analysing the relationship between one social actor (in this case a disabled person) and other social actors in their lives (family, friends, co-workers, physicians and other care providers) with whom they have relationships (Pescosolido

2006). Analysis of social networks concentrates on three components: structure, content and function. Structure concerns the size of the network, the different types of relationships that people can have with others and the strength and frequency of contact. Content includes the substance of what is addressed in relationships, be it information, emotional support, healthcare, rehabilitation activities, economic activity and/or sharing attitudes, values and a world view. Function indicates that social networks serve different and multiple purposes such as providing emotional support, assistance, economic and social support, transport and feelings of belonging and importance.

In social-network theory, there is a distinction between external social networks, comprised of a disabled person's family, friends and co-workers, internal networks within healthcare organizations, rehabilitation centres, medical and care teams that determine how interventions and support are delivered, and boundary-spanning networks that bridge the gaps between personal and disability-care networks. Social-network analysis maps the relationships between actors within and between each of these types of networks. The structure, content and function of these networks is recorded and analysed for directions and patterns of behaviour centred around one or more episodes. In the case of the disabled person, the analysis could, for instance, focus on how care was sought and delivered to a person who had experienced an arthritis flare-up, an asthma attack, a denial of healthcare insurance or a reduction in disability benefits. From a physician's perspective, attention would be given to what the structure, content and function of the doctor's relation was to the disabled person seeking help with a disability episode. What professional social networks would the physician employ to address this episode? This activity in multiple social networks would be focused on the health status, activity level and ability of the disabled person to participate independently in life.

Social networks are embedded in physical and social environments. The neighbourhoods in which we live and places that we work and play shape our view of the world and our behaviour (Bartels 2008; Massey 2007). The social, political-economic and physical environments characterizing these locations determine how we see ourselves, whom we interact with and how we treat others. For example, Sampson and colleagues report that 'neighbourhood effects', consisting of level of resources, physical conditions, institutions in the area, amount of poverty and social-interaction patterns, are powerful predictors of such diverse outcomes as delinquency, violence, depression, high-risk behaviours, educational performance and racial inequality (Sampson *et al.* 2002; Sampson and Sharkey 2008). Sampson *et al.* (1997) further argue that collective efficacy among friends and neighbours, defined as social cohesion, combined with their willingness to intervene on behalf of the common good, is related to reduced violence. In another context, Christakis and Fowler (2007) show how social networks of family and friends were quite influential in predicting whether or not a person would be obese. Their longitudinal analysis of social networks of 12,067 people followed regularly from 1971 to 2003 as part of the Framingham Heart Study revealed that obesity tends to spread through social ties. In a study of the social connectedness of older adults, Cornwell *et al.* (2008) suggest that successful ageing is related to the number and size of social contacts and the amount and type of social interactions that individuals have. This body of literature in diverse areas underlines the power of social networks and social relationships in situating and predicting behaviour.

For disabled persons, the utility and effectiveness of specific social networks will depend on whether or not the individual is recognized and included or marginalized. For physicians, the quality of the care they deliver will depend on their knowledge of and access to the types of social networks that will permit them to gather the best information, make informed decisions and refer the disabled person on to others that can provide the support and services required for the problems at hand. To lay down the infrastructure necessary for physicians to be able to recognize, understand and respond to the problems presented by disabled clients, they need to develop social networks beginning in medical school that will enable them to perform comfortably, effectively and in a timely fashion.

'Nothing about us without us'

Social network theory and the research evidence suggests that if physicians and care providers are to be knowledgeable about and effective in working with disabled people, they must engage with them in more than a perfunctory, episodic-oriented manner. This implies that disabled people should be intimately involved in medical education, training and practice as students, staff, doctors, patients, administrators, care reviewers and in the financial side of the business. Given the range and diversity of impairments, healthcare professionals need exposure to physically, mentally and developmentally disabled people. Inclusion of disabled people in medical education, training and practice addresses the worldwide protest from disability activists, 'Nothing about us without us' (Charlton 1998).

The effects of limited knowledge and exposure to disabled people lead to prejudice and discrimination towards disabled people and expensive, inappropriate and ineffective planning and care for them on the part of medical staff. In the present state of medical education, medical students and practising physicians are ill prepared to work with disabled people (Crotty *et al.* 2000). A study of 381 medical students in the UK found that they associated 'disability' with negatively and depersonalized descriptive words such as wheelchair-dependent, handicapped, impaired, disadvantaged, difficult, prejudice and stigma (Bryon *et al.* 2005). These negative attitudes and lack of exposure to disabled people result in doctors appearing to be insensitive and patronizing (Bryon and Dieppe 2000). In fact, some physicians who have firsthand experience with disabled persons observe that 'doctors can contribute to the discrimination, social exclusion and stigma experienced by disabled people' (Melville 2005: 122). These discriminatory attitudes and behaviours are particularly apparent in the treatment of mentally ill people. In a recent study in Turkey, medical students were seen to be more prejudiced against the mentally ill than was a sample of second-grade children (Ay *et al.* 2006). Such negative attitudes and perceptions are likely to constitute a barrier preventing patients from receiving appropriate care. Aulagnier *et al.* (2005), for example, report in a study of 600 General Practitioners in South-Eastern France that 21.3 per cent were uncomfortable with treating people with mental impairments and 8.2 per cent of people with physical impairments. In assessing the problems associated with patient impairment and disability, few physicians and the general public realize that disabled people can have a perceived high quality of life in spite of being seen by others as 'different' and experiencing restrictions in physical and social activities (Albrecht and Devlieger 1999). Furthermore, neither physicians nor their patients are fully aware of how healthcare services and resources are tightly rationed and poorly allocated to disabled people, often resulting in ineffective and even harmful outcomes (Albrecht 2001).

This complex of background factors influencing care for disabled people exerts increasing pressure on and produces confusion among physicians who are addressing their disabled clients' end-of-life decisions and care. End-of-life decisions are difficult enough when dealing with the general population but adding disability to the equation makes the exercise particularly contentious and knotty. Christakis points out (1999) that of the three core clinical tasks of the physician (diagnosis, treatment and prognosis), prognosis is the most overlooked. The major actors in end-of-life decisions (patients, family, insurance companies and care providers) rely heavily on the physicians' judgement in predicting and planning for the end of life. Decisions that are difficult under the best of circumstances are exacerbated by the complications of disability. Do disabled people and their families prefer them to die without extraordinary interventions to prolong their lives or do they desire to prolong their lives as much as possible? Do they think and behave like the more general population of patients or are they different? How do the families and caretakers of disabled persons influence the end-of-life decisions? Are there differences between people's conditions and wishes according to their particular type of disability and stage in life or not? Can people change their minds after they have signed 'Do Not Resuscitate' documents? What is ethical and moral care for disabled people? These issues indicate the imperative of better understanding and managing healthcare interventions for the terminally ill especially in the case of disabled people (Ross and Albrecht 2000).

Clearly, the only way for better and more appropriate care to be delivered to disabled people is to involve them centrally in the process. Disabled people must be included in the social networks of service and care if they and their needs are to be understood and effectively addressed. Medical educators are beginning to sound the clarion call to remedy this situation. DeLisa and Thomas (2005), for example, point out that the technical standards and core competencies taught in medical schools have not kept pace with the changing nature of medical practice and the types of patients seen. They suggest that medical education in the twenty-first century focus considerable attention on the inclusion and needs of medical students with disabilities as well as training all students to be comfortable with and competent in treating disabled patients. This implies that more disabled students should be accepted into medical school, making these institutions physically and socially welcoming and providing adapted environments and accessible instruction and training experiences.

Inclusion of disabled people in medical education

Acceptance of and inclusion of disabled students in medical, nursing, therapy and pharmacy schools would reshape the environment and training of healthcare professionals. Carroll (2004) argues that the inclusion of disabled students into nursing schools is feasible and desirable. She addresses the potential concerns of nurse educators regarding physical access, a decrease in the quality of care, meeting technical standards, practising care in a safe manner, meeting professional and licensure requirements and being accepted by patients. Addressing each concern in turn, she states that an important principle of the Americans with Disabilities Act of 1990 and its amendments (ADA) is that an individual must be qualified to meet the entry requirements of nursing, and by implication, medical schools, to be admitted. Furthermore, they must demonstrate the skills and competencies required to practise the profession before graduating and must pass the same licensure and medical-specialty boards as other students.

While the high standards of nursing and medical education and apprenticeship are not to be compromised, the ADA directs that reasonable accommodations are made for disabled students, professionals and other employees in schools and professional settings. Physical and social barriers are to be removed and necessary aids and services provided to allow disabled professionals to perform in their studies and jobs. Such environmental adjustments employing the principles of universal design are beneficial to disabled providers and consumers alike. Ramps in buildings, wheelchair-accessible restrooms, elevators and doors with easy-to-reach buttons and handles, signs and instructions that are easy to read for low-vision people, examination tables and imaging equipment that is adjustable for wheelchair users and individuals with prostheses and information on websites that is readily available make the practice of medical care easier and more humane for children, the elderly and other patients as well as disabled people.

Standards need not be lowered nor quality of care compromised if quality students are admitted and reasonable accommodations to their disabilities put in place. Hartman and Harman (1981), Carroll (2004) and DeLisa and Thomas (2005) suggest that medical and nursing students can function at high levels of competence and indeed bring exceptional insights to medical practice, if basic accommodations are made to their individual differences. As with any students, it is important to encourage a good fit between disabled professionals, their specialties and their working conditions so that they maximally utilize their abilities and strengths. Physically, emotionally and in terms of interest, some professionals are more suited than others to working with trauma patients, people with mental-health problems, children, individuals at the end of life, immigrants, prisoners, in wellness clinics or in public health. Therefore, part of medical training is sorting through the goodness of fit between students and what, where and how they might practise. So it is with disabled professionals. A key component of the socialization process is helping students find the best place for them and for their future clients.

Equally important, the inclusion of qualified disabled people into medical and nursing schools has many benefits. Medical schools have generally been slow to incorporate diversity into their student bodies, faculties, administration and support staff. As a consequence, medical schools do not reflect the range and diversity of the people that they were established to serve. Only in the last few decades have women been included in any sizeable numbers in the student populations and only more recently have they appeared in senior positions. Many schools are still struggling to recruit qualified, culturally diverse students from poor, African-American, American Indian, Hispanic, Asian and Russian communities where an understanding of culture, language and tradition is vitally important in the delivery of competent care. These problems are exacerbated by the increased health disparities between the rich and the poor and between minority groups and the majority population. These same patterns are evident in the general exclusion of disabled people from medical schools at a time when understanding and managing chronic illnesses and disabilities is becoming one of the major problems in the health of populations worldwide. The professionals that we train do not have personal experience of many of the people and problems they will be facing.

The inclusion of disabled people into all levels of medical schools will expose health professionals to disability personally and establish social networks that would be invaluable in the future. Numerous studies have shown that close interaction is an effective way to alter negative attitudes and perceptions, promote understanding and build good personal relationships. This adds strength and experience to the profession. In a global world, medical professionals need experience with diverse populations and what better way to do so than have people from diverse communities represented among the professionals, administrators and staff who deliver care. Disabled students and physicians are going to have insights into patients' life situations, abilities and the barriers they confront that others will not. This increased understanding is likely to translate into increased empathy and better communication with patients and more appropriately designed and delivered care.

By including disabled people as students, faculty and staff in medical schools and professional practices, the entire orientation of care will by force be modified. Much clinical education is directed at episodes and is focused on specific problems. In addition, few young physicians go into family or geriatric medicine, their interests tending to lead to specialty care concerned with one area of the body, organ system or disease and western medicine practice is organized around groups of specialists who only see one set of problems (Weisz 2006). This leads to serious lapses and breakdowns in care when an individual with multiple problems is seen by a string of specialists who do not communicate well with each other (O'Young *et al.* 2007). Insurance companies generally do not encourage nor pay for the time physicians spend discussing an individual's problem or treatment with other healthcare providers (Light 2007). So, when this does occur, it is rarely in a timely fashion. As a consequence, treatment for complex conditions associated with disability is often specialist-specific, uncoordinated and short- or medium-term oriented (Frontera and Silver 2001; Iezzoni 2006). On many occasions, disabled people are frustrated, demoralized and even refrain from returning to physicians after being led around in circles or given conflicting advice and treatment. At best, these circumstances lead to ineffective outcomes but in some instances, the results can be life-threatening. Albrecht (2001), for example, recounts how a post-polio patient in a wheelchair was suffering serious pulmonary distress but was mistakenly assumed to be a spinal-cord injury patient by young attending physicians who had little experience with polio and did not take an adequate history nor call the patient's primary-care physician before administering drugs which exacerbated his respiratory problems. Only intervention by his knowledgeable wife prevented a possible death. After the acute episode, it took two weeks in intensive rehabilitation for the patient to recover function.

Inclusion of disabled people in medical schools and clinical practices would sensitize physicians and healthcare staff to the problems, perspectives, conditions and daily lives of disabled people. Such contact with and intimate knowledge about disabled people would also improve diagnoses and prognostic abilities (Christakis 1999). It would become quickly apparent that disabled persons' health problems are frequently life-long, complex and require the coordinated efforts of numerous professionals to achieve the optimal solution. This emphasis on holistic care and a lifespan view of the patient are sorely needed in medical schools and clinical practice (Martin 2006; Mechanic *et al.* 2005). Daily contact with disabled people would help to drive the reforms necessary to re-orient healthcare delivery (Hirsh *et al.* 2007).

Broad-based patient outcomes for disabled patients

The central inclusion of disabled people in medical education would also support the current emphasis on organizing patient care, clinical practice and population interventions around evidence-based medicine and evaluating patient care and healthcare interventions according to the outcomes achieved (Goldenberg 2006; Gunderman 2007). Influenced by management research, physicians are increasingly interested in applying continual quality improvement techniques to healthcare delivery. In such a context, competence is seen as contextual, 'reflecting the relationship between a person's abilities and the tasks he or she is required to perform in a particular situation in the real world' (Epstein 2007: 387). Competence has typically been addressed on the level of the individual practitioner performing specific tasks. The critical question on the individual level has been: in this instance, did the physician competently execute the appropriate set of focused activities (usually judged by the individual physician based on her clinical experience or by peers)? Here the structure and process of the individual practising physician are assessed by the individual herself or by peers in the professional community.

The emphasis on evidence-based healthcare first moves the judgement of performance from the assessment of structure and procedures to focus on measurable illness and health outcomes such as mortality, morbidity, functional status, complications, side-effects and patient well-being. Second, judgements about performance are not based on individual self-assessments nor on the generally accepted, standard operating procedures of peers but on the results of outcomes from large clinical trials or population-based research. The effects of interventions on thousands of patients with problems similar to the one being observed receiving this type of care from many physicians in different practice settings becomes the 'gold standard' of evidence. If treatments are efficacious in terms of health outcomes over time for thousands of patients representative of larger populations and the side-effects are tolerable, the treatment protocol is considered beneficial and effective. On the group and population levels the critical question is: did this set of activities performed consistently over time improve population health, extend life, limit morbidity and complications and improve well-being when compared to doing nothing or another treatment protocol?

Third, attention to evidence-based practice and outcomes research often shifts the time perspective from short-term consequences to a longer timeframe of years or even decades without recurrence of the cancer, with improved cardiovascular functioning, or successful management of diabetes and, on a more general level, with higher levels of physical and mental functioning, fuller participation in society and better self-perceived quality of life. While attention continues to be given to individual medical problems concerning organ systems and disease management, additional importance is accorded to how these specific interventions affect the patient's general health and well-being over time.

Fourth, evidence-based and outcomes-oriented practice compels physicians to look at how the work of multiple healthcare providers and teams operating independently or in concert combine to affect patient outcomes. From this perspective, it is not enough to successfully treat an individual problem. The patient's general health status, life expectancy and years without disability are equally important considerations. Finally, an evidence-based and outcomes perspective draws attention to the costs of care. Extensive research indicates that problem-specific, episodic care delivered by different practitioners who often do not communicate well with each other is much more expensive and inefficient than coordinated, holistic care delivered and monitored over time. From this perspective, the cost horizon is extended beyond the charges associated with a particular procedure such as coronary-bypass surgery or pharmacological treatment of osteoarthritis to the direct, indirect and opportunity costs to the patients, their families, healthcare providers and healthcare system.

Establishing social networks during medical school and post-graduate training that includes disabled people is critical to preparing healthcare workers for the types of patients and problems they will see in their professional lives. These social networks result from their being in contact with disabled fellow students, faculty and staff and by training in settings where numerous types of disabled people are seen. Membership in these inclusive social networks in conjunction with a growing emphasis in clinical practice on evidence-based medicine and outcomes research will result in a better understanding of disabled people and in better care because medical personnel will be sensitized to the necessity of providing coordinated, integrated interventions, dealing with the whole person to achieve a long-term positive outcome.

In discussing how to improve patient care and outcomes in surgical settings, Gawande (2007) makes a series of observations that can be equally applied to improving care for disabled persons. He advocates considering the person in the context of their entire lives and asking unscripted questions of the patients and their families to better understand their life experiences and definition of their problems. For example, an attending physician can ask questions like: 'What would it take to improve your life?' He encourages colleagues to seek information from and listen to family members and other health professionals who know the patient. He encourages healthcare professionals to stand back and consider how they work and to ask whether or not their activities are best designed to accomplish the larger patient goals. He suggests that keeping careful records of what one did and observing the consequences stimulates reflection and encourages behavioural changes to enhance the quality of and reduce the cost of care. He follows his patients over time and charts their progress to ascertain the relation between interventions and outcomes. These suggestions target the reflective and efficient use of resources to enhance care and patient outcomes. In terms of dealing with disability, each of these proposals would be made easier to accomplish if disabled students, professionals and patients were included in the decision-making process and the evaluation of outcomes.

Team approach and continuity of care

Boundary-spanning skills and activities are paramount in managing complex projects. Boundary-spanning in management refers to those individuals, units and activities that serve to coordinate and integrate the work of multiple individual, specialized units. For example, some medical centres assign care managers to all patients who are admitted. Their job is to ensure that all the elements of service and multiple interventions occur in sequence, are coordinated, that nothing essential is omitted and that there is preparation to ensure that appropriate care is delivered and proper follow-up pursued to maximize the likelihood that the treatment is effective and long-lasting. In the case of a spinal-cord injury (SCI), the care coordinator is assigned to an individual immediately after a trauma such as an automobile accident on arrival at a specially designed, high-level trauma centre. The care coordinator oversees this person from arrival at the emergency service, through surgery, intensive care, hospital stay, transfer to a rehabilitation centre, preparation for and training of the person and his family for the return home, architectural modification of the home and rebuilding of a social life.

Since the care of an SCI patient is quite complex, lengthy and often entails setbacks like urinary-tract infection, the specialized Spinal Cord Injury Systems (integrated, multidisciplinary networks of care focused on spinal-cord injury patients) are structurally designed to incorporate boundary-spanning mechanisms in their operations. Each centre typically has an interdisciplinary team composed of trauma experts, orthopaedic surgeons, neurologists, nurses, physical and occupational therapists and social workers who meet regularly to coordinate and integrate care around the patient's needs and to monitor progress. The family is also included at critical points in this process. In addition, there are specially trained people in the financial office who know how to best utilize the mix of possible insurance benefits to pay for the individual's care and supplement these with charity funds when available. While such boundary-spanning activities and structures facilitate coordinated and continuous care and produce high-level outcomes, unfortunately, they are unusual in most medical-care centres. The point to be made here is that because of the complicated and long-term nature of many disabling conditions, exposure to disabled students, professionals, staff and patients early in medical-school training serves to orient thinking towards the overall picture and to long-term outcomes for patients.

To be cost-effective, the entire approach to healthcare delivery for and management of disabled patients must be different from the acute care, episode-oriented and speciality-focused care found in most western medical practices. Delivering comprehensive and coordinated care is expensive in the short term but has been demonstrated to result in long-term beneficial outcomes and be less costly over time. These data have persuaded some insurance companies in the US to generously fund care for many seriously disabled people because they know that their costs per case will be lower in the long run. In addition, such care results in higher levels of function, activity, participation and quality of life for disabled persons than the piecemeal approach to each sub-problem that they would typically encounter. An integrated system also directly includes disabled people in decision-making about their own care (Taylor and Bury 2007). This empowers people and allows them to be more independent.

To change the way that healthcare is conceptualized, taught and delivered, it is necessary to redesign the way that medical schools teach students and organize their staff and clinics. To encourage students to work together, a team approach to healthcare needs to be emphasized and taught. Students could be assigned to a family in the community where they will serve as healthcare ombudsmen. They would visit the family at home to take a family-health history, assess the environment, living conditions and health behaviours. The family could be followed over time to understand how public-health interventions and behaviours can prevent illness and how following up with chronic conditions can partially alleviate future disability. When illness episodes occur, the medical student would serve as the care coordinator. Similar techniques could be used to shadow a disabled person for a year to get an idea of what the natural history of a disability might look like and how to manage it effectively. In each of these examples, the intent is to change the perspective of doctors in training so that they better understand the social and health situations in which their future patients find themselves and to re-orient their thinking from acute episodes addressed by specialists to an understanding of the larger picture, appreciating the long-term nature of chronic illness and disability, valuing the importance of coordinated and integrated care and evaluating their work on health outcomes achieved.

Changes in the orientation and practice of healthcare can be facilitated by constituting new social networks for doctors in training. These include recruiting and retaining increased numbers of disabled students, faculty and staff in medical schools, assigning students to work in teams on complicated medical cases, making certain that each student has the experience of working with a disabled person in their medical training and seeing them in the individual's home. A version of medical-mortality conferences could be instituted in which experts would discuss and analyse how and why some disabled people lost function and perhaps even died because their cases were not handled well in a system of coordinated and integrated care and others had the opposite experience. Lessons could be drawn for assessment and management of similar cases in the future. Physicians with broad-based experience of disabled people could be assigned as resources for young physicians who are managing specific aspects of a case and might not see the whole picture. Students could sit in on conferences about how to manage the costs of care for an individual disabled person. These and similar steps to expose students to new ways of thinking about disability and allowing them the opportunity to build social networks to help them in their future work should result in more cost-effective health outcomes.

Disability disparities

In recent years, increasing attention has been given to the consequences of health disparities within and between populations. While the mechanisms are not completely understood, it is clear that growing gaps in income and assets between the rich and poor in wealthy and low-income countries alike are related to increases in mortality and morbidity indicators (Massey 2007; Meara *et al.* 2008). These have been related to decreases in public-health measures such as the percentage of children vaccinated for smallpox and measles, prenatal care, 'well baby' check-ups, adequate nutrition, availability of medication for diabetes and heart disease and increases in unhealthy environments characterized by pollution and violence (Gehlert *et al.* 2008). While much has been written about health disparities, less attention has been given to the effect of these inequalities on disabled people. Health disparities translate into disability disparities because poverty and disability are inextricably linked. Poor people experience a larger share of disability than do wealthier people and if people are not poor when they become disabled, they are likely to become poor as they pay for healthcare and deal with the consequences of being disabled.

Because of both health and disability disparities, medical students ought to be exposed to patients and families from a variety of social classes and ethnic backgrounds. Such experiences would illustrate the health consequences of being poor and, in user-pays systems such as that of the US, of having inadequate or no health insurance. In the case of disability disparities, following a disabled person over time would show the interactive dynamics between poverty and disability. These experiences during training and socialization could be of benefit when considering how healthcare delivery should be arranged and paid for and how best to organize medical practices to fit the needs and circumstances of disabled people.

Conclusion

Disability is an increasingly common phenomenon in every country of the world. At any one time, over 15 per cent of national populations report having a disability, as measured by limitations in function, activity and participation in social life. The training for and practice of medicine has not evolved well to prepare healthcare workers for the world of complex chronic illnesses and disability. Including significant numbers of disabled students, teachers and staff in medical schools and exposing students to the range and diversity of people with impairments and disabilities would better prepare them to work with this growing population. First-hand, repetitive contact with disabled people would also serve to make students comfortable and familiar with disabled people and break down stigma, negative attitudes and perceptions towards disabled people. Changing the structure of medical-school education to involve students with patients in their homes and communities would also better prepare them to work in a world where understanding the communities where patients live and function is critical to designing and implementing effective healthcare interventions. Training students to work in collaborative teams where communication across specialities and disciplines is important and ensure they develop a focus on evidence-based and outcomes-oriented practice will also prepare them to enter a world where performance indicators and closer evaluation of outcomes are a reality. The establishment of formal and informal social networks during these formative years provides a resource for future work with disabled people.

Iezzoni and O'Day (2006) suggest that these are the requirements for competent physicians of the future. Coordination of care across specialities and over time represents the future for healthcare delivery but students need to be trained how to do this. Bodenheimer (2008) states that this aim is not being achieved currently so we must train the healthcare practitioners of the future to do this work and convince national governments and insurance entities that these are essential delivery activities that must be insisted on and reimbursed. These approaches fit well with the international disability studies movement that draws attention to the interrelationship between the body, the physical, social, political and economic environments and individual function, activity and participation (Davis 2006; Shakespeare 2005, 2006). Such initiatives are also sensitive to the call for more humane care, rediscovering soul in the medical profession and seeing disability as a human-rights as well as a medical issue (Wear and Bickel

2000; Hafferty 2003). Finally, including disabled people fully in medical education, the healthcare professions and in clinical practice and policy discussions takes advantage of lay expertise and generates a set of cooperative rather than adversarial relationships (Fisher and Goodley 2007).

Note

1 This paper was written while the author was a Fellow in Residence at the Royal Flemish Academy in Belgium for Science and the Arts, Brussels, 2006–2008. The author is grateful to Professors Niceas Schamp and Marc De Mey and the Academy staff for providing a productive environment in which to work.

References

Albrecht, G. L. (2001) 'Rationing healthcare to disabled people', *Sociology of Health and Illness*, 23: 654–77.

Albrecht, G. L. and Devlieger, P. J. (1999) 'The disability paradox: high quality of life against all odds', *Social Science and Medicine*, 48: 977–88.

Albrecht, G. L., Devlieger, P. J. and Van Hove, G. (2008) 'The experience of disability in plural societies', *ALTER: European Journal of Disability Research*, 2: 1–13.

Albrecht, G. L., Gureje, O., Mont, D., Kostanjsek, N., Chatterji, S., Mathers, C., Fujiura, G. T., Kosen, S., Loeb, M., Martinho, M., Soliz, P., Diamond, M., Üstün, B. and Wen, X. (in press) 'Disability: a global picture', in *World Report on Disability and Rehabilitation*, Geneva and Washington, D.C.: World Health Organization and World Bank.

Aulagnier, M., Verger, P., Ravaud, J.-F., Souville, M., Lussault, P.-Y., Garnier, J.-P. and Paraponaris, A. (2005) 'General practitioners' attitudes towards patients with disabilities: the need for training and support', *Disability and Rehabilitation*, 27: 1343–52.

Ay, P., Save, D. and Fidanoglu, O. (2006) 'Does stigma concerning mental disorders differ through medical education?', *Social Psychiatry and Psychiatric Epidemiology*, 41: 63–7.

Bartels, L. M. (2008) *Unequal Democracy: the political economy of the new gilded age*, New York: Russell Sage Foundation.

Bodenheimer, T. (2008) 'Coordinating care – a perilous journey through the healthcare system', *New England Journal of Medicine*, 358: 1064–71.

Bryon, M. and Dieppe, P. (2000) 'Educating health professionals about disability: attitudes, attitudes, attitudes', *Journal of Research in Social Medicine*, 93: 397–8.

Bryon, M., Cockshott, Z., Brownett, H. and Ramakalawan, T. (2005) 'What does disability mean for medical students? An exploration of the words medical students associate with the term disability', *Medical Education*, 39: 176–83.

Carroll, S. M. (2004) 'Inclusion of people with physical disabilities in nursing education', *Journal of Nursing Education*, 43: 207–12.

Charlton, J. I. (1998) *Nothing about Us without Us: disability oppression and empowerment*, Berkeley: University of California Press.

Christakis, N. A. (1999) *Death Foretold: prophecy and prognosis in medical care*, Chicago, IL: University of Chicago Press.

Christakis, N. A. and Fowler, P. (2007) 'The spread of obesity in a large social network over 32 years', *New England Journal of Medicine*, 357: 370–9.

Cornwell, B., Laumann, E. O. and Schumm, L. P. (2008) 'Happiness and older Americans', *American Sociological Review*, 73: 185–203.

Crotty, M., Finucane, P. and Ahern, M. (2000) 'Teaching medical students about disability and rehabilitation: methods and student feedback', *Medical Education*, 34: 659–64.

Davis, L. (ed.) (2006) *The Disabilities Studies Reader*, 2nd edn, London: Routledge.

DeLisa, J. A. and Thomas, P. (2005) 'Physicians with disabilities and the physician workforce', *American Journal of Physical Medicine and Rehabilitation*, 84: 5–11.

Epstein, R. M. (2007) 'Assessment in medical education', *New England Journal of Medicine*, 387: 387–96.

Fisher, P. and Goodley, D. (2007) 'The linear medical model of disability: mothers of disabled babies resist with counter narratives', *Sociology of Health and Illness*, 29: 6–81.

Frontera, W. R. and Silver, J. K. (2001) *Essentials of Physical Medicine and Rehabilitation*, St Louis, MO: Hanley and Belfus.

Gawande, A. (2007) *Better: a surgeon's notes on performance*, New York: Picador.

Gehlert, S., Sohmer, D., Sacks, T., Mininger, C., McClintock, M. and Olopade, O. (2008) 'Targeting health disparities: a model linking upstream determinants to downstream interventions', *Health Affairs*, 27: 339–49.

Goldenberg, M. J. (2006) 'On evidence and evidence-based medicine: Lessons from the philosophy of science', *Social Science and Medicine*, 62: 2621–32.

Gunderman, R. B. (2007) *Achieving Excellence in Medical Education*, London: Springer.

Hafferty, F. W. (2003) 'Finding soul in a "medical profession of one"', *Journal of Health Politics, Policy and Law*, 28: 133–58.

Hartman, D. W. and Harman, C. W. (1981) 'Disabled students and medical school admissions', *Archives of Physical Medicine and Rehabilitation*, 62: 90–1.

Hirsh, D. A., Ogur, B., Thibault, G. E. and Cox, M. (2007) 'Continuity as an organizing principle for clinical education reform', *New England Journal of Medicine*, 356: 858–66.

Iezzoni, L. I. (2006) 'Going beyond disease to address disability', *New England Journal of Medicine*, 355: 976–9.

Iezzoni, L. I. and O'Day, B. L. (2006) *More Than Ramps*, Oxford: Oxford University Press.

Latour, B. (2007) *Reassembling the Social: an introduction to Actor-Network Theory*, Oxford: Oxford University Press.

Light, D. (2007) 'Struggling for the soul of academic medicine', *American Journal of Bioethics*, 7: 61–3.

Martin, T. (2006) 'Going blind on our watch: why doesn't the US health system keep people with preventable disabilities – such as diabetes-related blindness from becoming disabled?', *Health Affairs*, 25: 1121–6.

Massey, D. S. (2007) *Categorically Unequal: the American stratification system*, New York: Russell Sage Foundation.

Meara, E. R., Richards, S. and Cutler, D. M. (2008) 'The gap gets bigger: changes in mortality and life expectancy, by education, 1981–2000', *Health Affairs*, 27: 350–60.

Mechanic, D., Rogut, L. B. and Colby, D. C. (eds) (2005) *Policy Challenges in Modern Healthcare*, New Brunswick, NJ: Rutgers University Press.

Melville, C. (2005) 'Discrimination and health inequalities experienced by disabled people', *Medical Education*, 39: 122–6.

O'Young, B. J., Young, M. A. and Stiens, S. A. (eds) (2007) *Physical Medicine and Rehabilitation Secrets*, St Louis, MO: Mosby.

Pescosolido, B. A. (2006) 'Social networks', in G. L. Albrecht (ed.) *Encyclopedia of Disability*, Thousand Oaks, CA: Sage.

Ross, J. and Albrecht, G. (2000) 'Understanding and managing healthcare interventions in the terminally ill', *Research in the Sociology of Healthcare*, 17: 3–29.

Sampson, R. J. and Sharkey, P. (2008) 'Neighborhood selection and the social reproduction of concentrated racial inequality', *Demography*, 45: 1–29.

Sampson, R. J., Morenoff, J. D. and Gannon-Rowley, T. (2002) 'Assessing neighbourhood effects: social process and new directions in research', *Annual Review of Sociology*, 28: 443–78.

Sampson, R. J., Raudenbush, S. W. and Earls, F. (1997) 'Neighborhoods and violent crime: a multilevel study of collective efficacy', *Science*, 277: 918–24.

Shakespeare, T. (2005) 'Review article: disability studies today and tomorrow', *Sociology of Health and Illness*, 27: 138–48.

—— (2006) *Disability Rights and Wrongs*, London: Routledge.

Taylor, D. and Bury, M. (2007) 'Chronic illness, expert patients and care transition', *Sociology of Health and Illness*, 29: 27–45.

Wear, D. and Bickel, J. (eds) (2000) *Educating for Professionalism: creating a culture of humanism in medical practice*, Iowa City: University of Iowa Press.

Weisz, G. (2006) *Divide and Conquer: a comparative history of medical specialization*, Oxford: Oxford University Press.

8 The status of complementary and alternative medicine (CAM) in biomedical education

Towards a critical engagement

Alex Broom and Jon Adams

Introduction

Complementary and alternative medicine (CAM) has become increasingly prominent over the last three decades with more individuals using CAM in combination with, or as an alternative to, biomedical treatments. In addition to this resurgence in consumer interest in CAM modalities, health-insurance companies in the US, Britain, Australia and New Zealand now fund selected CAM therapies such as chiropractic, osteopathy, acupuncture, homoeopathy and healing-touch therapy for certain medical conditions (Cassileth 1999). While there is still only limited and sporadic provision of CAM in mainstream western medical contexts, consumer interest, health-insurance rebates and political impetus have provided some degree of momentum toward the development of 'integrative' approaches to patient care. Progress has been slow in terms of actual mainstream integration of CAM practices, yet doctors are increasingly faced with patients wanting to discuss CAM-related issues. In areas such as cancer care or the treatment of other chronic illness, CAM use is traditionally high (Thorne *et al.* 2002) and discussions about non-biomedical options are frequent and are valued by patients (Tovey and Broom 2007). However, the skill and knowledge base of practising clinicians in relation to CAM is generally limited and paradigmatic divergences between CAM and biomedicine can complicate patient–doctor discussions regarding what constitutes 'effectiveness', 'evidence' and 'risk' (Broom and Tovey 2007b).

As such, there remains an urgent need for some form of CAM education at an undergraduate level for medical students. Specifically, there is increasing awareness within the biomedical community that in order to produce multiskilled and reflexive doctors, medical education must, at least in part, incorporate elements of CAM practice within its training programmes (CAHCIM 2004). While CAM education in medical curricula is an important development amid recent changes, there has been little sociological or critical social-science analysis to date on this topic. Much of the debate regarding educational integration has been conducted and led by those in the practice field and has tended to promote one of a number of partisan positions and failed to subject the issue to wider cultural and political analysis.

In response, we here provide an introductory framework for exploring and appraising the status of CAM in medical undergraduate education.[1] The chapter is divided into two sections. Section 1 provides a critical sociological engagement with CAM education in the medical curriculum, including an overview of key issues and developments on the international scene. Section 2 examines the need for critical sociological teaching within such integrative educational programmes. This teaching should be offered as a means to improve successful communications and facilitate potential collaboration across different medical paradigms as well as to create better understanding and contextualize patient decision-making and motivations regarding CAM use for medical students.[2]

Thus, this chapter examines key issues concerning the teaching of CAM in undergraduate medical education, including those related to: epistemology and paradigmatic commensurability; theoretical ideas that can inform CAM education; existing empirical research on doctors' and medical students' perspectives on CAM; and key models of integrating CAM into medical education. In doing so, it aims to present both a critical discussion of the principal theoretical ideas as well as an overview of the state of play of CAM in medical education.

1 CAM in undergraduate medical education: an overview

Attempts to educate medical students about CAM

There have been sporadic attempts to educate medical students about CAM in most developed countries and surveys appear to suggest that CAM incorporation into the medical undergraduate curriculum is growing apace (Wetzel *et al.* 2003). For example, Cook *et al.* (2007) piloted an online CAM course for medical students and residents in the US and found that as a result participants felt more comfortable discussing CAM with patients, recognized a greater role for CAM, and knew better where to find information on CAM. Similarly, Owen and Lewith (2001) developed a special-study module on CAM as part of the Southampton (UK) Medical School undergraduate curriculum. Focusing on homoeopathy, chiropractic, osteopathy and acupuncture, the module explored different models of healthcare, encouraged students to question their own assumptions about illness, and examined the evidence base for CAM. According to the results of a follow-up questionnaire, while some students became more sceptical about CAM, many others reported that they had developed an increased interest in CAM as a result of completing the module.

While providing a breakthrough in the coverage of CAM in such programmes (that would have appeared unimaginable a few decades ago), these CAM teachings, in electives or other compartmentalized offerings, do nevertheless tend to marginalize the significance of CAM. Such teachings also help bolster a medical culture where CAM is considered more a fringe activity engaging only a select few within the profession rather than exploring the possibility of CAM providing a set of complementary core values that can guide and refine broader conventional medical education and practice in the future. Indeed, CAM, and the wider values that it embraces, has long been promoted as one possible means by which conventional medicine may improve its effectiveness and relationship to patients and may be the necessary antidote to what are sometimes seen as the invasive and insensitive (and ultimately unpopular) procedures and approaches to patient care (Berman 2001; Frenkel and Ben-Arye 2001; Park 2002; Pietroni 1992; Weil 2000).

More recent years have seen the drive towards full integrative medical programmes (primarily within US medical faculties) as opposed to the compartmentalized teaching of CAM (CAHCIM 2004). Such integrative programmes are founded upon an aim to provide a rich, in-depth and broad teaching in not only CAM but also a wider 'healing-orientated medicine that re-emphasizes the relationship between patient and physician and integrates the best of CAM with the best of conventional medicine' (Maizes *et al.* 2002: 851).

One key difference of such programmes is that they provide an opportunity for students to be educated in not only the practical application and clinical considerations but also the wider context and more fundamental underpinnings of the modality/ies. Compartmentalized CAM teaching (whereby CAM is introduced in a piecemeal and excessively time-starved fashion) promotes an educational climate with a focus upon narrowly defined hard end points that may not necessarily take into account some 'alternative' CAM practices, approaches and philosophies considered more esoteric and challenging from the perspective of the biomedical paradigm.

Unfortunately, the vast majority of the integrative programmes developed to date have been focused upon those at postgraduate and professional levels (Maizes *et al.* 2002) and of those pitched at undergraduate level, the bulk has been concentrated within Bachelor of Health Science and Bachelor of Arts curricula programmes (Burke *et al.* 2004). Exceptions to these rules are, however, beginning to emerge – with a small number of medical colleges in the US moving towards educational initiatives whereby CAM is woven seamlessly throughout the pre-clinical, clinical and graduate medical curricula (Sierpina and Kreitzer 2005; Wetzel *et al.* 2003).

Despite all these advances and developments in recent years, there is still an acknowledgement that programmes to effectively educate large numbers of up-and-coming medical students about CAM are desperately needed (Cook *et al.* 2007; Wetzel *et al.* 2003) and it does seem that such integration is highly likely, perhaps inevitable, given the exponential rise of CAM over recent years. A more interesting and pertinent range of questions facing such integration revolves around the future nature of such developments: who will provide the CAM teaching?; to what extent will CAM be incorporated?; how will integrative teachings sit alongside other professional educational movements such as evidence-based medicine (Marcus 2001; Sampson 2001)?; and, given the time-starved nature of the medical undergraduate curriculum, what will be the potential casualties of such educational integration (what will be omitted from the syllabus)? (Wetzel *et al.* 2003).

Medical students' attitudes to CAM

Just as attitudes to CAM are constantly evolving in the wider population, so too are those of medical students. Over the last decade there has been some research, particularly in the US, on the perceptions medical students and their educators have of CAM. For example, in their study, Lie and Boker (2006) found that medical educators were likely to have more positive attitudes towards CAM than interns and students. However, they also found that medical-student attitudes to CAM (and CAM use) remained stable and largely positive and did not deteriorate over the course of training (such as through exposure to negative attitudes to CAM or immersion in the biomedical model). In another US study, Chaterji *et al.* (2007) found that, of the 266 first- and second-year medical students surveyed, nearly all (91 per cent) agreed that biomedicine could benefit from CAM ideas and methods, and significantly, greater than 85 per cent agreed that knowledge about CAM was crucial for their future as a health professional. Three-quarters also felt that CAM should be included in the medical curriculum. Clearly more research is needed within different sociocultural contexts, but in general, support for CAM among medical students seems surprisingly high.

There is also some empirical work to suggest support for CAM may not be uniform across all student groups. For example, gender may play a role in mediating students' tendencies to utilize or indeed support CAM practices and CAM education. In a study by Greenfield *et al.* (2006), female medical students were significantly more likely than males to feel CAM has an important role in healthcare – a pattern potentially linked to wider CAM usage in the female population (Adams *et al.* 2003). This difference *increased* through their medical education. Female medical students gave a more positive rating than males to the use of five CAM modalities, and moreover, females were more positive than males about learning the theory and practice of CAM and about increasing CAM curriculum time. Thus, just as preferences for CAM (and support for science) are differentiated in wider societal terms, so too, it seems, are attitudes and perspectives among medical students. Increased diversity in terms of culture and religion of students in medical training contexts will no doubt influence such patterns, with further research needed on the ways in which different types of students respond to CAM practices.

Doctors' views on CAM and medical education

Lessons can also be learnt from the experiences of existing clinicians in terms of their education on CAM-related issues. In Winslow and Shapiro's study (2002), 751 physicians were asked about their experience with CAM and 59 per cent were asked about specific CAM treatments: 48 per cent had recommended CAM to a patient; and 24 per cent had personally used CAM. Few of these physicians felt comfortable discussing CAM with their patients, and 84 per cent thought they needed to learn more about CAM to adequately address patient concerns.

In the authors' research on CAM in oncology in Australia which aimed to examine doctors' perspectives on CAM and their interactions with cancer patients, none of the 13 oncology consultants interviewed had received any meaningful education (undergraduate or postgraduate) on CAM (other than being told patients use it). For these clinicians, who regularly face patients who are active (if not intensive) CAM users, this gap in baseline knowledge about available CAM interventions, as well as lack of continuing education once in a clinical setting, posed numerous problems for patient care and doctor–patient communication as these excerpts illustrate:

CONSULTANT ONCOLOGIST: At least one thing in my training experience is information on complementary and alternative medicines was never part of my [course] ... for people of my generation, one of the problems from our end is that we've never actually been educated on alternative medicines ... all these myths ... we rarely approach alternative medicine in an upfront way and so our exposure is often when there is an adverse effect – whether it be someone selling their house [to go to Mexico] or something else. But the reality is, as I say, most patients are taking or thinking about taking them and the adverse events we see related to alternative medicines are relatively rare.

Another respondent

CONSULTANT ONCOLOGIST: Sure, medical training should include information about alternatives but who's going to teach it and what will they teach? It's complicated and is it *really* that important?

Another respondent

INTERVIEWER: In terms of your medical training, did it involve much discussion about complementary medicines?
CONSULTANT ONCOLOGIST: In medical school I guess we were introduced ... [pauses to try to remember]. Never went into much depth about it. It's just awareness I think and they've probably changed that in some respects.
INTERVIEWER: Do you actually think it should be a part of the medical training, whatever shape and form it may be?
CONSULTANT ONCOLOGIST: I don't think it should be compulsory post-medical school.
INTERVIEWER: No?
CONSULTANT ONCOLOGIST: Well ... I mean you can have education sessions about it but I don't think you can force a cardiologist to come to a session on alternative medicines. I think it would be interesting to go through some of the things that were out there in the oncology setting.

While there was broad support among these clinicians for some form of CAM education in undergraduate medical education, the prospect of continuing professional education about CAM produced mixed views, with some viewing the imposition of CAM training on already time-constrained consultants as an unnecessary burden. However, it was interesting to note that each of the 13 clinicians interviewed viewed lack of CAM discussion in undergraduate medical education in Australia as a significant problem.

While limited, there is some other research available that examines clinicians' perspectives on CAM training in medical education. In the context of primary care, perspectives on the value and need for CAM education have been shown to be quite varied. In an Australian study by Pirotta *et al.* (2000), most General Practitioners (93 per cent) agreed that there should be some education on complementary therapies in core medical-undergraduate curricula. However, in this same study, the doctors surveyed were divided about the relative importance of this education for students versus conventional training modules.

One general theme throughout the literature in this area is the broad consensus that effective doctor–patient discussion about CAM is crucial *and* that adequate training on the part of doctors regarding CAM is the only way to achieve this. As noted by Caspi *et al.* (2000), the current scarcity of thorough exposure of biomedical practitioners to the diversity of CAM therapies and their fundamental concepts *and* of students of CAM to biomedicine and its related sciences, is far from ideal.

2 A critical sociology within CAM medical education

As explored in this chapter so far, sociology can help illuminate key social, cultural, professional and political issues relating to CAM in medical undergraduate education. In the discussion below we argue that CAM could and should also be an integral component of any such integrative teaching. While sociology has a firm place in any well-rounded medical education, it is particularly useful, given the explicitly temporal and cultural variation and fluidity of the border between the two medicines, that the discipline is maximized to contextualize CAM teaching. Below, we highlight key issues and opportunities that the discipline of sociology holds for CAM teaching in medical undergraduate education.

Epistemological and ontological issues related to CAM and biomedicine

There are some key issues and barriers in the introduction of CAM to biomedical education. The first, and the one most engaged with by medical sociologists (Coulter 2004), is the issue of therapeutic paradigms, and the seemingly divergent ontological and epistemological positions of CAM versus those espoused by the biomedical model of disease. Indeed, much of the debate in the sociological and biomedical literature over the last two or three decades in relation to CAM has centred on 'models of care' and the supposedly divergent perspectives of CAM and biomedicine on such things as: the nature of disease, the importance of the individual in therapeutic effect, key mechanisms of action and so on. These divergences, as far as we can meaningfully typologize CAM and bio-medicine, engender key ontological and epistemological positionings that medical students *must* understand in order to develop critical awareness of thera-peutic pluralism. Moreover, in addition to ideological divergence, there are key language differences in CAM (for example, meridians, chakras or energy fields) which do not fit with the lexicon of biomedicine as currently taught to medical students, although this is not the case in all CAM (for example, osteopathy and chiropractic have increasingly framed their practices through a biomedical lens). As such, a genuine understanding of, say, naturopathy and homoeopathy, is very difficult to achieve due to divergent views of the body and disease (Caspi *et al.* 2000). In order to bridge language barriers, teaching a critical approach to ideo-logical framing is crucial.

So what are the key ontological and epistemological issues and how might we make sense of the differences in ideological approach between CAM and bio-medicine? Ontology, in this context, refers to the study of the nature of reality and epistemology refers to the study of knowledge or how we get to know certain things. CAM practice and biomedicine, in some cases, pursue quite dif-ferent approaches to the reality of disease (ontology) and prioritize different ways of creating knowledge about disease and the body (epistemology). As shown in Table 8.1, the biomedical model (the broad therapeutic approach espoused within biomedicine), entails a *functionalist* approach to illness, with an emphasis on the body as an organism that can be treated symptomatically. The biomedical model constructs illness as a breakdown or dysfunction of a particu-lar organ. Medicine, especially hospital-based, is broadly mechanistic, with doctors viewing the body as a machine made of many parts, with the respective individual parts treated separately. This mechanistic approach, crucially, stresses the centrality of the doctor in the healing process. The doctor's intervention is active, and, in general, downplays the role of any psychological or metaphysical factors that may cause the disease or play a role in its natural evolution or treat-ment. The biomedical model is thus characterized as *materialist* in its focus on the corporeal body, yet at the same time abstract in its removal of the body from the soul and from the person. It is important at this point to stress that this is a model of healthcare, *not* a description of the actual approach taken by biomedi-cal practitioners. However, in saying this, the centrality of this model in biomed-ical training and organizational culture does strongly influence how doctors

Table 8.1 The biomedical model

Mechanistic	The body is compartmentalized
Symptomatic	A condition is reduced to a category, a single disease entity, which exhibits a distinctive set of symptoms
Objectivity	The practitioner is separate and detached from the patient, maintaining objectivity, assisted by scientific evidence
Quantification	Information is derived from what can be quantified
Determinism	Phenomena can be predicted from knowledge of scientific laws

approach treatment and is key within the curricula of medical-education programmes internationally.

Ontologically speaking, CAM practices tend to focus on disease as an issue of (im)balance and as a reflection of systemic (rather than organ-centred) pathologies. As such, the body is viewed in a holistic rather than compartmentalized manner, and disease is viewed as specific to the individual person and body rather than abstractable in any meaningful way. As shown in Table 8.2, a key factor in many CAM practices is the therapeutic relationship and the importance of interpersonal elements within the therapeutic process. Conceptualized as 'placebo' within biomedicine, interactional dynamics are viewed as core facets of the treatment process. Moreover, 'disease' is often viewed as natural rather than pathological per se, and treatment aimed at 'healing' rather than cure.

To integrate discussion of and debate about CAM into biomedical education, the examination of these ideological differences is a key point of departure. Providing a critical understanding of the embeddedness of 'best practice' in ideological positioning is critical for giving doctors insight into why their patients may use CAM, and as a means of encouraging debate about the nature of disease, therapeutic effect and wider divisions in healthcare provision.

In saying this, we should emphasize that while these broad typologies are useful to a degree, they also tend to reify distinctions that can be blurred in practice. Thus, as pedagogical tools they can, if deployed simplistically, be regressive in attempts to enhance medical students' understandings of therapeutic practices. Biomedicine, for example, does not always present a simplistic, coherent and linear ideological front. In fact, in grassroots clinical practice, individual practitioners and sub-specialities can present (and employ) quite different approaches to disease and to the patient. There are, for example, biomedical clinicians (and specialities) which broadly maintain a self-defined, patient-centred and holistic approach to patient care (for example, factions within palliative medicine). Moreover, some CAM practitioners pursue a largely mechanistic and positivist approach to the treatment of disease. For example, while some within chiropractic market themselves as holistic, others are relatively mechanistic in their clinical approach. Likewise, while homoeopathy is seen by many as a system of medicine that fundamentally contradicts and challenges a biomedical perspective, in certain circumstances it can be approached and employed in a less challenging, standardized, first-aid fashion (this has been identified as a style

Table 8.2 The complementary and alternative medicine (CAM) model

Self-healing	The body has a 'natural' ability to heal itself and maintain homoeostasis
Holism	A person is a subtle and complex blend of body, mind and spirit
Patient-centred	Treating root causes is more important than just managing symptoms – each person is unique
Self-help	The patient must take responsibility for his or her own wellness
Intimacy	The client/practitioner relationship is seen to aid healing through intimacy, intentionality and awareness of multiple variables in illness

of homoeopathy employed by General Practitioners (Adams 2004)). Similarly, acupuncture is, in some cases, utilized as a technical skill, rather than a system of healing, and is deployed with little ideology in clinical practice. As such, teaching medical students oversimplistic paradigmatic divergences is inaccurate, in terms of what occurs in clinical contexts, and furthermore, may function to reify such differences and overstate incommensurability. We are thus left with a difficult choice: to teach philosophical difference and further compartmentalize CAM and biomedicine, or to reflect on the irreconcilability of such typologies in practice. In all probability, a combination of both is the best solution, emphasizing difference and conflict but also interplay and cross-over where appropriate.

Understanding the ideologies underpinning therapeutic modalities is a critical component of medical education. However, there is also a need to understand why patients are utilizing CAM practices, why there are sometimes conflicts between CAM and biomedicine and why some biomedical practitioners/organizations are against CAM integration. It is here that work done in the sociology of CAM can help medical students make sense of such questions.

Theoretical approaches to CAM: conceptualizing patient engagement

It can be difficult, from a biomedical (or medical-student) perspective, to understand the varying reasons why people may actually use or gain benefit from CAM. Sociologists have been fascinated by the rise in popularity of CAM despite resistance from biomedical organizations and many practitioners and a virtual absence of state funding. To provide some explanation, sociologists have been delving into the sociocultural factors influencing this recent proliferation of the non-biomedical therapeutics. This work has drawn on a range of theoretical traditions with numerous attempts to highlight: a societal shift to 'postmodernity'; processes of reflexive modernization; and the emergence of new forms of 'selfhood', to help conceptualize and explain CAM popularity (for example, Siahpush 1998; Sointu 2006; Tovey *et al.* 2001). These conceptual arguments, and others, may be useful in providing medical students and educators with useful frameworks for understanding the recently increased popularity of CAM.

The postmodernization thesis has been popular among some CAM sociologists as an explanation for the increased presence of CAM. Its proponents view CAM use as reflecting wider patterns related to the 'postmodernization' of social life (for example, Siahpush 1998). In this context postmodernization is broadly seen to denote an increased fragmentation of experience, consumerism, individualization and aestheticization of social life. In the context of healthcare, metanarratives (for example, the biomedical model) are subsumed by subjective individualized knowledges that inform social practices and identity work. CAM use, within this model, is viewed as a rejection of the metanarratives related to disease and the selection, and production, of individualized understandings of disease-and-treatment regimes. Implicit in such arguments is the increased prioritization of lay knowledge of disease and, importantly, the rejection of the superiority of scientific knowledge and expertise.

Social theorizations of late modernity have also been drawn on in attempts to conceptualize patients' preferences for CAM (Low 2004; Tovey *et al.* 2001). Moving beyond the rather oversimplistic 'fragmentation of experience' and 'individualization' themes implicit in the postmodernization thesis, authors like Beck (1992) and Giddens (1991) have focused on increased reflexivity in modern societies, and the tendency of 'consumers' to be more critical of expert knowledges. The result, it has been argued, is that people have become more sceptical of the judgements or advice of (scientific) experts (Lupton and Tulloch 2002), actively assessing the merits of particular claims. This in turn, it has been postulated, has opened up the potential for the proliferation of CAM – a backlash against the perceived failings of science and biomedical technologies (Kaptchuk and Eisenberg 1998).

There have also been some recent attempts to theorize the potential implications, at an individual level, of new therapeutic models of care and their implications for changing notions of selfhood (for example, Doel and Segrott 2003; Sointu 2006). This work has examined the degree to which CAM use represents a significant shift in conceptions of disease and selfhood. In particular, the notion of well-being has emerged recently as a potentially useful concept for characterizing what CAM offers to the individual. Departing from biomedical notions of being 'cured', 'healthy' or 'disease-free', well-being encapsulates notions of authenticity, recognition and self-determination, restructuring 'health' as a subjective and individualized process (Bishop and Yardley 2004; Sointu 2006). CAM use is thus conceptualized as a project of the self – an individual search for recognition as being an authentic self that is both 'discovered' by the individual and shaped by the nature of individual therapeutic practices.

Broom and Tovey (2007a) argue that while these theoretical ideas have some merit, what characterizes patients' engagement with CAM is a complex dialectical tension between the appeal of individualization and depersonalization. Alternative models of healing, they argue, are valued, primarily, for their subjectified (rather than abstracted) and individualized (rather than depersonalized) approach – an approach seen to allow for and promote agency, self-determination and, ultimately, hope (Broom and Tovey 2007a). CAM practitioners, they argue, promote a 'project of the self' – a reclaiming of hope, subjectivity and control – elements that were largely perceived to be neglected in biomedical care.

As sociologists, we argue for a critical distanced approach to teaching about CAM within biomedical education. This involves teaching about the benefits *and* limitations of both CAM and biomedical models of care. Not all writing on CAM has focused on the positive liberating elements of non-biomedical therapeutics. Moreover, teaching about CAM will benefit from a critical examination of how CAM-derived models of care may have limitations for some patients with certain disease trajectories.

Theoretical approaches to the potential limitations of self-healing and self-help

The potentially restrictive, disciplinary or digressive aspects of CAM therapeutics have received some attention in the biomedical and psychotherapeutic literature, where there has been some discussion of the potentially pathological discursive deployment of notions of self-healing and self-responsibility in CAM therapeutic models. Permeating some CAM practices are discourses of positivity and self-responsibility, engendering quasi-metaphysical notions of self-actualization, and self-healing. What is interesting, as sociologists, is the degree to which CAM-related ideological and rhetorical devices contain and deploy potentially restrictive (or even spurious) models of therapeutic process. There is, as mentioned above, an emerging critique within the psychotherapeutic literature regarding the promotion of pseudo-spiritual ideas of self-healing and self-responsibility. In this literature the ideals engendered in some CAM approaches have been critiqued as toxic to patients' psychological and physical health.

While some CAM practices (and models of care) are clearly extremely helpful to patients, there may also be certain problems endemic in new discourses around self-help and (spiritually mediated) self-actualization. An example is the ontological view, evident in some CAM practices, that one can actively shape or change one's reality and that to heal oneself necessarily involves an active reconstructing of one's worldview and view of the self. Such therapeutic frameworks ultimately denote a degree of self-responsibility for disease or disease progression, and place the burden of 'reconceptualization of reality' squarely on the individual patient. It is not posited here that such conceptions are indeed prima facie negative or positive for patients. Rather, what it does point to is a repositioning of responsibility (and potential guilt) for those who find this state impossible to achieve or indeed maintain. Such criticisms of CAM-related models of care should also be included in teaching about CAM in undergraduate medical education. Specifically, such possibilities should be placed alongside representations of CAM models of healing as potentially useful and liberating for patients.

Theorizing the relationship of CAM to biomedicine: inter- and intra-professional issues

There has been a lot of sociological work undertaken on the inter- and intra-professional boundary disputes between CAM and biomedicine (for example, Adams 2004; Hirschkorn and Bourgeault 2005; Mizrachi *et al.* 2005; Tovey and Adams 2001) with an emphasis placed on the complex dominance/subordination of various therapeutic modalities (for example, Mizrachi *et al.* 2005), shifts over time in public deference to biomedicine and increasing support for non-biomedical therapeutics (for example, Adams 2004). For example, Social Worlds Theory has been developed as a useful explanatory tool for understanding the dynamics between CAM and biomedicine and this sociological framework can act as a highly effective conceptual tool for clinicians/students (both conventional and CAM) in their studies of CAM and wider social, cultural, professional and political contexts.

Social Worlds Theory (SWT) is useful in the case of educational CAM integration because it allows medical students to locate and contextualize the behaviours, practices and motivations of different professional groups (none more so than CAM and conventional medicine). The formalizing of ideas about social worlds has largely been carried out by Strauss, building upon the work of the key thinkers from the early Chicago tradition (Strauss 1993). Central to the approach is the idea that society is constituted by multiple social worlds which 'both touch and interpenetrate' (Clarke 1990: 19). What is crucial to the perspective, however, is the fluidity of these worlds: how they are formed and re-formed by social action and how their fragmentation and proliferation into numerous subworlds is an inevitable consequence of processes within and between groups. A social world will characteristically be dominated by one main activity, have sites for that activity, involve technologies of one form or another, and be structured around some form of organization. In these terms we can begin to approach CAM as one medical or healing world (incorporating many subworlds modelled around modalities) and conventional medicine as another medical world (also made up of subworlds such as General Practice, rural healthcare, nursing and others).

At the heart of the SWT approach is a focus upon communication and language (both within a world and between worlds). Medical worlds can be conceptualized as universes of language whereby world members sanction and legitimate the actions and expressions of others within their world. Similarly, each world can also be approached as a paradigm that promotes and embodies its own language code. In terms of CAM and the conventional medical worlds (of which medical undergraduate education is a central component) there is indeed often a perception of divergent key concepts and ways of expressing and understanding health, illness and healing. Also of importance here is the SWT concept of intersection – the process through which subworlds overlap with a consequent transmission of knowledge – recognized by Strauss as being crucial in contemporary society, and one which has clear application to CAM in medical-undergraduate education. The incorporation of CAM into medical-undergraduate education is itself a prime example of a process of intersection whereby two worlds are moving towards an overlap of shared territory. In this case, the interesting features yet to be finalized relate to the nature and extent of such intersection. It appears from current trends that the intersection will be 'weak' – some of the territory and practices of CAM may be incorporated into the medical curricula but this will not necessarily encourage or permit direct involvement from CAM practitioners and educators. Instead, CAM integration will be piecemeal and potentially secured in terms comfortable for and managed exclusively by medical-world members. While we have only provided a brief overview of key features, SWT (with necessary refinements and revisions) can provide an effective tool for medical students to appreciate and anticipate the cartography of contemporary healthcare organization and its influence upon both cross-practitioner communications and clinical dynamics with the patient.

CAM and the deprofessionalization of medicine

Understanding the potential impacts of the emergence of CAM for biomedicine as a profession and form of expertise could also form a key element of CAM-related medical undergraduate education. Again, sociologists have focused on both the dominance of biomedicine (over, say, CAM) and the potential threat of CAM to biomedical hegemony (Saks 1994). Specifically, although the biomedical community has to a certain degree maintained much of its control over healthcare delivery, a perceived relative waning in the dominance and professional autonomy of biomedicine has driven some sociologists to reflect on whether previous conceptualizations of 'medical power' and 'medical dominance' are actually relevant to contemporary healthcare organization (Broom 2006). Such debates have been prompted by such things as: increased public scepticism towards scientific and technological development; lack of recent progress in biomedicine in the treatment and prevention of disease; increased public questioning of 'expert' knowledges; and, increased use of CAM (for example, Calnan *et al.* 2005). Structural processes occurring within medicine, such as increased managerialism, have also prompted questions regarding the relevance of previous conceptualizations of the dominance of biomedicine in contemporary healthcare contexts (Gray 2002). Specifically, this has resulted in the development of theorizations of a so-called waning in medical power and autonomy including the deprofessionalization and proletarianization theses. Proletarianization represents the process whereby organizational and managerial changes divest professionals of the control they have enjoyed over their work (McKinlay and Arches 1985). Deprofessionalization, in the context of the medical profession, is associated with a demystification of medical expertise and increasing lay scepticism about health professionals. However, there is emerging evidence that the idea that CAM is a threat (see Broom and Tovey 2007b) and that it might have a potentially deprofessionalizing impact within medicine may be inaccurate, with processes of strategic enlistment and translation occurring and the intersections of CAM and biomedicine (see Broom 2006; Broom and Tovey 2007b). Thus, models espousing a linear, power-based theorization of CAM and biomedicine may create the illusion of a waning in biomedical power and patient support for biomedical expertise. Moreover, there is potential for CAM integration to bolster biomedical legitimacy and expert status (Broom and Tovey 2007b), rather than CAM merely being viewed as a threat. Similarly, we argue that in teaching about CAM and biomedicine, while conflict and division may enhance understanding, students may begin to appreciate the interplay and potential commensurability of CAM and biomedicine by learning about the complex intersections and alignments existing between them.

Conclusion

Medical education on CAM is in its infancy and much work is needed before CAM can be included as a meaningful and useful element in undergraduate medical education. In an increasingly pluralistic contemporary healthcare context, medical students must receive the necessary knowledge base to allow them to engage with patients regarding CAM. A key point to emphasize here is that CAM integration into the medical curriculum is not about CAM advocacy or clinical integration. Rather, it is about promoting debate and dialogue about the variety of therapeutic practices patients use and arming future doctors with the critical skills necessary to navigate such complex terrain. While for some, teaching medical students about practices that are not 'evidence-based' may seem inappropriate, medical education necessarily involves creating a skill and knowledge base for dealing with complex subjects who utilize multiple therapeutic systems and support varied models of disease and the body. Thus, integration of CAM into medical curricula is an essential step forward in providing society with doctors who have had the opportunity to develop critical perspectives of therapeutic models. Sociology, we argue here, is well placed to bridge the gap between advocates of CAM and those supporting the biomedical model, providing a set of critical perspectives for students to think about the nature of disease, the body and the subject in contemporary society.

Notes

1 This chapter focuses upon the undergraduate medical curriculum but it is important to note that much literature is also emerging that focuses upon CAM as part of continuing professional education for medics and other health professionals.
2 We are not here promoting CAM uncritically as a necessary component of undergraduate medical education but we are keen to explore all potential options and perspectives as a means of helping produce best practice and care for health consumers.

References

Adams, J. (2004) 'Demarcating the medical/non-medical border: occupational boundary-work within GPs' accounts of their integrative practice', in P. Tovey, G. Easthope and J. Adams (eds) *The Mainstreaming of Complementary and Alternative Medicine: studies in social context*, London: Routledge.

Adams, J., Sibbritt, D., Easthope, G. and Young, A. (2003) 'The profile of women who consult alternative health practitioners in Australia', *Medical Journal of Australia*, 179: 297–300.

Beck, U. (1992) *Risk Society*, London: Sage.

Berman, B. (2001) 'Complementary medicine and medical education', *British Medical Journal*, 322: 121–2.

Bishop, F. and Yardley, L. (2004) 'Constructing agency in treatment decisions', *Health*, 8: 465–82.

Broom, A. (2006) 'Reflections on the centrality of power in medical sociology: an empirical test and theoretical elaboration', *Health Sociology Review*, 15: 55–70.

Broom, A. and Tovey, P. (2007a) 'The dialectical tension between individuation and depersonalisation in cancer patients' mediation of complementary, alternative and biomedical cancer treatments', *Sociology*, 41: 1021–39.

—— (2007b) 'Therapeutic pluralism? Evidence, power and legitimacy in UK cancer services', *Sociology of Health and Illness*, 29: 551–69.

Brownlie, J. (2004) 'Tasting the witches' brew: Foucault and therapeutic practices', *Sociology*, 38: 515–32.

Burke, A., Peper, E., Burrows, K. and Kline, B. (2004) 'Developing the complementary and alternative medicine education infrastructure: baccalaureate programs in the United States', *Journal of Alternative and Complementary Medicine*, 10: 1115–21.

Calnan, M., Montaner, D. and Horne, R. (2005) 'How acceptable are innovative healthcare technologies?', *Social Science and Medicine*, 60: 1937–48.

Caspi, O., Bell, I., Rychener, D., Gaudet, T. and Weil, A. (2000) 'The tower of Babel: communication and medicine', *Archives of Internal Medicine*, 160: 3193–5.

Cassileth, B. (1999) 'Complementary and alternative cancer medicine', *Journal of Clinical Oncology*, 17: 44–52.

Chaterji, R., Tractenberg, R., Amri, H., Lumpkin, M., Amorosi, S. and Haramati, A. (2007) 'A large-sample survey of first- and second-year medical student attitudes toward complementary and alternative medicine in the curriculum and in practice', *Alternative Therapies in Health Medicine*, 13: 30–5.

Clarke, A. (1990) 'A social worlds research adventure', in S. Cozzens and T. Gieryn (eds) *Theories of Science in Society*, Bloomington: Indiana University Press.

Consortium of Academic Health Centers for Integrative Medicine (CAHCIM) (2004) *Curriculum in Integrative Medicine: a guide for medical educators*, Minnesota, MN: CAHCIM.

Cook, D., Gelula, M., Lee, M., Bauer, B., Dupras, D. and Schwartz, A. (2007) 'A webbased course on complementary medicine for medical students and residents improves knowledge and changes attitudes', *Teaching and Learning in Medicine*, 19: 230–8.

Coulter, I. (2004) 'Integration and paradigm clash: the practical difficulties of integrative medicine', in P. Tovey, G. Easthope and J. Adams (eds) *The Mainstreaming of Complementary and Alternative Medicine: studies in social context*, London: Routledge.

Doel, M. and Segrott, J. (2003) 'Self, health, and gender: complementary and alternative medicine in the British mass media', *Gender, Place and Culture*, 10: 131–44.

Frankl, V. (1992) *Man's Search for Meaning*, Boston, MA: Deakin.

Frenkel, M. and Ben-Arye, E. (2001) 'The growing need to teach about complementary and alternative medicine: questions and challenges', *Academic Medicine*, 76: 251–4.

Giddens, A. (1991) *Modernity and Self-identity: self and society in the late modern age*, Palo Alta, CA: Stanford University Press.

Gray, D. (2002) 'Deprofessionalising doctors? The independence of the British medical profession is under unprecedented attack', *British Medical Journal*, 324: 627–9.

Greenfield, S., Brown, R., Dawlatly, S., Reynolds, J., Roberts, S. and Dawlatly, R. (2006) 'Gender differences among medical students in attitudes to learning about complementary and alternative medicine', *Complementary Therapies in Medicine*, 14: 207–12.

Hirschkorn, K. and Bourgeault, I. (2005) 'Conceptualising mainstream healthcare providers' behaviours in relation to complementary and alternative medicine', *Social Science and Medicine*, 61: 157–70.

Kaptchuk, T. (2002) 'The placebo effect in alternative medicine: can the performance of a healing ritual have clinical significance?', *Annals of Internal Medicine*, 136: 817–25.

Kaptchuk, T. and Eisenberg, D. (1998) 'The persuasive appeal of alternative medicine', *Annals of Internal Medicine*, 129: 1061–5.

Lie, D. and Boker, J. (2006) 'Comparative survey of complementary and alternative medicine (CAM) attitudes, use, and information-seeking behaviour among medical students, residents and faculty', *BMC Medical Education*, 9: 58.

Low, J. (2004) 'Managing safety and risk', *Health*, 8: 445–63.

Lupton, D. and Tulloch, J. (2002) ' "Risk is part of your life": risk epistemologies among a group of Australians', *Sociology*, 36: 317–35.

McClean, S. (2005) ' "The illness is part of the person": discourses of blame, individual responsibility and individuation at a centre for spiritual healing in the North of England', *Sociology of Health and Illness*, 27: 628–48.

McKinlay, J. and Arches, J. (1985) 'Towards the proletarianization of physicians', *International Journal of Health Services*, 15: 161–95.

Maizes, V., Schneider, C., Bell, I. and Weil, A. (2002) 'Integrative medical education: development and implementation of a comprehensive curriculum at the University of Arizona', *Academic Medicine*, 77: 851–60.

Marcus, D. (2001) 'How should alternative medicine be taught to medical students and physicians?', *Academic Medicine*, 76: 224–9.

Mizrachi, N., Shuval, J. and Gross, S. (2005) 'Boundary at work: alternative medicine in biomedical settings', *Sociology of Health and Illness*, 27: 20–43.

Owen, D. and Lewith, G. (2001) 'Complementary and alternative medicine (CAM) in the undergraduate medical curriculum: the Southampton experience', *Medical Education*, 35: 73–7.

Park, C. (2002) 'Diversity, the individual, and proof of efficacy: complementary and alternative medicine in medical education', *American Journal of Public Health*, 92: 1568–72.

Pietroni, P. (1992) *The Greening of Modern Medicine*, London: Victor Gollancz.

Pirotta, M., Cohen, M., Kotsirilos, V. and Farish, S. (2000) 'Complementary therapies: have they become accepted in general practice?', *Medical Journal of Australia*, 172: 105–9.

Saks, M. (1994) 'The alternatives to medicine', in J. Gabe, K. Keheller and G. Williams (eds) *Challenging Medicine*, Routledge: London.

Sampson, W. (2001) 'The need for educational reform in teaching about alternative therapies', *Academic Medicine*, 76: 248–50.

Siahpush, M. (1998) 'Postmodern values, dissatisfaction with conventional medicine and popularity of alternative therapies', *Journal of Sociology*, 34: 58–70.

Sierpina, V. and Kreitzer, M. (2005) 'Innovations in integrative healthcare education', *Explore*, 1: 140–1.

Sointu, E. (2006) 'Recognition and the creation of wellbeing', *Sociology*, 40: 493–510.

Strauss, A. (1993) *Continual Permutations of Action*, New York: Aldine de Gruyter.

Thorne, S., Paterson, B., Russell, C. and Schultz, A. (2002) 'Complementary/alternative medicine in chronic illness as informed self-care decision-making', *International Journal of Nursing Studies*, 39: 671–83.

Tovey, P. and Adams, J. (2001) 'Primary care as intersecting social worlds', *Social Science and Medicine*, 52: 695–706.

Tovey, P. and Broom, A. (2007) 'Oncologists' and specialist cancer nurses' approaches to complementary and alternative medicine use and their impact on patient action', *Social Science and Medicine*, 64: 2550–64.

Tovey, P., Atkin, K. and Milewa, T. (2001) 'The individual and primary care: service user, reflexive choice maker and collective actor', *Critical Public Health*, 11: 153–66.

Weil, A. (2000) 'The significance of integrative medicine for the future of medical education', *American Journal of Medicine*, 108: 441–3.

Werneke, U., Earl, J., Seyde, C., Horn, O., Crichton, P. and Fannon, D. (2004) 'Potential health risks of complementary alternative medicines in cancer patients', *British Journal of Cancer*, 90: 408–13.

Wetzel, M., Kaptchuk, T., Haramati, A. and Eisenberg, D. (2003) 'Complementary and alternative medical therapies: implications for medical education', *Annals of Internal Medicine*, 138: 191–6.

Winslow, L. and Shapiro, H. (2002) 'Physicians want education about complementary and alternative medicine to enhance communication with their patients', *Archives of Internal Medicine*, 162: 1176–81.

9 Evidence-based medicine and medical education

Stefan Timmermans and Neetu Chawla

The Medical School Objectives Project is an initiative of the Association of American Medical Colleges (AAMC) listing the skills that medical students should possess at graduation. Its first report specified that 'in caring for individual patients, [physicians] must apply the principles of evidence-based medicine and cost effectiveness in making decisions about the utilization of limited medical resources' (AAMC 1998: 8). Even before the AAMC endorsed evidence-based medicine (EBM) in medical education, medical schools began to integrate EBM in training programmes. For example, 95 per cent of US internal medicine residency programmes have journal clubs and 37 per cent of US and Canadian internal medicine programmes have dedicated time for EBM (Green 2000), while other medical specialties have also incorporated EBM in curricula. It is little surprise that medical schools have shown interest in EBM since its aim is to provide a stronger scientific foundation for clinical work in order to achieve consistency, efficiency, effectiveness, quality and safety in medical care. Evidence-based medicine is commonly defined as 'the conscientious, explicit, and judicious use of current best evidence in making decisions about the care of individual patients' (Sackett *et al.* 1996). The term is rather loosely employed and can refer to anything from conducting a statistical meta-analysis of accumulated research, promoting randomized clinical trials, supporting uniform reporting styles for research, to a personal orientation towards critical self-evaluation. Initially, EBM was defined in opposition to clinical experience but later definitions emphasized its complementary character and aimed to improve clinical experience with better evidence (Sackett *et al.* 2000). Yet, while medical schools now offer courses in EBM, it is unclear whether this actually makes a difference in the educational experience. Does EBM create better doctors?

In this chapter, we will review the sociological and biomedical literature on EBM as it pertains to medical education. To expand the sociological frame, we situate the emergence of EBM in the professionalization literature and evaluate the track record of EBM in teaching students to practise medicine. The professions literature tangentially touches upon the role of education and we can deduce some theoretical suggestions about the possible effect of introducing EBM in medical education. We then examine the available medical literature for evidence supporting or contradicting these predictions. The topic of EBM in education potentially covers any aspiring and established clinician from undergraduate students, medical-school students, residents to practising physicians who are exposed to mandatory continuing medical-education requirements. In addition, EBM has spilled over to allied professional fields (where it is usually referred to as EBP for evidence-based practice). We will follow the leads of the literature and focus mostly on medical students and residents training in clinical settings.

EBM and education in professionalization theory

Profession theories aim to explain the emergence and fate of specific occupational groups in contemporary late-modern societies. Eliot Freidson's theory of professional dominance and Donald Light's theory of countervailing powers offer opposite assessments of the current situation of the medical profession, including different motivations for clinicians to engage in EBM, and a different view of the opportunities and pitfalls of EBM for medical education.

As the main proponent of the theory of professional dominance, Freidson argues that professions claim that their work is special and valuable for the broader collective, requiring protections from the state and safeguards from economic competition. Once granted these protections through formal institutional mechanisms such as educational, licensing and credentialling requirements, the profession regulates itself through peer review and a code of ethics. The challenge for the profession is not to let standards relax within a protective institutional environment but to fulfil its collective mission.

Medical education features in two different ways in clinicians' ascent to professionalism: historically, as a site where power was consolidated, and contemporaneously, as a place where novices are socialized into a medical-professional perspective. Observers argued that conferring professional powers to medicine was key in the reforms of medical education in the aftermath of the Flexner report (Wolinsky 1988). As Starr elaborates (1982: 112–27), initiatives from within elite medical schools to lengthen the curriculum and raise admission standards and the reforms following the Flexner report led many weak medical schools to close their doors. The surviving schools became more selective and instituted a basic science-based curriculum. These educational reforms generated greater uniformity among medical professionals as well as increased specialization and geographic concentration of physicians.

Freidson emphasized how a body of highly specialized, esoteric medical knowledge formed the cornerstone for professional autonomy, but held a dim view of medical schools' ability to transfer such knowledge. Professions distinguish themselves from other occupations by the special character of the knowledge required to perform their tasks and the autonomy they have over their work (Freidson 1986). Only certain types of knowledge beget professional power: Freidson emphasized that professional knowledge needs to be exclusive, esoteric, theoretical and discretionary to advance professional interests. Some of this knowledge is picked up in medical schools and graduates of medical schools obtain employment based on the strength of their educational credentials. Various sociological studies have explored how the professional self is shaped during a lengthy socialization process in medical schools (Becker *et al.* 1961; Merton *et al.* 1957). Based on these studies, Freidson doubted that faculty members had great influence even on student attitudes toward medicine, let alone the medical knowledge they received. He repeatedly noted the gap between what physicians are taught and what they do in medical practice. For Freidson, the true realm of medical knowledge is clinical care:

> If medical education molds the medical man, the exigencies of practice are likely to be the proof of the mold.... And it is in the realities of practice rather than in the classroom that we find the empirical materials for clarifying and articulating the actual rather than the imputed or hoped-for nature of the professional role.
>
> (1970: 18)

Freidson, however, allowed for the possibility that medical-school socialization and the long-term investment in medical training provided some inertia against bureaucratic rationales (Freidson 1986: 99).

Writing about the nexus between power and knowledge, Freidson did not anticipate the emergence of EBM (Timmermans and Kolker 2004). He observed that professionals exercised power in the political economy by formulating technical product standards and developing personnel standards. In passing, he mentioned the danger of standardizing the actual content of medical work:

> it is true that there are generally recognized standards of procedure that exist in medicine and law, for example, and that they become the focus of attention (...), but they are rarely officially codified. Nor are service outcomes. If they were, of course, professionals would have considerably less discretion in performing their work.
>
> (1986: 203–4)

By the time that Freidson's 1970 treatise on professional dominance gained a privileged place in theories of the medical profession, significant structural changes had already taken place in both the organization and delivery of healthcare services that challenged Freidson's hegemonic perspective. The changes included the corporatization of medicine, increased involvement of the government in the financing and regulation of healthcare, unprecedented growth in biomedical technologies, the emergence of 'defensive medicine', the growth in physician administrators, ongoing specialization within medicine, an end to medicine's exemption from antitrust law, the codification of medical knowledge and the public's increased distrust and critical stance toward medical authority (Clarke *et al.* 2003; Haug 1973, 1975; Light and Levine 1988). The rise of the internet and increase in direct-to-consumer advertising are also important factors that have changed the knowledge base of the patient population, and shaped patient demand for services and medications. These changes have resulted in increased challenging of medical authority and have shaped the interactional components of the patient–doctor relationship.

Taken together, these changes had implications for the medical profession's autonomy. In various works, Freidson (1986, 1994) held steadfast the notion of professional dominance, arguing that these changes may have stratified the medical profession and put more pressure on practising clinicians, but that they had not lost control over their work. Freidson also noted the increased formalization of the methods through which professions control their own members, with EBM as an example of this formalization (Armstrong 2002). While being challenged, physicians still dominated professionalism.

Other social scientists were not persuaded. To account for the structural and organizational changes that seemed to erode the power of professionals, Light developed the cybernetic conflict theory of countervailing powers (Light 1991). According to Light, when one player in the healthcare field dominates, other players will react and redress the 'excessive' power base of the dominator. Healthcare thus takes place in a market of 'interdependent yet distinct' parties vying for resources, favourable public opinion, territory and control (Light 1995). The so-called 'golden age' of professional dominance during the 1950s and 1960s was a period of excess when the medical profession dominated the healthcare market. As a consequence, other parties (Light distinguishes government, consumers, corporate buyers, corporate sellers and other healthcare providers (Light 1993)) attempted to chip away at the control of the medical profession. The rise of managed care, cost-containment and the broader 'buyer's revolt' together constitute one of the 'ironies of success' (1993: 73). It was precisely because the profession was so powerful in setting up protected markets for healthcare providers that it created ideal markets for pharmaceutical and other health-related, for-profit corporations. A high level of clinical autonomy may have led to the decline in trust in medical professionals in recent decades, as the lack of external controls led to spiralling costs and inefficient or even incompetent care. The weakening of professional power is thus to some extent the profession's own doing, or at least an unintended consequence of its dominance.

The theory of countervailing powers allows Light to detect a downward momentum in professional power, in part because of the erosion of the monopoly over medical knowledge in recent years (Hafferty and Light 1995). While most observers agree that the medical profession maintains general cultural authority in the healthcare field, Hafferty and Light argue that professionals have lost ground in the detailed aspects of their daily activities. They agree with Freidson's observations that medicine is increasingly becoming bifurcated with a cadre of elite physician-administrators separate from the rank-and-file clinicians. These elite physicians increasingly identify with administrative mandates, loosening ties with their MD degree to focus on administrative issues such as utilization reviews.

Writing before the big influx of EBM, Hafferty and Light speculated about some of the potential consequences of introducing standardized instruments in a profession that greatly valued autonomy. Whether or not EBM led to a reduction or increase of professional medical power depended on which of the countervailing powers was able to create EBM and who was able to enforce compliance to these guidelines. Light imagined two opposite scenarios. First, EBM and guidelines could provide a more secure scientific footing that might enhance the overall professional authority of medicine because physicians remain in charge of deciding what counts as evidence-based medicine. Second, guidelines created by third parties could threaten professional interests because third parties have fundamentally different interests (for example, economic versus professional interests). Hafferty and Light considered this second scenario most likely because they imagined a decline of clinical autonomy guided by principles of cost control:

> The arrival of medical effectiveness research raises the very real possibility that medicine's longstanding claim to a professional status based on its scientific expertise is about to be hoisted by its own petard.... It appears clear that the payer-driven movement to assess effectiveness clearly threatens the autonomy of individual physicians.
>
> (1995: 143)

Light consequently reconceptualized the centrality of autonomy to professional power; autonomy is only one pole on a continuum of control in the medical profession.

How does the theory of countervailing forces relate to medical education? Light remains silent about the role of physicians' training but Hafferty speculated about some possible effects. Within medical training, Hafferty (2000) has argued that the influx of evidence-based medicine, standards, protocols and guidelines has led to a broad-scale standardization of clinical practice, leading not only to greater uniformity of the knowledge taught to medical students but also to a shift in values. Medical students' exposure to standardization may lead to subtle changes in the nature of medical uncertainty (Fox 1980), the difference between technical and normative errors (Bosk 1992), and especially the value of personal, hands-on experience. In addition, the rise of EBM also restratifies sub-areas within medicine because some areas may be more compatible with the focus on randomized clinical trials (RCTs) than other areas and data from these trials are often seen as better forms of evidence than other types of studies.

The professionalization literature suggests several areas of enquiry for the incorporation of EBM in medical education:

1 What form does EBM take in medical education and how much has EBM penetrated medical education? With Freidson, we would expect that most EBM initiatives would remain under the control of clinicians, while Light and Hafferty predicted that EBM may be imposed on medical education from stronger outside forces.
2 Does the introduction of EBM shift the normative focus of medical education? Specifically, Hafferty suggested that EBM may change medical

students' management of uncertainty and their personal experience with patients, shifting the emphasis from patient-specific knowledge to more general, population-based knowledge. EBM may also affect physicians' autonomy because it implies a restriction of professional discretion.

3   Finally, since the goal of EBM is to improve decision-making, we should also look at how EBM training affects decisions in clinical situations both within medical training and beyond.

We will consider each of these issues in turn.

1 Origins of EBM – its form in education

For many clinicians, medicine has always been 'evidence-based'. For others, the current turn to EBM privileges specific kinds of evidence that have been less emphasized in the past. EBM represents a break with a time when the most reliable evidence in medicine was pathophysiological (Evidence-Based Medicine Working Group 1992). Since the late 1980s, the goal of EBM has been to inform clinical decision-making with an evaluation of a clearly defined hierarchy of available evidence. EBM elevated population-based, epidemiological studies with randomized controlled double-blind clinical trials to the top of medical knowledge (Sackett *et al.* 1996). The new knowledge was disseminated through formalized tools such as utilization reviews, clinical-practice guidelines, and protocols. This reshuffling of epistemics came after various high-profile researchers in Canada, the UK and the US expressed dissatisfaction with the basis of medical decision-making, noting that many common medical interventions and therapies lack a scientific foundation of their efficacy (Daly 2005). Medical interventions were authority-based rather than evidence-based. This dissatisfaction gained notoriety in the small-area variation studies that showed that the kind of care clinicians provide varies tremendously over geographical areas. In some areas, prostate surgeries were eight times as common as in other parts of the US (Wennberg 1999). EBM was embraced by medical professional groups concerned that practice variation may lead to a loss of trust, by payers in the healthcare system looking to reform clinical practice, by allied professionals aiming to capture medical jurisdictions and by educators looking for a stronger curriculum (Timmermans and Mauck 2005).

In medical education, the role of EBM was to encourage students to ask 'what's the evidence?' (Eisenberg 1999: 1868) when contemplating therapeutic interventions. Researchers at McMaster University, Ontario, have further developed this question into five key components: translation of uncertainty into an answerable question; systematic retrieval of the best evidence available; critical appraisal of evidence for validity, clinical relevance and applicability; application of the results into practice; and evaluation of performance (or Ask, Acquire, Appraise, Apply and Assess) (Sackett *et al.* 2000). Proponents of evidence-based medicine suggest that learning EBM skills will allow practitioners to deal more directly and effectively with gaps in their knowledge and will allow them to develop an approach that is more self-directed and patient-centred (Bordley *et al.* 1997).

Current medical literature describes a range of methods and formats for teaching these skills: required coursework in EBM, journal clubs, faculty development and training in EBM, workgroups, use of the internet and laptops in clinical settings, use of PDAs (personal digital assistants) or smart phones, electronic medical records, research mentors, EBM clerkships or rotations, grand rounds, peer discussion groups, use of the librarian or medical school/library partnerships, and creating organizational and infrastructural support for EBM on an institutional level. The internet is a fundamental component of both teaching evidence-based medicine and practising EBM principles in clinical settings and the many information sources available online include: MEDLINE; Cochrane Database of Systematic Reviews; Best Evidence; ACP Journal Club; Ovid Technologies; PUBMED; and the National Guideline Clearinghouse. In addition, technologies such as 'smart phones' (Leon *et al.* 2007) – hybrid devices that combine mobile phones with PDAs and the electronic medical record (Stewart *et al.* 2007) – containing reminders of guidelines and contraindications for medications, have been used in teaching EBM.

A consideration in the nature of teaching EBM is the level of intensity with which it is incorporated into the medical curriculum, which varies widely across international medical schools and residency programmes. Mount Sinai Medical School in New York provides an example of extensive engagement with EBM (Barnett *et al.* 2000). The faculty created a multidisciplinary Evidence-Based Medicine Working Group in 1995 to assess the extent to which EBM was taught in the traditional curriculum and to infuse the curriculum with EBM. Their assessment showed that faculty needed education in EBM and the university organized retreats with members from McMaster University. Faculty then trained medical students through both coursework and clerkship opportunities. The courses included teaching in information retrieval and epidemiology. The curriculum for the clinical years was based upon the five principles developed at McMaster University described earlier. It focused upon clerkships that involved each department teaching one of the McMaster modules, preceptor-led presentations and group meetings, and student demonstration of proficient application of EBM practice to clinical care. The evaluation of this programme demonstrated that students had significantly increased skills in search strategies, including use of keywords, subheadings, MeSH (medical subject heading) headings, combining multiple headings and limiting search strategies. The programme illustrated the gradual process of improvement of students in employing EBM skills and the level of intensity required to achieve long-term success in application of EBM principles in clinical situations.

The implementation of evidence-based medicine faces several logistical barriers to do with infrastructure and personnel. In a study with 417 programme directors of US internal medicine residency programmes, Green *et al.* found that the primary barriers to incorporating EBM principles into practice were that only about half (51–64 per cent) of the programmes had onsite electronic information and only about one-third (31–45 per cent) had site-specific faculty development (Green *et al.* 2000). Less than half of curricula incorporated evaluations and many did not include important sources of medical information such as well-regarded EBM databases. Furthermore, Green *et al.* recognized the lack of documentation of actual EBM behaviours among residents for all major areas, particularly in the emergency departments, weekly rounds led by attending physicians and interdisciplinary daily bedside rounds. Limited information exists on the effectiveness of existing faculty-training programmes, including computing capacity. David Nierenberg and Patricia Carney suggest that sustaining medical curricular change requires a focus on clinical research and a supportive infrastructure at each educational level (Nierenberg and Carney 2004).

Other key obstacles to the implementation of evidence-based medicine can be broadly categorized as lack of evidence and cognitive barriers. Many clinical outcomes in medicine are uncertain or do not have current research to direct clinical decision-making. Furthermore, several researchers have questioned the state of 'the evidence' in current medical research, given issues such as publication bias, poor validity and reliability of studies, and unclear recommendations for practical application. In clinically uncertain circumstances with little, poor or no evidence to guide clinical decision-making, physicians will probably turn to their own clinical experience or 'gut reactions' to resolve problems (Porzsolt *et al.* 2003).

In the opposite situation, where there is extensive evidence, cognitive barriers exist for students and practitioners of EBM because of the volume of literature pertaining to certain medical outcomes. Extensive literature for common conditions, such as heart disease, may overwhelm students faced with challenges in sifting through available information to determine which studies constitute 'the best evidence'. Several studies have also indicated that medical students and residents experience difficulty in understanding and applying the principles of biostatistics and epidemiology in order to critically appraise research articles. Windish *et al.* (2007) evaluated the ability of residents to understand statistical principles and interpret research findings. They administered a survey to 277 residents and found that only 41 per cent could correctly understand statistical concepts and research results. In addition, they found that 75 per cent of residents did not understand all statistics they read in journal articles, though 95 per cent felt it was important to understand these concepts to intelligently navigate the literature.

Even if infrastructural problems are overcome and the necessary skills are acquired, the implementation of EBM still faces the obstacle of simply being one concern in a very hectic and high-stakes educational environment. Green and Ruff (2005) explored reasons why residents failed to pursue answers to their clinical questions, using focus groups with 34 internal medicine residents. The predominant barriers included access to medical information, skills for searching, time, clinical-question tracking and priority, personal initiative, team dynamics and institutional culture. The authors concluded that educators should pay increased attention to attitudes towards learning EBM and the influence of institutional cultures. In a different study also exploring unanswered clinical questions by residents, Green *et al.* (2000) interviewed 64 residents after 401 patient encounters. In this study, authors found that residents had approximately two questions for every three patients, but only pursued questions 29 per cent of the time. Questions were typically related to therapy (38 per cent) or diagnosis (27 per cent). The most common reasons for failure to pursue answers were lack of time (60 per cent) and forgetting the question (29 per cent). In order to answer questions, residents typically turned to textbooks, original articles or attending physicians.

Thus, while there is a strong consensus that EBM is beneficial for medical education, the implementation of EBM has run into the same problems that plague the macro healthcare field. Light and Hafferty predicted that third parties would use EBM to wrestle control away from clinicians over the content of medicine. Clinicians have in fact remained in charge of curricula in medical schools but the problem of practice variation continues. Practice variation in the broader field trickles down to disparities in computer infrastructure and research orientation in medical schools, different capacities in urban and rural areas, and varying pedagogical priorities. This situation is further complicated by an uneven evidence base with some conditions: most highly prevalent chronic conditions requiring drug treatment are well researched, but other therapies, conditions, or even patient populations are under-researched. Implementing EBM may have exposed the lack of strong evidence in medicine.

2 Impact of EBM on healthcare norms: uncertainty and autonomy

In the 2000 edition of the *Handbook of Medical Sociology*, Frederic Hafferty noted that the rise of EBM might have repercussions for the study of uncertainty in medical education:

> We might want to revisit the writings of Renée Fox, Donald Light, Jack Haas, and William Shaffir, and others on the nature and impact of uncertainty in medical work and question whether the deployment of research protocols and the use of report cards is generating a new definition of uncertainty in medical practice.

(2000: 252)

Timmermans and Angell (2001) took up Hafferty's suggestion by studying how residents in two paediatrics programmes used EBM to manage the uncertainty of medical knowledge and to balance EBM knowledge against first-hand experience.

The topic of uncertainty in medical education is one of the oldest in sociological scholarship. Based on research in Cornell medical school during the early 1950s, Renée Fox argued that medical knowledge is inherently uncertain because it is riddled with gaps and unknowns and because the amount of medical facts is ever-expanding and impossible to completely master (Fox 1957). The dilemma for students in medical school consists of managing the limitations of their own cognitive ability and the vast medical literature. During the clinical-training years, medical uncertainty emerges when students apply textbook knowledge to clinical situations and handle both the physiological and psychological aspects of patient care. Fox's sociology of knowledge consists of a gradual socialization in medical confidence; instead of blaming oneself for clinical mistakes, the aspiring doctor learns to successfully manage the limitations of medicine. Training for uncertainty serves to imprint a professional attitude of objective expertise and detached concern on the next generation of physicians. Other authors have questioned the primacy of 'uncertainty' and instead highlighted that 'training for control' closely follows 'training for uncertainty' (Atkinson 1984; Katz 1984; Light 1979). Instead of being imbued with scientific scepticism, for example, Atkinson portrays medical students as pragmatists, 'content to work within the conceptual bounds of a given "paradigm"' (Atkinson 1984: 954). In her most recent update of the 'uncertainty' literature, Fox addresses the rise of EBM. Fox contends that EBM reinforces collective-oriented approaches in medicine at the expense of individualized patient–doctor interactions (Fox 2000). Siding with the critics of EBM, Fox remains apprehensive of EBM's narrow biomedical positivism and its threat to clinical expertise.

Timmermans and Angell (2001) found that residents in the two paediatrics programmes were exposed to EBM but they engaged with this scientific evidence in different ways. About two-thirds of the residents interviewed interpreted EBM to mean consulting the medical literature (these were designated by Timmermans and Angell as 'librarians'), while the remaining third believed that EBM required an active evaluation of the research literature (designated 'researchers'). Timmermans and Angell found that EBM foremost created a new source of research-based uncertainty to be mastered by medical residents: learning the skills to retrieve and evaluate the research literature. Whether EBM instilled an attitude of scientific scepticism or increasing medical dogmatism, depended on the researcher's mode of using scientific evidence. To inform clinical decision-making, 'librarian' residents tended to become frustrated with evaluating individual studies and used summaries of the medical literature to gain confidence. They could become more dogmatic from their uncritical and instrumentalist take on the literature or avoid consulting the literature for a lack of clear answers. 'Researcher' residents, in contrast, appreciated the contradictions and uncertainties of the medical knowledge base and learned when not to follow guidelines or published recommendations. They turned the critical attitude fostered by EBM to EBM itself, sharpening discriminatory powers in decision-making. Even researchers, however, ran into trouble if they attempted to contradict superiors based on EBM. Attending physicians' understanding of the literature and scientific evidence prevailed in training situations and every resident agreed that it was more important to know what your supervisor expected than to be familiar with the latest literature.

How does EBM mediate the tension between personal first-hand experience and external (book) knowledge? Timmermans and Angell argue that the difference between these two realms of experience is exaggerated because any consultation of the literature is already influenced by clinical observations while any observation is steeped in book knowledge. They came to this observation because no resident seemed to be able to implement EBM unproblematically. At each point, they ran into problems with attending physicians, patient preferences, allied professionals and organizational constraints. Clinicians in training ultimately draw on evidence-based clinical judgement, an inevitable mixture of hard-won experience from watching others, personal tryouts, mistakes and admonishments and various forms of evidence gathered from lectures, various written sources, and their own attempts to summarize the literature. Over time, the knowledge base of both experience and published evidence expands and may shift when, for example, residents move from consumers to producers of knowledge over their careers.

Besides uncertainty, EBM is also presumed to affect a physician's autonomy. Evidence-based medicine promises to preserve the professional autonomy of clinicians by committing to high scientific standards of care. Yet, this same autonomy may be under attack since EBM aims to restrict clinical discretion on scientific grounds. Whether or not individual discretion gives way to standardization depends on how clinicians learn and modify their behaviour. In a study of how primary-care clinicians determine what kind of drugs to use in the treatment of depression, David Armstrong (2000) found that clinicians conducted personalized 'clinical trials' with individual patients to check the effectiveness of new drugs and to match drugs with particular groups of patients, and remained attentive to patient choice and their general relationship with patients. He noted that 'a formalized approach to patient care, especially one based on trial evidence derived from populations of patients, was far removed from the individualized clinical decisions being made by these doctors' (Armstrong 2002: 1775). Armstrong's study focused on General Practitioners who have medical degrees but are expected to keep abreast of ever-changing therapeutic innovations. This situation is different from the typical pedagogical situation where teachers have more power over students and can offer various incentives and punishments. Like their peers in training, General Practitioners also relied on senior academic colleagues for the most updated information but the information exchange followed a particular etiquette where seniors made suggestions without undermining the professional autonomy of the first-line practitioners (Armstrong and Ogden 2006).

Armstrong's study shows that trying to ward off external pressures for cost containment and consumerism with a strategy that undermines the clinical autonomy of practising care providers may backfire as a professional strategy. The danger remains that when physicians claim scientific superiority with greater uniformity but practice variation continues unabated, they open themselves up to cost-control measures developed by external parties (Timmermans and Berg 2003: Chapter 3).

Rather than a seismic shift in medical norms and values, sociological research suggests that the effect of EBM on the values acquired in medical education is modest. An emphasis on EBM in medical training may reinforce certain skill sets but does not undermine, for example, the authority of attendings or of elite academic researchers. EBM does not level the playing field in medicine but it may slightly narrow the gap between student and teacher. At best, EBM works as a value catalyst, allowing residents to either develop greater scepticism or dogmatism. EBM then does not decisively solve or redefine the issue of managing uncertainty but adds a new set of skills to be mastered by novice clinicians.

3 Impact on medical care

While EBM may have been one factor in a continuing stream of factors reshaping the uncertainties of learning medicine and professional autonomy, what have been the effects of evidence-based medicine on how and what physicians learn? Evidence-based medicine supports and presumes a positivistic science of behaviour modification: if only physicians knew about the best evidence, they would be compelled to implement this knowledge. The literature on outcomes of EBM in medical education suffers from similar gaps, biases and weaknesses as the overall biomedical literature. EBM is generally accepted as effective, but precious little research supports this presumption (Green 2006). Ironically, many of the evaluation studies do not meet the highest evidentiary standards of EBM because randomized controlled trials (RCTs) are notoriously difficult to run in educational settings (Hatala and Guyatt 2002). Yet, EBM advocates have turned to RCTs to grapple with the implementation gap of EBM in education and clinical practice in general.

In the last five years, educators and biomedical researchers have aimed to improve the available methodology and evidence. One of the few studies with a control group of an EBM educational intervention showed a statistically significant increase in awareness of EBM principles and their use in the experimental group (Ross and Verdieck 2003). Yet the researchers were unable to demonstrate changes in patient care or improved health outcomes and this research may thus lack face validity. The same problem occurred in a study where residents were asked about their familiarity with recent journal articles relevant to primary care (Stevermer et al. 1999). More promising may be the attempt to have medical students maintain evidence-based learning portfolios, representing a student's work to address clinical problems. Studies have shown that working on these portfolios leads to greater 'self-directed learning readiness' (Crowley et al. 2003; Fung et al. 2000).

These evaluation studies reflect the distinction between 'researchers' and 'librarians'. Studies where students are tested on their familiarity with formal EBM tools and databases interpret EBM in the librarian mode, while studies where students are evaluated on their ability to put a research portfolio together are more likely to check for critical appraisal researcher skills. The studies thus contain different conceptual models of learning centred around EBM and of EBM itself (see also Straus et al. 2004). An observational study of how residents use EBM after receiving training showed that 'librarians' are more numerous than 'researchers': residents are most likely to consult with summarized EBM sources for answers to clinical questions. The study's authors noted that 'residents operated more as information managers within the constraints of time limitations and job responsibilities' (McCord *et al.* 2007: 301). The most important information resource remained consulting their superiors (McCord *et al.* 2007). Launching a critical appraisal of the literature was often not performed owing to simple logistical barriers, such as having to go to a different room to access a computer. Other studies have confirmed that residents only pursue about a quarter of their clinical questions, often consulting non-evidence-based information sources (Green *et al.* 2000).

The key question is whether this influx of EBM has actually resulted in improved patient outcomes. This question should be easy to measure because researchers can review therapeutic decisions based on chart reviews by assigning primary diagnoses and interventions and determine whether the resident reached a decision backed up by the best available evidence. Ellis *et al.* (1995) introduced this methodology by classifying the evidence in three broad categories: intervention with evidence from RCTs; intervention with convincing non-experimental evidence; and intervention without substantial evidence. While this method has indeed been employed in various medical subspecialties such as surgery, anaesthesiology and other fields (Green 2006), it has only been used sporadically in medical education. In one study (Straus *et al.* 2005), patients were significantly more likely to receive EBM-derived therapy than those treated before the intervention (82 per cent versus 74 per cent; $P = 0.046$). Even in this study, the researchers focused on process outcomes rather than clinical outcomes such as mortality. Thus, EBM interventions can indeed change physician behaviour, but we still do not know whether patients benefit from recommendations grounded in the best available evidence.

We have thus some evidence that EBM teaching modules may change some clinical decision-making, but physicians in training are more likely to rely on authoritative EBM sources than to conduct their own critical appraisal of the literature. While some decisions seem to have a stronger scientific foundation as defined by EBM proponents, the question is still open as to whether training in EBM-saturated environments benefits patients.

Conclusion

EBM has made inroads in medical education. It is difficult to find either students, residents or faculty who believe that strengthening the scientific base of medical decision-making has no place in education. Over the past years, EBM has gradually been incorporated into pedagogy through journal clubs, workshops, specialized reference materials, clinical practice guidelines, PDAs and other tools. While some of the logistical barriers have been fixed – especially in well-funded academic centres – other important barriers remain, such as the acquisition of scientific skills and finding the time to practise EBM in clinical settings. Consequently, we see a bifurcation of EBM use: for some students, practising EBM means consulting different authoritative sources, while for others it implies conducting a critical appraisal of the literature. Most studies suggest that EBM has not replaced the traditional, hierarchical authority of checking in with superiors.

The effect of EBM on medical education is thus subtle rather than revolutionary. EBM explicitly aims to address the uncertainty of medical decision-making and it may have provided some guidance in how to tackle clinical dilemmas, but it has also posed new sources of uncertainty, such as translating findings from research using population-based data sources or randomized clinical trials to the individual patient sitting in front of the clinician. EBM may theoretically undermine a practising clinician's professional discretion and autonomy by substituting individualized decisions with standardized guidelines, but the reality is that most clinicians have been able to hold on to their autonomy even if that means ignoring or disregarding the 'best' scientific evidence.

Sociologists and social scientists more generally have been slow to intellectually engage with EBM in medical education. The journals *Health, Social Science and Medicine*, *Biosocieties* and *Perspectives in Biology and Medicine* have devoted special issues to the phenomenon of EBM and science-studies scholars in particular have examined the epistemic qualities of randomized clinical trials. But there has been little interest in the sociological area of education. Still, the research possibilities are promising. Among topics of interest is the key question of whether evidence-based medicine actually leads to better patient outcomes. Biomedical research up to now has shown that EBM training may generate awareness of EBM and even obtain some intermediate, process-oriented outcomes, but the more fundamental question of whether EBM affects patient outcomes has rarely been queried. A second issue of research is broached by David Armstrong: how do you change the behaviour of professionals whose occupational distinguishing characteristic is exactly autonomy in medical decision-making? Here, an observational or records review study that combines learning from EBM or other traditional educational sources with the techniques used by pharmaceutical companies to convince clinicians to prescribe their products should produce fascinating results. A third possibility is to conduct one of the classical long-term ethnographies where researchers follow a cohort of medical students through their educational trajectory to see how EBM changes the socialization process in medical school.

References

AAMC (Association of American Medical Colleges) (1998) *Report 1: Learning Objectives for Medical Student Education: Guidelines for Medical Schools*, Washington, DC: AAMC.

Armstrong, D. (2002) 'Clinical autonomy, individual and collective: the problem of changing doctors' behaviour', *Social Science and Medicine*, 55: 1771–7.

Armstrong, D. and Ogden, J. (2006) 'The role of etiquette and experimentation in explaining how doctors change behaviour: a qualitative study', *Sociology of Health and Illness*, 28: 951–68.

Atkinson, P. (1984) 'Training for certainty', *Social Science and Medicine*, 19: 949–56.

Barnett, S. H., Kaiser, S., Morgan, L. K., Sullivant, J., Siu, A., Rose, D., Rico, M., Smith, L., Schechter, C., Miller, M. and Stagnaro-Green, A. (2000) 'An integrated program for evidence-based medicine in medical school', *Mount Sinai Journal of Medicine*, 67: 163–8.

Becker, H. S., Geer, B., Hughes, E. C. and Strauss, A. L. (1961) *Boys in White: student culture in medical school*, Chicago, IL: University of Chicago Press.

Bordley, D. R., Fagan, M. and Theige, D. (1997) 'Evidence-based medicine: a powerful educational tool for clerkship education', *American Journal of Medicine*, 102: 427–32.

Bosk, C. L. (1992) *All God's Mistakes: genetic counseling in a pediatric hospital*, Chicago, IL: Chicago University Press.

Clarke, A. E., Shim, J. K., Mamo, L., Fosket, J. R. and Fishman, J. R. (2003) 'Biomedicalization: technoscientific transformations of health, illness, and US biomedicine', *American Sociological Review*, 68: 161–94.

Crowley, S. D., Owens, T. A., Schardt, C. M., Wardell, S. I., Peterson, J., Garrison, S. and Keitz, S. (2003) 'A web-based compendium of clinical questions and medical evidence to educate internal medicine residents', *Academic Medicine*, 78: 270–4.

Daly, J. (2005) *Evidence-Based Medicine and the Search for a Science of Clinical Care*, Berkeley: University of California Press.

Eisenberg, J. M. (1999) 'Ten lessons for evidence-based technology assessment', *Journal of the American Medical Association*, 282: 1865–9.

Ellis, J., Mulligan, I., Rowe, J. and Sackett, D. L. (1995) 'Inpatient general medicine is evidence based. A-Team, Nuffield Department of Clinical Medicine', *Lancet*, 346: 407–10.

Evidence-Based Medicine Working Group (1992) 'Evidence-based medicine: a new approach to teaching the practice of medicine', *Journal of the American Medical Association*, 268: 2420–5.

Fox, R. C. (1957) 'Training for uncertainty', in R. K. Merton, G. Reader and P. L. Kendall (eds) *The Student-Physician*, Cambridge, MA: Harvard University Press.

—— (1980) 'The evolution of medical uncertainty', *Milbank Memorial Fund Quarterly*, 58: 1–49.

—— (2000) 'Medical uncertainty revisited', in G. L. Albrecht, R. Fitzpatrick and S. C. Scrimshaw (eds) *The Handbook of Social Studies in Health and Medicine*, London: Sage.

Freidson, E. (1970) *Professional Dominance: the social structure of medical care*, New York: Atherton Press.

—— (1986) *Professional Powers: a study of the institutionalization of formal knowledge*, Chicago, IL: Chicago University Press.

—— (1994) *Professionalism Reborn: theory, prophecy and policy*, Chicago, IL: Chicago University Press.

Fung, M. F., Walker, M., Fung, K. F., Temple, L., Lajoie, F., Bellemare, G. and Bryson, S. (2000) 'An internet-based learning portfolio in resident education: the KOALA multi-centre programme', *Medical Education*, 34: 474–9.

Green, M. L. (2000) 'Evidence-based medicine training in internal medicine residency programs: a national survey', *Journal of General Internal Medicine*, 15: 129–33.

—— (2006) 'Evaluating evidence-based practice performance', *Evidence-Based Medicine*, 11: 99–101.

Green, M. L. and Ruff, T. R. (2005) 'Why do residents fail to answer their clinical questions? A qualitative study of barriers to practicing evidence-based medicine', *Academic Medicine*, 80: 176–82.

Green, M. L., Ciampi, M. A. and Ellis, P. J. (2000) 'Residents' medical information needs in clinic: are they being met?', *American Journal of Medicine*, 109: 218–23.

Hafferty, F. W. (2000) 'Reconfiguring the sociology of medical education: emerging topics and pressing issues', in C. E. Bird, P. E. Conrad and A. M. Fremont (eds) *Handbook of Medical Sociology*, 5th edn, Upper Saddle River, NJ: Prentice Hall.

Hafferty, F. W. and Light, D. (1995) 'Professional dynamics and the changing nature of medical work', *Journal of Health and Social Behavior* (Extra issue): 132–53.

Hatala, R. and Guyatt, G. (2002) 'Evaluating the teaching of evidence-based medicine', *Journal of the American Medical Association*, 288: 1110–12.

Haug, M. R. (1973) 'Deprofessionalization: an alternative hypothesis', in P. Hamos (ed.) *Professionalisation and Social Change*, Keele: University of Keele.

—— (1975) 'The deprofessionalization of everyone?', *Sociological Focus*, 8: 197–213.

Katz, J. (1984) *The Silent World of Doctor and Patient*, New York: Free Press.

Leon, S. A., Fontelo, P., Green, L., Ackerman, M. and Liu, F. (2007) 'Evidence-based medicine among internal medicine residents in a community hospital program using smart phones', *Biomed Central: Medical Informatics Decision Making*, 7: 5.

Light, D. W. (1979) 'Uncertainty and control in professional training', *Journal of Health and Social Behavior*, 20: 310–22.

—— (1991) 'Professionalism as a countervailing power', *Journal of Health Politics, Policy and Law*, 16: 499–506.

—— (1993) 'Countervailing power: the changing character of the medical profession in the United States', in F. W. Hafferty and J. B. McKinlay (eds) *The Changing Medical Profession: an international perspective*, New York: Oxford University Press.

—— (1995) 'Countervailing powers: a framework for professions in transition', in T. Johnson, G. Larkin and M. Saks (eds) *Health Professions and the State in Europe*, London and New York: Routledge.

Light, D. W. and Levine, S. (1988) 'The changing character of the medical profession: a theoretical overview', *The Milbank Quarterly*, 66 (Supp 2): 10–32.

McCord, G., Smucker, W. D., Selius, B. A., Hannan, S., Davidson, E., Schrop, S. L., Labuda, M., Rao, V. and Albrecht, P. (2007) 'Answering questions at the point of care: do residents practice EBM or manage information sources?', *Academic Medicine*, 82: 298–303.

Merton, R., Reader, G. and Kendall, P. (eds) (1957) *The Student-Physician: introductory studies in the sociology of medical education*, Cambridge, MA: Harvard University Press.

Nierenberg, D. W. and Carney, P. A. (2004) 'Nurturing educational research at Dartmouth Medical School: the synergy among innovative ideas, support faculty, and administrative structures', *Academic Medicine*, 79: 969–74.

Porzsolt, F., Ohletz, A., Thim, A., Gardner, D., Ruatti, H., Meier, H., Schlotz-Gorton, N. and Schrott, L. (2003) 'Evidence-based decision making – the 6-step approach', *American College of Physicians Journal Club*, 139: A11–12.

Ross, R. and Verdieck, A. (2003) 'Introducing an evidence-based medicine curriculum into a family practice residency – is it effective?', *Academic Medicine*, 78: 412–17.

Sackett, D. L., Rosenberg, W. M. C., Gray, J. A., Haynes, B. R. and Richardson, W. S. (1996) 'Evidence-based medicine: what it is and what it isn't', *British Medical Journal*, 312, online at www.bmj.com/cgi/content/full/312/7023/71 (accessed December 2008).

Sackett, D. L., Straus, S. E., Richardson, W. S., Rosenberg, W. and Haynes, R. B. (2000) *Evidence-Based Medicine: how to practice and teach EBM*, 2nd edn, Toronto: Churchill Livingstone.

Starr, P. (1982) *The Social Transformation of American Medicine*, New York: Basic Books.

Stevermer, J. J., Chambliss, M. L. and Hoekzema, G. S. (1999) 'Distilling the literature: a randomized, controlled trial testing an intervention to improve selection of medical articles for reading', *Academic Medicine*, 74: 70–2.

Stewart, W. F., Shah, N. R., Selna, M. J., Paulus, R. A. and Walker, J. M. (2007) 'Bridging the inferential gap: the electronic health record and clinical evidence', *Health Affairs (Millwood)*, 26: w181–91.

Straus, S. E., Ball, C., Balcombe, N., Sheldon, J. and McAlister, F. A. (2005) 'Teaching evidence-based medicine skills can change practice in a community hospital', *Journal of General Internal Medicine*, 20: 340–3.

Straus, S. E., Green, M. L., Bell, D. S., Badgett, R., Davis, D., Gerrity, M., Ortiz, E., Shaneyfelt, T., Whelan, C. and Mangrulkar, R. (2004) 'Evaluating the teaching of evidence-based medicine: conceptual framework', *British Medical Journal*, 329: 1029–32.

Timmermans, S. and Angell, A. (2001) 'Evidence-based medicine, clinical uncertainty, and learning to doctor', *Journal of Health and Social Behavior*, 42: 342–59.

Timmermans, S. and Berg, M. (2003) *The Gold Standard: the challenge of evidence-based medicine and standardization in health care*, Philadelphia, PA: Temple University Press.

Timmermans, S. and Kolker, E. (2004) 'Evidence-based medicine and the reconfiguration of medical knowledge', *Journal of Health and Social Behavior*, 45 (extra issue): 177–93.

Timmermans, S. and Mauck, A. (2005) 'The promises and pitfalls of evidence-based medicine', *Health Affairs*, 24: 18–28.

Wennberg, J. E. (1999) *The Dartmouth Atlas of Health Care 1999*, Chicago, IL: American Hospital Publishing.

Windish, D. M., Huot, S. J. and Green, M. L. (2007) 'Medicine residents' understanding of the biostatistics and results in the medical literature', *Journal of the American Medical Association*, 298: 1010–22.

Wolinsky, F. D. (1988) 'The professional dominance perspective, revisited', *The Milbank Quarterly*, 66 (Suppl. 2): 33–47.

10 Crisis or renaissance?

A sociology of anatomy in UK medical education

Samantha Regan de Bere and Alan Petersen

Teaching anatomy to both under- and postgraduates is in the midst of a downward spiral.

(Older 2004)

Anatomy teaching in the UK is in crisis.

(*Surgery* 2006)

I have no doubt that Anatomy is beginning to undergo a renaissance.
(President of the Anatomical Society of Great Britain and Ireland 2007)

Introduction

Anatomy has a distinctive history in medicine and clinical training. Its story is one of great achievements, but also drama, its narratives redolent with Enlightenment, scandal, professional rivalries and technological innovation. A series of medical controversies surrounding the illegal collection and storage of body tissues in the UK has recently underscored the sensitivities that shroud this field of medical knowledge and practice. Given its colourful and contentious history, it is perhaps unsurprising that anatomy and its practices have come under critical scrutiny. The two quotations that open this chapter would appear to signal something of a watershed in relation to the perceived role of anatomical knowledge in medical education, and fundamental questions have been raised about the content and manner of teaching anatomy. In a series of debates about anatomy, educators have asked: how are subjectivities shaped by knowledge and methods of instruction? How does the manner of teaching and learning anatomy affect practitioners' views on the body, health and illness? Do established methods contribute to the purported lack of empathy or 'poor bedside manner' ascribed to doctors? What are the implications of curricula heavily dominated by anatomy teaching for how doctors practise?

Some anatomists have begun to speak about a renaissance in their discipline, reaffirming the importance of those approaches and practices that have defined the field and arguably served the profession well. This includes rigorous training in anatomical dissection – seen to fulfil multiple purposes, such as allowing the student to become familiar with the fleshy body, to become desensitized to death and to be initiated into the profession. The debate in recent years has become one of dissection versus non-dissection, with proponents of the latter championing the relevance of new approaches based on living and virtual models. In this chapter, we step aside from such arguments to offer a more nuanced, sociological analysis of developments in the pedagogy of anatomy in medical education, and assess the implications for a profession that is purportedly under scruting.

Adopting a broadly genealogical approach, developed by philosopher and historian Michel Foucault (1979, 1981) to explore the character and influence of various discursive practices and forms of knowledge at different periods of time and in different spaces, we examine the conditions that render certain approaches to anatomy teaching both possible and desirable. Tracing the history of anatomy from its development as an opportunistic endeavour to a formalized profession within an autonomous scientific medicine and then a clinically relevant, interdisciplinary and socially accountable field of medical education, one can begin to understand the factors that underpin the profession's rise to prominence and its responses to change.

We argue here that, historically, anatomical instruction can be seen to have played a central role in forging the identity of biomedicine. Recent shifts in medical pedagogic practice occasioned by far-reaching social and technological changes, have presented a significant challenge to the anatomy profession's self-conception. In this chapter, we outline the nature of these changes, and offer an interpretation of the responses that have been made within the profession and beyond. In particular, we contend that evidence of resistance from within the anatomy profession to changes in pedagogy can be seen as indicative of a perceived threat to professional identity and ultimately to medical dominance. We illustrate how anatomy has been called upon to adapt itself to a changing curriculum that is aimed at training a new, socially relevant breed of doctors. Such adaptation is especially evident within the new generation of medical schools within the UK. In this chapter we offer some critical reflections on the direction of pedagogic innovation in anatomy, focusing particularly on the development of scientific medicine and the recent turn towards the so-called humanistic approach.

Learning anatomy: a history of understanding the human

Current discussions about the appropriate content and teaching and learning practices of anatomy can only be fully understood in the light of historically contingent knowledge about the body, its health and vitality and human identity. The different approaches that have been used to understand the human body, and the changing motivations to learn about its health and workings, are of enduring sociological interest. The sociology of health and illness and the sociology of the body have been centrally concerned with epistemological questions about how 'the body' has been variously understood through time and across societies. Both their preoccupations have been with revealing how particular ways of knowing the body are used to shape institutional arrangements and categories (such as 'healthcare' for 'the sick'), social relations (such as between doctors and other healthcare workers and patients) and conceptions of self (such as being ill or well).

Social constructionism has initiated new ways of understanding embodiment. Some constructionists appear to deny the materiality of the body. More sophisticated analyses do not dispense with corporeal matters, but rather draw attention to the implications of changing ideas about the body – and categories of body classification (Williams and Bendelow 1998). Analyses of shifts in epistemologies reveal much about changing conceptions of the human. For example, the rise of the so-called mind–body (Cartesian) dualism during the modern period is seen to represent a fundamental shift from the 'holistic' conception of the person. Such epistemological departures have been integral to the objectification of the body, the development of classificatory systems for understanding the nature and localization of its 'dis-ease' and the practices that constitute the 'medical gaze' (Foucault 1975: Chapter 1).

Given its focus on the detailed structure, functioning and movement of the biophysical body and its lack of reference to the person and their milieu, modern anatomy – perhaps more obviously than other fields of medical knowledge and practice – provides a key site for examining cultural assumptions about what it means to be human, what constitutes normality, and the malleability or otherwise of ourselves and environments. The history of anatomical illustration and imaging techniques and technologies provides a rich source for investigating changing constructions of the body and body ideals through time and space (for example, see Moore and Clarke 1995; Petersen 1998). Discourses and practices of anatomy have changed dramatically over time, and between groups, in line with changing economic, political and social conditions. However, it is widely agreed among scholars that the rise of the scientific worldview has been fundamental to the modern anatomical imagination.

The science of the body: anatomy in modernity

Since its emergence, scientific medicine was strongly wedded to a particular conception of anatomy teaching and learning and of the relationship between the practitioner (the knower) and the patient's body (the known). This conception was reinforced by the rise of germ theory in the nineteenth century, which postulated that disease could be objectively understood as a biophysical phenomenon (Foucault 1975). The epistemology of scientific anatomy was oriented to making up a particular kind of practitioner: the detached, disembodied, rational mechanic of the body-machine.

Foucault talked about the significance of dissection for scientific medicine: his seminal *Birth of the Clinic* described how the rise of biomedicine brought to light that which was previously below the threshold of visibility (Foucault 1975: xii). As Foucault explains:

Generally speaking, it might be said that up to the end of the eighteenth century medicine related much more to health than to normality; it did not begin by analysing a 'regular' functioning of the organism and go on to seek where it had deviated, what it was disturbed by, and how it could be brought back into normal working order; it referred, rather, to qualities of vigour, suppleness, and fluidity, which were lost in illness and which it was the task of medicine to restore.... Nineteenth-century medicine ... was regulated more in accordance with normality than with health; it formed its concepts and prescribed its interventions in relation to a standard of functioning and organic structure, and physiological knowledge – once marginal and purely theoretical knowledge for the doctor – was to become established ... at the very centre of all medical reflexion.

(1975: 35)

Pre-modern medicine had operated under a holistic model of human physical and mental health (Persaud 1967), but the scientific ideal began to separate anatomical and social questions into the different universalistic principles of science-based medicine. In contrast to pre-modern disciplinary spheres of medicine and social science/the humanities, anatomy began to reflect anatomy. Where schematic representations often displayed the body in motion and in its environment, naturalistic explanations disposed with any notions of mediating spirits or governing social laws, and established representations of the body as passive and decontextualized vessels. Thus, the gulf between artistic and expressive depictions of the body, and the factual and scientifically 'real' diagrams institutionalized in formal anatomical study widened (Kemp and Wallace 2000).

While pre-modern 'anatomists' had relied on rather more opportunistic and voyeuristic methods of exploring the body, modern medicalized understanding was supported by technological advance. First, scientific logic had informed the production of sophisticated surgical instruments, which allowed for complex and precise dissection (Dyer and Thorndike 2000). Second, artificial materials provided for the relatively unobtrusive preservation of dead bodies (embalming) and body parts (prosection), and specimen displays were made possible by the use of new artificial media.

Increased communications facilitated the dissemination of anatomical knowledge to a growing medical profession. A profusion of early anatomical imagery was enabled by the advent of the printing press, and the lessons learned from subsequent dissections were made increasingly available during the following five centuries. Sixteenth- and seventeenth-century medical research utilized this widespread information, testing the emerging theories of anatomical endeavour against the 'factual' findings of cadaveric dissection. It was this development that signified a shift in the training of doctors, away from exclusively theoretical and spiritual concerns and towards a formalized education in the structures, functions and pathologies of the human body. The teaching of anatomy by dissection became the mainstay of modern medical education, a symbolic initiation that distinguished medical professionals from practitioners of other established sciences. This approach endured for some while, and latterday reactions to the appearance of alternatives to dissection might well be taken as a sign of its legacy as the defining feature of the profession.

The formal study of the anatomical body in modernity thus became associated with the art of understanding the internal structure and functioning of the body in order to provide insight into the normal and the pathological (Canguilhem 1978). The objective knowledge of static bodily material was quite different to any creative or culturally meaningful observation of the living, breathing and messy performances that were played out by embodied human beings in their social and physical environments.

This mechanistic, as opposed to humanistic, approach to knowing the body was strengthened by the formalizing of medical education in the early twentieth century, particularly as manifest in the Flexner Report of 1910 (Flexner 1910). Flexner's report originated as an indictment of American medical education, but it reflected a medical culture akin to that of the UK, and the climate in which anatomy was to operate for the following hundred years was clearly shaped by its principles. Here, an emphasis on allopathic medicine (based on the scientific method, evidence-based practice and clinical trials), placed mainstream science at the very heart of medical training, and discredited other more holistic forms of healthcare (Beck 2004; Wheatley 1989). Importantly for anatomy, medical training became predicated upon two years of formal study of human anatomy and physiology, followed by two years of clinical practice (Willis 1983).

The challenge of 'postmodern' medicine

Since Flexner, sociologists and other social scientists have increasingly drawn attention to the implications of a reductive understanding of the body-as-machine for how biomedicine is practised. Their critiques have highlighted the limitations this has placed on understanding the multidimensional bases of health and illness, including: inadequate attention to the social and physical environmental determinants of disease; a lack of concern for the person and their embodied experiences; inattention to cultural differences; iatrogenesis (the overuse of drugs and surgery, hospital infections); and burgeoning healthcare costs in modern healthcare systems. That a variety of sociologists and critical theorists (such as Townshend, Illich, Doyal, Navarro, Gorz) have written on these subjects, demonstrates their dominance in contemporary medicine.

At the end of the twentieth century, in the midst of these criticisms, government reforms elevated the social and psychological aspects of clinical education and practice – at (what some described as) the expense of medical 'science'. The policy document *Tomorrow's Doctors* (GMC 1993), and other reports (BMA 1991, 1995; Department of Health 1989), slowed the apparent progression of the 'doctor as scientist', and refocused medicine as a moral, as well as a technoscientific, pursuit. As Corrigan and Pinchen state (this volume), curriculum designers became less concerned with learning biological facts and more focused on dealing with the complexities and uncertainties inherent in medical practice.

Whether developments such as the above represent a significant transformation in the epistemological foundations of anatomy is questionable. On the one hand, recent shifts in emphasis from purely positivistic endeavours to an appreciation of social and political contexts may seem to signal a break with the scientism of modern medicine. On the other, they can be viewed from a non-linear perspective to indicate continuities with a pre-modern past which very much placed the human and his/her (usually his) environment at the centre of the clinical encounter.

The nature of anatomy teaching and the science that underpinned it were thus subject to change in 'late modern' or 'postmodern' medicine. One of the most highly debated influences on anatomy teaching was the introduction to medical education of 'problem-based learning' (PBL). This development was celebrated by many educationalists as a superior pedagogic strategy, and lamented by many anatomists as a threat to the anatomical knowledge acquisition necessary for proficient medical practice. Some anatomical educators argued that PBL was a more suitable approach to the learning of anatomy than the traditional method of cadaveric dissection (Dinsmore *et al.* 1999; Scott 1994). This was a direct reflection of the strong emphasis on the clinical contexts of contemporary medical practice as defined in the UK by the General Medical Council (GMC) in *Tomorrow's Doctors* (1993), whereby learning and developing clinical skills came more to rely on an understanding of surface, clinical and radiological anatomy. Such perspectives advocated learning that developed around areas of clinical importance, supported by anatomical resources such as peer examination, the use of prosections and computer-generated images and simulations.

With *Tomorrow's Doctors*, the GMC effectively brought the focus back to relating the study of human anatomy to the clinical encounter with the patient under observation. This represented an apparent departure from the 'pure knowledge' imperative that had long motivated modern anatomy teaching. New programmes of medical education began to integrate subjects (including anatomy) into problem-based learning (Bligh 1995). For critics of 'traditional' dissection-based anatomy, and proponents of living and virtual anatomies, this was important. PBL was heralded as the most appropriate way of instilling in students a capacity for critical reflection on interpersonal skills and ethics (Leider 1984). It was also considered vital to students' ability to reflect on their own feelings and beliefs about morbidity and mortality – the 'messy' human aspects of anatomical existence.

Avowedly challenging medical dominance, the patient-centred approach of contemporary biomedicine emphasized the relevance of the person's possession and occupation of a personalized and individualized body. Doctors were incited to consider not just structure and function, but also people's sensuous, psychological and social experiences (GMC 1993). The increasing questioning of the traditionally disengaged practitioner led medical trainers to incorporate purportedly humanistic issues into teaching based on a new bio-psycho-social model. In truth, this in itself was not new: the hospice movement in particular demonstrates that such issues have played a role in palliative healthcare for many years. But now it had become a mainstream preoccupation.

One result of these changes in attitude was the General Medical Council's stipulation that significant cuts should be made to the time and resource budgets previously devoted to basic science, and specifically anatomy, courses. Unsurprisingly, the 'mainstream' medical profession resisted this change. Older, providing a much debated article for the *Journal of the Royal College of Surgeons*, stated:

> This reform has lead [*sic*] to a reduction in both time and content of gross anatomical instruction, more than 50% compared with 25 years ago. In some centres, the pendulum has swung so far that gross cadaver-based anatomy is no longer taught. Teaching anatomy to both under- and postgraduates is in the midst of a downward spiral, so their lack of knowledge has become a steady exponential curve.
>
> (2004: 79)

Reactions from within the medical profession were accompanied by a number of responses from external commentators, including educationalists, sociologists and historians, scholars in other academic fields, media journalists, politicians and the general public. Their concerns with the more social and political aspects of anatomy teaching provide the foundations for most of the criticisms that have plagued the profession, not just recently but ever since its conception in antiquity. Though the recent furore has been prompted by reduced curriculum time and resources, ensuing debate became primarily focused around a single issue: the replacement of the traditional method of anatomical instruction – cadaveric dissection – with other approaches to teaching and learning gross anatomy. But underpinning many discussions were more economic, political and sociocultural considerations including:

- Challenges to the dualistic and reductionist thinking about human bodies (posed by postmodern theories, feminist deconstruction, alternative and humanistic medicine).
- Technological innovations that altered how we view, act upon and intervene into the body, and facilitated new methods of instruction that challenged the age-old tradition of cadaveric dissection.
- Commodification, and growing interest in popular cultural portrayals of the body, which to some extent contributed to the demystification of anatomy among the broader population.
- Public reaction against what some had come to see as excesses and abuses in medical practices (demonstrated in government responses to the profession).

These changes provided the backdrop to the purported 'crisis' in the teaching and learning of anatomy in medicine that manifested in the early years of the twenty-first century. We therefore consider next the epistemological issues relating to the possible 're-humanizing' of medicine and the impact of technological advancement on methodological approaches, public and government engagement with the profession, and the notion of a threat to medical dominance, in order to help assess whether anatomy in the UK is indeed in a critical 'downward spiral' or if what it is experiencing might be appropriately described as a 'renaissance'.

Reviewing notions of humanness: the implications for anatomy

We have outlined the development of the mechanistic 'body-as-machine' paradigm of medical science and anatomical learning. The naturalistic body framed by modern anatomists provided doctors and society at large with an essentialist vision of corporeality. An archetypal (typically male) human body filled the pages of anatomy atlases and formed the basis of the standardized models that populated anatomy labs and doctors' consulting rooms (Schiebinger 1986). Any sign of 'difference' came to be perceived as a deviation from the norm – despite the unfixing of the body from its environments for purposes of medical examination, discourses defining abnormality or pathology were increasingly extended to ordering the social and political world. And the sociocultural differences of individuals inhabiting those worlds were explained according to these discourses, along highly politicized and exploitative lines.

Eighteenth- and nineteenth-century social discourses on the body drew upon epistemologies that frequently reduced social organization to the biological bases of those individuals and groups so ordered (Shilling 2003). Gender relations became characterized by reference to biological differences that justified largely patriarchal distributions of roles and power relationships between men and women (Kaplan and Rogers 1990; Martin 1989). Notions of biological 'race' were used to understand and legitimize colonialism, slavery and unequal race relations (Jordan 1982). Sexuality and gender became two-dimensional, whereby previously accepted bodies that lay between male and female ideals were now formally pathologized by what Laqueur refers to as the emergence and dominance of the 'two-sex model' (Laqueur 1990).

Medicine was not free from these discourses; indeed its own discourses frequently *framed* the interpretation of anatomical and aesthetic 'differences' in these terms. Here 'the social' informed 'the medical', and vice versa. Modern anatomy was located within a cultural and political milieu that could adhere to the new scientific and humanistic, egalitarian principles of the Enlightenment project, while at the same time maintaining the unequal treatment of bodies that varied according to gender, race, sexuality, class, age and so on. And, because anatomy had been detached from the study of the social, such inequalities became naturalized – a process for which medicine was not deemed accountable. As a result, unchallenged socially constructed categories found their way into medico-nursing discourses and into the treatment of patients within medical environs.

Anatomy as a profession, practice and field of interest has reflected this naturalization of difference. Through its history, biomedicine has been a deeply gendered profession and field of practice. From the eighteenth to the twentieth century, those relatively few women who were admitted to medical schools were largely excluded from the dissection room, this gendering being only recently challenged during the 1970s (Sappol 2002). The teaching of anatomy has thus been a rite of male passage and a key means of engendering sociability among male recruits and of defining the identity of the mostly male recruits. Women who undertook dissection were often ostracized and masculinized (Petersen and Regan de Bere 2006). The masculinity–femininity dualism that characterizes the practices of anatomical dissection is part and parcel of the more general dichotomization that characterizes the biomedical approach to understanding the body: the separation of mind and body, nature and culture, and object and subject (Shilling and Mellor 1996; Turner 1984).

The implications of biomedical reductionism and dichotomization, however, have become increasingly evident in recent years. Social-constructionist perspectives, in particular, have unsettled the notion of the pre-social or natural body (Shilling 2003; Turner 1992). While contemporary doctors are unlikely to ever refute the fact that bodies clearly have a corporeal reality – they grow, move, decay and ultimately die – they are also beginning to embrace the view that they are social and cultural entities (GMC 1993; NLM 2008). This reflects a contemporary re-connecting of the social with the anatomical, and of the cultural with the biological. At the same time, the increasingly popular holistic view of health acknowledges the inextricable links between mind and body and the importance of patients' lived experiences of health and illness. Today's students consider, for example, the view that people presenting the same symptoms will interpret and respond to them differently, for personal and cultural reasons, and often with implications for the future of the condition (Freund 1982, 1988, 1990).

In a highly individualized society, consideration of how people variously interact with their bodies and experience illness is deemed crucial. More widely, the contemporary body has become viewed as a source of social identity: a site on which we can inscribe who we are, or who we wish to be (Featherstone *et al.* 1991; Turner 1984). This is quite distinct from the body that was long subject to the pathological labelling that derived from modern anatomical discourses – those notions of abnormality that were institutionalized, applied by an apparently objective profession, and served to shape both the medical and social experiences of those so diagnosed (Canguilhem 1978).

This is not merely an indictment of society – the apparent shift towards personalization and individualization in culture and medicine is important for anatomy, in so far as it requires students to assess critically the implications of social and cultural phenomena in addition to learning the established processes of diagnosis, prognosis and treatment. Furthermore, the shift parallels changes in conceptions of contemporary bodies that are themselves a result of technological advancement: the body has become a mirror for the cultural mores of contemporary, technological societies. Postmodern critiques focus on technological change and its facilitation of 'dehumanized', 'post-human', 'technological' or even 'cyborg' bodies. The impact of technological appliances (mobile telephones, PCs, portable CD and MP3 players, virtual reality, gaming devices and so on), alongside developments in health technologies (such as clinical and cosmetic surgery, artificial body parts, reproductive technologies, contraceptive devices) and other technology or technology-induced innovations (GM foods, genetic cloning, synthetic diseases and 'superbugs') all have implications for the ways in which society has come to view bodies and embodied identities.

One particularly significant line of thought has centred on how technologies have changed or are changing our bodies to the extent that our 'embodied' identities have become unstable (Baudrillard 1993; Kelly 1994). Philosophers talk of 'the death of the subject' and the end of the fixed natural body: the idea that in a postmodern world there can be no such thing as a real or core self or an unchangeable body. From the extreme of this point of view there is no underlying human or embodied essence beyond its construction via the diversity of our social roles. Just as their predecessors in pre-medicalized anatomy explored these dimensions of human life, medical scholars have begun to note collaborations between artists, scientists and social scientists, as well as medical educators, in coming to terms with how best to approach the teaching and learning of human anatomy. Educators have argued that it is therefore time for anatomical education to be seriously and rigorously reviewed, in order that it can best serve these transformations.

As we have seen, dissection was historically viewed as a supreme tradition that developed in students a detailed understanding of the structures and functions of the human body. But in the late 1990s and the early twenty-first century, proponents of living anatomy began to champion the use of more live and virtual methods of learning (McLachlan *et al.* 2004; McLachlan and Regan de Bere 2004). This emerged for several reasons. On a practical level, many of the objections levelled at cadaveric dissection were based on quite straightforward disadvantages: dissection is labour intensive and requires skilled anatomy tutors; cadavers are expensive and donated corpses scarce; dead bodies may carry disease (CJD, HIV, hepatitis and tuberculosis), their tissues are dead and therefore unlike living tissues; and the student experience is generally aesthetically unpleasant and stress provoking (Aziz *et al.* 2002).

New technologies have enabled those teaching anatomy to employ a number of sophisticated alternatives to cadaveric dissection. Alongside traditional methods of peer review and prosection, students are now able to learn from highly accurate, often 3D, imaging of various anatomical structures (McLachlan *et al.* 2004). In addition, anatomical simulation has now been made available in the form of patient 'dummies': lifelike models that can allegedly communicate the idea of living, breathing human beings more effectively than real, but dead, human corpses (Aziz *et al.* 2002). Reflecting the individualization of the body, such dummies come in various shapes and sizes, including different genders, ages, skin tones and even hairstyles. Many are fitted with audio systems that reproduce human 'noises', such as coughing, complaining, vomiting and so on. Reports from anatomy tutors employing these dummies demonstrate that students often responded as they would to real patients, holding the models hands and developing a sense of empathy for their hypothetical suffering (BBC News 2002). Developments in anatomy have thus reflected the growing use of simulation in medical education more generally (McLachlan *et al.* 2004), although recent research has suggested a mixed economy of methods should feature simulation as a supplement to dissection, rather than a method to be used on its own (Moxham and Patel 2008).

The variety of non-dissection methods of teaching anatomy is broad non-dissection methods of teaching anatomy is broad and widely discussed in anatomical and medical education literatures. Their importance here is that they appear to signal a major discursive shift in medical training, to a much more serious emphasis placed on identity, cultural politics and human emotion (BMA 1991; GMC 1993). Medical educators, both in the UK and abroad, have responded accordingly (Aziz *et al.* 2002; Dangerfield *et al.* 1996; Dyer and Thorndike 2000), embracing, to a greater or lesser extent, the alleged humanizing of doctors via the introduction of the social sciences and medical humanities to curricula. This has involved exploration of the sociohistorical and political meanings inherent in anatomical understandings as applied to medical knowledge, and the celebration of aesthetic medicine: the 'creative and uncertain art' – as opposed to the previously precise but destructive process – of working with human bodies (Bleakley *et al.* 2006).

Of course, attitudinal change has been far from straightforward and the idea of humanistic, social medicine has certainly been received with a less-than-universal welcome within some medical spheres. However, the social relevance of the departure from the fixed, machine body is clear in contemporary constructions of multiple 'bodies'. Sociological and cultural theories of the body have made reference to pluralism, difference and hybridization (Featherstone 2000), and this has serious implications for how students learn, teach and practise medicine. If the body has been portrayed as a site for 'the life project' – a key site for identity construction and, by implication, lived experience – then viewing the anatomical body as a passive, mechanical object is no longer sufficient. Tutors and students of anatomy are thus increasingly faced with the task of incorporating social relevance into their programmes of teaching and learning.

The selection of various anatomical teaching methods is typically related to clinical and very often practical questions that we lack adequate expertise to discuss. However, anatomy departments have also now begun to frame their curriculum design in more psychological and social terms than was typical in the past. While few educators would reject the use of cadavers as a method fit for education and practice, they have nevertheless debated the 'dehumanizing' nature of cadaveric dissection, whereby students are required to learn about the living from the dead. Although dissection is useful in preparing raw recruits to medicine for developing 'defence mechanisms' against the stress of working with deep anatomy, research has demonstrated that it also imbues new medics with a clinically disengaged approach to their work. In the extreme, this can lead to a lack of empathy for the patient and his or her individuality as a human person (Dinsmore *et al.* 1999; McLachlan *et al.* 2004).

This in itself fits with the scientific conception of anatomy and detached, dualistic medicine that we have already discussed. Popular imagery has frequently involved disengaged and inhumane pioneers, the 'mad scientist' uncluttered by any regard for human life or death and, as an extension of this, a lack of respect for the body itself. This is more poignant when the notion of the body as the prime site for identity is taken into account. The extent to which biomedicine has objectified the body became apparent with the Alder Hey report of 2001, which revealed the unethical and illegal removal and retention of body parts at the Liverpool children's hospital. The ensuing controversy and the regulatory policies that have followed in its wake and that of other medical controversies around the same time (such as the Bristol Royal Infirmary controversy and the Harold Shipman case) underlined the extent to which taken-for-granted biomedical practices are now under close scrutiny.

For example, the Bristol Royal Infirmary Inquiry report included the recommendation that greater priority be given to non-clinical aspects of care and that healthcare professionals be educated in communication skills which 'include the ability to engage with patients on an emotional level, to listen, to assess how much information a patient wants to know, and to convey information with clarity and sympathy' (Recommendation 59, Bristol Royal Infirmary Inquiry 2001). It also recommended that there be a change in the culture of the NHS where much of medicine is practised in the UK. This included 'tribalism' and 'a hierarchical approach' within and between professional groups which potentially compromised the safety and quality of care (2001: 266–77). This has become a central issue for contemporary anatomists, whose dwindling supply of cadaveric resources has resulted primarily from government policies (particularly the 2004 Human Tissue Act), brought about by a perceived decline in public trust and an increased emphasis on politico-legal discourses (Regan de Bere and Petersen 2006).

Anatomy, governance and public trust

The emergence in the early twenty-first century of a potentially damaging dichotomous relationship that served to divide anatomists who supported dissection and those who did not, is significant. It is important not only pedagogically, but also in terms of reinforcing a split within a profession that had already suffered from pressures exerted by perceived government intrusion into their field of expertise. *Tomorrow's Doctors* (2003) signified a shift in the types of doctors government policy had defined as desirable. It also represented a potential threat to the autonomy of a profession that had for at least a century defined the nature and scope of its training itself. This relative loss of autonomy has been strongly linked to calls for greater accountability within the medical profession.

A shift towards a more critical and litigious culture has rendered the current medical profession more open to question (Phillips 2004). The negative media reporting that has dogged recent events, such as occurred at Alder Hey and

Bristol Royal Infirmary, has provoked a reconsideration of anatomical pedagogic endeavours, albeit in relation to a new set of social conditions, including: a greater receptivity to ethics and human rights; technological innovations (for example, routine use of MRIs, CAT scans, lifelike plastinated models); and changes in the nature of healthcare, with a greater focus on chronic conditions, community-based care and self-care. In the UK, one development contributing to the growing receptivity to alternative approaches to the teaching and learning of anatomy, especially in the new-generation medical schools, was the new Human Tissue Act, enacted in June 2004, which followed in the wake of public responses to the above events. This Act arguably contributed to a shortage of body donations and the search for newer approaches that do not involve dissection.

The methods employed by anatomists throughout history have been alternately revered and feared, celebrated and discredited. Since its beginnings, anatomical dissection has been contentious, within the church and among some sections of the public, including the families of those who were subject to dissection. As is well known from the histories of anatomy, the anatomy profession dissected the cadavers of the poor, the destitute and the criminally insane in order to further anatomical knowledge (Richardson 2001; Sappol 2002). Public responses to such practices have always been noted, but in earlier days had lesser impacts on the work of a profession that now operates within a highly litigious culture. For eighteenth-century anatomists, although political governance had become rationalized and bureaucratized, medicine relied on a more autonomous legitimacy than most contemporary institutions.

Nevertheless, the difficult relationship between dissection and popular opinion has always been an issue. The original Human Tissue Acts for example, were the result of declining public trust following the media-provoked 'Burkophobia' of the nineteenth century, and the association of anatomy with unethical procedures:

> scarcely a day passes but reports are circulated of the supposed sacrifice of fresh victims to the 'interests of science'. We suppose in future, this epidemic [Burkophobia] will as regularly make its appearance in winter as the hydrophobia does in the summer.
>
> (*York Chronicle 1831*, cited in Richardson 2001)

The mass media have arguably played a key role in heightening public concerns about medical practices. In the public imagination, the more controversial activities of anatomists (such as 'body snatching') have always been 'exposed' by a sensational media, public scandals and panic-inspiring crusaders outside of the field (Richardson 2001). By framing issues in particular ways – by attention to certain facts, values and images and the use of particular voices – the media are likely to play an important role in setting the agenda for public debate and policy action. Regan de Bere and Petersen's study of UK media coverage highlighted how both the broadsheet and tabloid press present anatomy via a number of frames, both positive (such as stories of awe and amazement, medical break-throughs, stories of heroism) and negative (for example, images of Frankenstein, Brave New World, 'rape of the body') (Regan de Bere and Petersen 2006). The latter included unscrupulous medical research and fears over the infringement of human rights.

Attention to such concerns is perhaps unsurprising, given the aforementioned controversies that preceded their study. Regan de Bere and Petersen argued that the contemporary news media represent a society more attuned than in the past to challenging medical-expert knowledge claims, and one in which litigation has far more influence than it had previously. However, their analysis also revealed that media coverage portrays anatomy teaching and research in a partial and in sometimes confusing and contradictory ways. The focus is on more emotive issues, with relatively little systematic attention given to other aspects of anatomy, such as pedagogical debates about the use or non-use of cadaveric dis-section, the use of peer assessment and virtual technologies in teaching and learning, and instruction through the use of performative and other artistic means (Regan de Bere and Petersen 2006: 86). This may lead to a public representation of anatomy that is partial, thus limiting debate on the range of issues of relev-ance to current anatomy practice, the training of new doctors, and the profession of medicine as a whole.

It is within these social, ethical and public contexts that critics of dissection have turned to the role of technological change in directing a more creative and 'living' science, shaping anatomy and medical education itself. Technological advances have precipitated the availability of a wide range of alternatives to cadaveric dissection for examining bodies and, at the same time, have trans-formed the nature of those very bodies we seek to understand, and the culture in which we try to understand them. But dissection remains a popular teaching methodology, and its relevance here is also in its role as victim to the same mys-tifying processes evoked in educational circles as those that have occurred as a result of sensational press coverage.

More recent academic and clinical papers have highlighted a growing consen-sus within the field that a combination of dissection and living and virtual anato-mies now offers the most educationally effective and clinically relevant approach to teaching doctors (Mattick and Regan de Bere 2008; Moxham and Patel 2008). Such studies have set out to debunk the myths brought about by dichotomizing approaches, in favour of exploring the virtues of a mixed economy of methods. The likely directions that these endeavours may take are yet to be discovered, but according to the most recent survey of anatomy tutors from a census of all the UK medical schools, perceptions on the ground are encouragingly positive (Mattick and Regan de Bere 2008).

Conclusions

The cautions that opened this chapter represented fears of a decline in anatomy as a medical field, and we have demonstrated that the last 15 years have indeed witnessed serious shifts in thinking about anatomical knowledge and practice. But shifts in emphasis do not herald the demise of anatomy as a key subject, discipline or profession. Conversely, historical analysis demonstrates that anatomy is resilient – it has consistently changed but it has continued to hold a central position in medical education and research, and retained elements of its character throughout time. Its major challenge is to adapt to the economic, political and sociocultural changes that shape the practices of medicine of which anatomy is still arguably the core. Thus the responses of those such as Older (2004) may not represent dying voices, or any clear sidelining of anatomists in the face of *Tomorrow's Doctors*. Reconfigured as a positive force, they may instead provide a counterpoint that signifies the reassertion of anatomy's power and professional autonomy.

The impact of *Tomorrow's Doctors*, the alleged humanistic turn and the distinction between the traditional and problem-based learning (PBL) approaches, the predominance of the dissection versus non-dissection debate, concerns about a decline in public trust and increased government intrusion into the field of anatomy can all be viewed as important features of anatomy's character in the early years of the twenty-first century. These can also be seen as manifestations of the profession's fears, and of a more medically aware and consumer-oriented public. In reflecting on the role of anatomy in medical education, our sociohistorical overview emphasizes that it is not so much the economic and sociocultural imperatives shaping developments in curricula that is interesting, but rather professional and public responses to change. Anatomy has been forced to adapt itself to the reality of a reduced portion of curriculum time, while at the same time, in the midst of internal debate and external pressure, to promote the importance of its role to medicine and the training of new doctors.

Sociologically, then, we can begin to appreciate that the profession of anatomy has been forced to articulate a clear role in the training of doctors. The high-profile reviewing of anatomy that engages anatomists, sociologists, the media and the public alike, demonstrates that anatomy still has a very strong position in medical culture and education, albeit one in which it must step up to the challenge of addressing sociocultural change. And all of this may in fact move anatomy rather more towards the 'renaissance' referred to by the President of the Anatomical Society of Great Britain and Ireland, than to the 'downward spiral' feared by many of its members.

References

Aziz, A., McKenzie, J., Wilson, J., Cowie, R., Ayeni, S. and Dunn, B. (2002) 'The human cadaver in the age of biomedical informatics', *Anatomical Record (New Anatomy)*, 269: 20–32.

Bauchner, H. and Vinci, R. (2001) 'What have we learnt from the Alder Hey affair?', *British Medical Journal*, 322: 309–10.

Baudrillard, J. (1993) *Symbolic Exchange and Death*, London: Sage.

BBC News (2002) 'University defends "corpse-free classes"', *BBC News On-line*, 30

September, online at http://news.bbc.co.uk/1/hi/health/2288631.stm (accessed December 2008).

Beck, A. H. (2004) 'The Flexner Report and the standardization of American medical education', *Student Journal of the American Medical Association* 291: 2139–40.

Bleakley, A., Marshall, R. and Brömer, R. (2006) 'Toward an aesthetic medicine: developing a core medical humanities undergraduate curriculum', *Journal of Medical Humanities*, 27: 197–214.

Bligh, J. (1995) 'Problem-based, small-group learning: an idea whose time has come', *British Medical Journal*, 311: 342–3.

Bristol Royal Infirmary Inquiry (2001) *Learning from Bristol: the report of the public inquiry into children's heart surgery at the Bristol Royal Infirmary 1984–1995*, online at www.bristol-inquiry.org.uk/final_report/rpt_print.htm (accessed June 2008).

British Medical Association (BMA) (1991) *Report of the Medical Academic Staff Working Party on the Undergraduate Curriculum*, London: British Medical Association.

—— (1995) *Report of the BMA Working Party on Medical Education 1995*, London: British Medical Association.

Canguilhem, G. (1978) *On the Normal and Pathological (Studies in the History of Modern Science)*, Dordrecht: Kluwer Academic Publishers.

Dangerfield, P. H., Bligh, J., Leinster, S. and Griffiths, R. (1996) 'Curriculum reform in Britain and its effects on anatomy', *Clinical Anatomy*, 6: 418 (abstract).

Department of Health (1989) *France Report: undergraduate medical and dental education 1st report 1989*, London: HMSO.

Dinsmore, C. E., Daugherty, S. and Zeitz, H. J. (1999) 'Teaching and learning gross anatomy: dissection, prosection or "both of the above?"', *Clinical Anatomy*, 12: 110–14.

Dyer, G. S. M. and Thorndike, M. E. L. (2000) 'Quidne mortui vivos docent? The evolving purpose of human dissection in medical education', *Academic Medicine*, 75: 969–79.

Featherstone, M. (ed.) (2000) *Body Modification*, London: Sage.

Featherstone, M., Hepworth, M. and Turner, B. (eds) (1991) *The Body: social process and cultural theory*, London: Sage.

Flexner, A. (1910) *Medical Education in the United States and Canada: bulletin number four*, New York: Carnegie Foundation for the Advancement of Teaching.

Foucault, M. (1975) *The Birth of the Clinic: an archeology of medical perception*, New York: Vintage Books.

—— (1979) *Discipline and Punish: the birth of the prison*, Harmondsworth: Penguin.

—— (1981) *The History of Sexuality, Vol. 1. An introduction*, Harmondsworth: Penguin.

Freund, P. (1982) *The Civilized Body: social domination, control and health*, Philadelphia, PA: Temple University Press.

—— (1988) 'Understanding socialized human nature', *Theory and Society*, 17: 839–64.

—— (1990) 'The expressive body: a common ground for the sociology of the emotions and health and illness', *Sociology of Health and Illness*, 12: 454–77.

General Medical Council (GMC) (1993) *Tomorrow's Doctors: recommendations on undergraduate medical education*, London: General Medical Council.

Jordan, W. (1982) 'First Impressions: initial English confrontations with Africans', in C. Husband (ed.) *'Race' in Britain*, London: Hutchinson.

Kaplan, G. and Rogers, L. (1990) 'The definition of male and female. Biological reductionism and the sanctions of normality', in S. Gunew (ed.) *Feminist Knowledge, Critique and Construct*, London: Routledge.

Kelly, K. (1994) *Out of Control: the new biology of machines*, London: Fourth Estate.

Kemp, M. and Wallace, M. (2000) *Spectacular Bodies: the art and science of the human body from Leonardo to now*, London: Hayward Gallery Publishing.

Laqueur, T. (1990) *Making Sex: body and gender from the Greeks to Freud*, Cambridge, MA: Harvard University Press.

Leider, S. R. (1984) 'An Australian approach to medical education – the Newcastle experience', *Medical Journal of Australia*, 140: 158–62.

Levin, D. M. (1990) 'The discursive formation of the body in the history of medicine', *Journal of Medicine and Philosophy*, 15: 515–38.

Martin, E. (1989) *The Woman in the Body: a cultural analysis of reproduction*, Boston, MA: Beacon Press.

Mattick, K. and Regan de Bere, S. (2008) *Is Anatomy Different? A survey of views of UK anatomy tutors*, Higher Education Academy Subject Centre for Medicine, Dentistry and Veterinary Medicine (MEDEV), online at www.medev.ac.uk/miniproject_resources/411/411_Final_report_31_Jul_08.doc (accessed December 2008).

McLachlan, J. C. and Regan de Bere, S. (2004) 'How we teach anatomy without cadavers', *Clinical Teacher*, 1: 49–52.

McLachlan, J. C., Aiton, J. F., Whiten, S. C. and Smart, S. D. (1997) '3-D modelling of human embryo morphology using QuickTime VR™', in T. Strachan, S. Lindsay and D. Wilson (eds) *Molecular Genetics of Human Development*, Oxford: Bios Scientific Publishers.

McLachlan, J. C., Bligh, J., Bradley, P. and Searle, J. (2004) 'Teaching anatomy without cadavers', *Medical Education*, 38: 418–24.

Moore, L. J. and Clarke, A. (1995) 'Clitoral conventions and transgressions: graphic representations in anatomy texts, c1900–1991', *Feminist Studies*, 21: 255–301.

Moxham, B. J. and Patel, K. M. (2008) 'The relationship between learning outcomes and methods of teaching anatomy as perceived by professional anatomists', *Clinical Anatomy*, 21: 182–9.

National Library of Medicine (2008) *Visionary Anatomies*, online at www.nlm.nih.gov/exhibition/dreamanatomy (accessed December 2008).

Older, J. (2004) 'Anatomy: a must for teaching the next generation', *The Surgeon: Journal of the Royal Colleges of Surgeons of Edinburgh and Ireland*, April: 79–90.

Persaud, T. (1967) *A History of Anatomy: the post-Vesalian era*, Springfield, IL: Charles C. Thomas.

Petersen, A. (1998) 'Sexing the body: representations of sex differences in *Gray's Anatomy*, 1858 to the present', *Body and Society*, 4: 1–15.

Petersen, A. and Regan de Bere, S. (2006) 'Dissecting medicine: gender biases in the discourses and practices of medical anatomy', in D. Rosenfeld and C. Faircloth (eds) *Medicalized Masculinities*, Philadelphia, PA: Temple University Press.

Phillips, S. (2004) 'The return of the body snatchers', *Times Higher*, 26 March, online at www.timeshighereducation.co.uk/story.asp?storyCode=187687&sectioncode=26 (accessed December 2008).

Porter, R. (1997) *The Greatest Benefit to Mankind: a medical history of humanity from antiquity to the present*, London: HarperCollins.

——— (2003) *Blood and Guts: a short history of medicine*, London: Penguin.

Regan de Bere, S. and Petersen, A. (2006) 'Out of the dissecting room: news media portrayal of human anatomy teaching and research', *Social Science and Medicine*, 63: 76–88.

Richardson, R. (2001) *Death, Dissection and the Destitute*, London: Penguin.

Sappol, M. (2002) *A Traffic in Dead Bodies: anatomy and embodied social identity in nineteenth-century America*, Princeton, NJ and Oxford: Princeton University Press.

Schiebinger, L. (1986) 'Skeletons in the closet: the first illustrations of the female skeleton in eighteenth-century anatomy', *Representations*, 14 (Spring): 42–82.

—— (1990) 'The anatomy of difference: race and sex in eighteenth-century science', *Eighteenth-Century Studies*, 23: 387–405.

Schon, D. A. (1987) *Educating the Reflective Practitioner: toward a new design of teaching and learning in the professions*, San Francisco, CA: Jossey-Bass.

Scott, T. M. (1994) 'A care-based anatomy course', *Medical Education*, 28: 68–73.

Shilling, C. (2003) *The Body and Social Theory*, 2nd edn, London: Sage.

Shilling, C. and Mellor, P. A. (1996) 'Embodiment, structuration theory and modernity: mind/body dualism and the repression of sensuality', *Body and Society*, 2: 1–15.

Starr, P. (1982) *The Social Transformation of American Medicine: the rise of a sovereign profession and the making of a vast industry*, New York: Basic Books.

Stillman, P. L., Ruggill, J. S. and Sabers, D. L. (1978) 'The use of live models in the teaching of gross anatomy', *Medical Education*, 12: 114–16.

Turner, B. (1984) *The Body and Society*, Oxford: Blackwell.

—— (1987*) Medical Power and Social Knowledge*, London: Sage.

—— (1990) 'The interdisciplinary curriculum: from social medicine to postmodernism', *Sociology of Health and Illness*, 12: 1–23.

—— (1992) *Regulating Bodies: essays in medical sociology*, London: Routledge.

Wheatley, S. C. (1989) *The Politics of Philanthropy: Abraham Flexner and medical education*, Madison: University. of Wisconsin Press.

Williams, S. and Bendelow, G. (1998) *The Lived Body: sociological themes, embodied issues*, London: Routledge.

Willis, E. (1983) *Medical Dominance: the division of labour in Australian healthcare*, Sydney: George Allen and Unwin.

11 Bioethics and medical education

Lessons from the United States

Carla C. Keirns, Michael D. Fetters and Raymond G. De Vries[1]

> In America ... we devise an ingeniously brutal and degrading way to train our doctors and charge them upwards of $100,000 for the privilege; we wilfully ignore the poor, and pay our doctors the highest incomes of any doctors in the world – and then try to correct the situation with an ethics consultation service and a few hours of humanities in the medical curriculum.... The suggestion might be funny if it were not made with such sincerity.
>
> (Elliott 1999: 22)

We know of a philosophy professor who, on the first day of his ethics class, announces to his students that Satan could easily get an 'A' in his course – his way of pointing out that rigorous study of moral theory and thorough deliberation on specific ethical dilemmas will do nothing to make one an ethical person. Our professor friend goes on to tell his students that in-depth understanding of moral philosophy may, in fact, equip students to be *less* ethical, providing them with a way to rationalize unethical behaviour. This idea – that one cannot teach others to be moral – has long been the fly in the ointment of ethics education, often used to resist the introduction of courses on ethics in professional schools and graduate programmes.

In spite of this general attitude about ethics education and legendary resistance to curricular change on the part of medical schools, bioethics has, over the course of the last 30 years, become a *required* part of the education of tomorrow's physicians. It is not easy for *any* new course to worm its way into the curriculum of a medical school. While the introduction of a new area of study may seem a routine event – after all, courses and course content must adjust as new knowledge is developed and as societies change – instructional hours in the medical-school curriculum are highly prized and fiercely contested (Bloom 1988; Christakis 1995). How did bioethics – a field that is decidedly not scientific or therapeutic – secure a place alongside clinical skills, anatomy, physiology and pharmacology as an essential content area and set of skills to be taught in medical school? What is the content of bioethics instruction? How (if at all) has the addition of bioethics training influenced the way medicine is practised? In order to answer these questions we need to know something of the history of bioethics.

A very short history of bioethics

Up until the 1960s, the ethical work of medicine was done under the rubric of 'medical ethics', an area of enquiry that was developed, taught and transmitted by the medical profession itself. In the 1960s and 1970s a series of scandals, together with unprecedented technological challenges in medicine, transformed the insider's game of medical ethics to an interdisciplinary project that came to be called 'bioethics'. The ethics of medicine became a topic, not just for medical practitioners, but for scholars from the humanities and social sciences; these 'strangers' to the clinic and the research laboratory began to make judgements about the moral problems of medicine (Jonsen 1998; Rothman 1991). Medical ethics – sometimes called 'medical morality' – focused on concepts like medical privacy, putting patient interests first, and relationships between and among the healing professions; bioethics expanded that focus, directing attention to patient autonomy, informed consent and shared decision-making, particularly for diagnoses such as cancer (Lerner 2004: 507–21).

Bioethics was born in the second half of the twentieth century, a period marked by rapid social and cultural changes, two of which have special significance for the move from medical- to bio-ethics: the proliferation of new medical technologies and the rise of the anti-war, civil and women's rights movements. In the 1960s, the Vietnam War and the oppression of minorities and women led to widespread questioning of governmental power and institutional authority. The medical establishment (and the doctors who ran it) did not escape the cultural critique of power. The authority of physicians and trust in medicine, already made suspect by this general challenge to society's institutions, suffered further as a result of several well-publicized scandals in medical research. A sceptical public was made more cynical after learning about research projects that exposed patients to illnesses and toxic treatments without their knowledge or consent.

In this cultural climate, old-style medical ethics – granting unilateral authority to physicians to make decisions about certain aspects of life, death and medical care – was deemed insufficient. New technologies such as the ventilator, incubator and artificial feeding tube brought the promise of success in medicine's long struggle with disease and death, but they also increased the risk of prolonged suffering and technological dependence. Doctors were not trusted to respond to the pressing questions created by the new machines of medicine. From the 'God committees' of 1960s' Seattle – groups of physicians and lay people charged with deciding who would and would not have access to highly expensive dialysis machines – to deliberations on brain-death criteria and organ transplant, to debates about genetic enhancement, physicians were (and are) no longer trusted to be the sole decision-makers on matters medical. Debates over these and other issues, including patient's rights, moved from bedsides and hospital conference rooms to newspapers and legislatures.

Forged in the United States, it is no surprise that the field of bioethics has a peculiarly American, individualist character where autonomy and empowerment play a central role (Wolpe 1998). Interestingly and often unnoticed, bioethics and the medical ethics it seeks to replace share a profoundly individualistic approach to the problems of medicine. Both medical ethics and bioethics assume a patient is a rational and autonomous individual whose relationships to family, community and society are essentially irrelevant to the decisions to be made at the bedside. Bioethics merely shifts the power to make decisions from the (paternalist) physician to the patient. This singular focus on the individual keeps economic and resource-allocation decisions out of (bio)ethical discussions, even though they have proved critical in many cases. For example, the ethical problem of who should have dialysis (and therefore be allowed to live), which led to the 1960s' 'God committees', was not ultimately solved by bioethics. Rather, the problem went away when the US Congress decided to pay for dialysis for all Americans. Similarly, the Quinlan and Cruzan cases – each involving a woman in a persistent vegetative state kept alive by artificial means – were manifestations of the fee-for-service medicine of the 1970s and 1980s, in which patients feared being forced to endure over-treatment, suffering and the bankrupting of their families in the course of their deaths. These cases led to judicial and legislative determinations that patients (or their legally designated decision-makers) can request removal of a ventilator or a feeding tube even if death will result.

Looking back on the twentieth century, public interest in medicine, technology and the goals of healthcare seems almost unavoidable. In fact, given the intersection of an ageing population, the proliferation of 'halfway' technologies that could ameliorate but not cure, crises in medical costs and social movements for civil rights, patients' rights, and disability rights, conflicts about the means and ends of medical care were inevitable. Most interesting to a sociologist in this turn of events is *how* this new-found public interest in medicine was channelled. Notice that problems such as the withholding of life-sustaining treatment, organ allocation and decision-making in neonatal intensive-care units came to be seen as questions of *ethics* rather than narrowly medical-technical questions. Notice, too, that ethics, as the dominant mode of understanding these problems, strips away the social, economic and political context in which these problems are generated and defined.

Working within American culture, early bioethicists such as Paul Ramsey (Princeton), John Fletcher (University of Virginia), Daniel Callahan (Hastings Center), and André Hellegers (Georgetown) framed these 'problems in medical care' as ethical problems. These men and the field they helped to create offered compromise solutions that could be accepted by the medical profession as workable, the legal profession as logical and the public as fair. Had bioethicists chosen a more social focus, calling on the disciplines of sociology, social work, economics and political science, the field would look quite different, seeking political reform, building public programmes and promoting social justice. As we will see, this individualist slant is an important part of the explanation of the acceptance of bioethics in medical-school curricula.

(Bio)ethics instruction in medical education

As we noted above, medical training has long included instruction on medical morality, the etiquette of practice and that old chestnut, 'the art of medicine'. Through the nineteenth century, the 'art of medicine' class usually meant practical advice about how to get and keep patients, matters of trust such as confidentiality, but also issues of practical concern such as the delicate matter of billing for services. Subjects such as medical jurisprudence and medical police – covering public health, the roles of physicians in public institutions and malpractice – were also sometimes included. Codes of ethics were part of the curriculum at some institutions, with Manchester (UK) physician Thomas Percival's code of 1803, the basis for many later codes of ethics, serving as a model for medical training. Sociologists have critiqued these nineteenth- and early-twentieth-century codes of ethics as self-serving and protectionist. In general these codes emphasized responsibility to care for the sick, but they also sought independence from outside regulation, prohibited consultation with homoeopaths and other 'irregular' medical practitioners, limited advertising of services, banned participation in abortion and allowed the splitting of fees with referring physicians.

The shift from medical ethics to bioethics that occurred in the 1960s changed the way ethics was taught to medical students. As early as 1972 the new field of bioethics had entered the medical curriculum at 17 American schools (Veatch 1973: 97–102). By 1974 this had expanded to 56 (Veatch and Sollitto 1976: 1030) and by the 1980s some training in ethics was required for *all* medical students in the United States. In 1985, a consensus conference identified the minimal content areas for an ethics curriculum to include identifying moral aspects of medical practice, obtaining valid consent for treatment, assessment of competence to consent, principles for managing patient refusals, justifications for withholding information and breaching confidentiality, and management of terminal illness (Culver *et al.* 1985: 233–56).

The current requirement in the US – set by the Liaison Committee on Medical Education (LCME), the accrediting authority for medical education programmes leading to the MD degree in the US – is specified in the 'Accreditation Standards', Educational Objective 23:

1 A medical school must teach medical ethics and human values, and require its students to exhibit scrupulous ethical principles in caring for patients, and in relating to patients' families and to others involved in patient care.
2 Each school should assure that students receive instruction in appropriate medical ethics, human values, and communication skills before engaging in patient care activities. As students take on increasingly more active roles in patient care during their progression through the curriculum, adherence to ethical principles should be observed and evaluated, and reinforced through formal instructional efforts.
3 In student–patient interactions there should be a means for identifying

possible breaches of ethics in patient care, either through faculty/resi-dent observation of the encounter, patient reporting, or some other appropriate method.

4   'Scrupulous ethical principles' imply characteristics like honesty, integ-rity, maintenance of confidentiality, and respect for patients, patients' families, other students, and other health professionals. The school's educational objectives may identify additional dimensions of ethical behavior to be exhibited in patient-care settings.

(www.lcme.org/standard.htm, accessed 5 May 2008)

The introduction of bioethics into medical education moved ethics training from an undifferentiated combination of ethics and etiquette – to separate instruction in:

1   Moral theory and the ethical dilemmas of medicine.
2   (Proper) professionalism.

Medical professionalism, shorn of the self-interested aspects found in earlier codes of ethics, is now taught in conjunction with the 'white-coat ceremony'. Begun in 1993 at Columbia University, this ceremony is seen as an opportunity for medical educators to teach the virtues of altruism, accountability, excellence, duty, honour, respect for others and compassion. The ceremony itself – now con-ducted in more than 100 US schools of medicine and osteopathy as well as many in the UK, Europe and Israel – typically involves first- or second-year medical students (and their families) gathered to hear an eminent physician role model speak on the professional obligations of physicians, the donning of the white coat, the symbol of physician authority, and the recitation of an oath (Hippocratic or some variation). Some schools use the white-coat ceremony as the culmination of a series of courses on 'professional responsibility'. Rhodes (2001: 504) describes the white-coat ceremony at the Mount Sinai School of Medicine in New York City as the 'centrepiece' of 'six medical ethics modules … designed to teach the central elements of professional responsibility and to explain how these requisite attitudes and behaviors are expressed in doctor–patient interactions, in interactions with peers, and in clinical decisions'. Rhodes is not alone in seeing this aspect of ethics education as a return to the medical-insider perspective of 'medical ethics' rather than the external watchdog role of 'bioethics'.

The white-coat ceremony, while increasingly popular, has been criticized by both medical educators and bioethicists. Robert Veatch (2002), a well-known American bioethicist, believes that first-year medical students are not prepared to take any sort of oath related to the *practice* of medicine, and that the 'robing' (or 'cloaking') aspects of the ceremony created an unhealthy separation between these would-be doctors and their communities of origin. Others worry that the ceremony 'fosters a sense of entitlement whereby authority is based on title and uniform' rather than on trust (Russell 2002: 56).

The teaching of *bioethics* to medical students has no ritual centrepiece like the white-coat ceremony. Although it is a required part of the medical-school curriculum, there is widespread disagreement and diversity in the content, form and goals of bioethics training. Bioethics is taught using lecture formats, discussions, role-modelling, debriefing and journalling. Sometimes it is taught within a context of medical humanities, medical law, moral philosophy and ethics, and other times as a branch of clinical medicine. Perhaps the most common method of teaching bioethics is a mix of 'moral philosophy light' and case-based discussions. Drawing on 'principlism' – an approach to ethics that distinguishes the principles of autonomy, beneficence, justice and non-maleficence – students are presented with a moral dilemma and taught to identify the critical ethical issues at stake and to find ways to resolve the dilemma respectfully. Less frequently students are taught a number of ethical theories ranging from virtue ethics, to casuistry, to care ethics (Cocking and Oakley 2001; Drane 1988). Textbooks intended for medical students include a smattering of moral theory and the review of high-profile controversies in bioethics involving the limits of technology, the right of refusal, the protection of confidentiality and informed consent.

In the past 15 years, bioethics education has been criticized for emphasizing the extraordinary rather than the typical case. Unusual and even bizarre cases add interest to bioethics discussion groups, but make bioethics instruction irrelevant to the ethical problems that medical students face in their clinical clerkships and unhelpful in responding to problems of routine clinical care. Feudtner *et al.* (1994) are among the advocates for making ethics training more relevant to the actual experiences of medical students, rather than focusing on ethical dilemmas they will not face until they are in independent practice. In response, an approach dubbed 'ward ethics' has been developed with case material relevant to the medical-student role such as disclosing one's student status, how to challenge one's clinical superiors and how to respond to a colleague's derogatory remarks about patients. While parallel to many of the issues in traditional textbooks of bioethics, the ward ethics approach is designed to be developmentally appropriate – presenting principles and scenarios relevant to medical students' day-to-day experience. Partly to address these challenges, some schools have instituted formal mechanisms for reflection during the clinical years, including narrative-writing and discussion groups (Charon 2006).

A wide body of evidence drawn from ethnographies, autobiographies and novels shows how ethics instruction competes with a clinical and training environment in which overwork, exhaustion, intimidation and inadequate resources constrain the actions of healthcare providers at all levels. Fred Hafferty (1998; Hafferty and Franks 1994; and with Castellani in Chapter 2 of this *Handbook*) emphasizes the importance of the hidden curriculum in shaping the experience of medical trainees. Hafferty makes the case that medical students learn what is *really* important from interpersonal interactions, institutional policies and institutional resource-allocation decisions. Brainard and Brislen (2007) put it more pointedly, arguing that professionalism education at their medical school was systematically undercut by unprofessional behaviour by faculty. In response to these kinds of critiques, the American Council on Graduate Medical Education has sought to improve the 'learning environment' as well as curricula, though it is uncertain how much it can be improved as long as steep hierarchies, inadequate hospital support services, and 30-hour work shifts remain the structural features that determine student lives.

Assessing ethics education: form, content and function

There are several ways to assess the introduction of bioethics education in medical schools. Most obvious, and most difficult, is a measure of how instruction in bioethics influences subsequent behaviour. The LCME requirement asks that students 'exhibit scrupulous ethical principles in caring for patients, and in relating to patients' families and to others involved in patient care'. Most would agree with this objective, but is it possible to measure the effect of bioethics instruction in exhibiting 'scrupulous ethical principles?' We can also assess the form, content and placement of bioethics instruction. Here we can learn something about the material presented to students, and, the attitudes about, and functions of, bioethics education.

The most telling feature of bioethics instruction is its chronological place in the curriculum. When is bioethics taught to medical students? The preference of most bioethicists would be for some didactic instruction in the pre-clinical years, preferably year two, and clinic-based instruction in years three and four where small group discussions are augmented by role-modelling by senior clinicians demonstrating difficult conversations and decisions. This preference makes pedagogic sense: bioethics instruction in year one of medical school, when students are inundated with memory-demanding courses like biochemistry, physiology, anatomy, pharmacology and pathology is ineffective. At that point, students are busy cramming their heads with information they hope will prevent them from killing their future patients. But, as we noted at the outset, time in the medical curriculum is precious, and bioethics, the newcomer, is frequently relegated to year one, though recently more US institutions are moving to longitudinal ethics curricula. As instructors in those courses, we have noticed a certain lack of seriousness in student attitudes about the material, an attitude that is abetted by the irrelevance of the material to the rest of the first-year curriculum and by evaluation methods that are less rigorous than those in their other courses. Medical students, who earned their places in school by assessing their teachers' priorities in high school and college, demonstrate those priorities clearly when medical-ethics lectures are given to empty auditoriums the day before an anatomy exam.

A casual attitude about bioethics instruction, on the part of both students and medical-school administrators, is encouraged by the LCME. While the LCME demands 'instruction in appropriate medical ethics, human values, and communication skills', it gives no hint as to the appropriate place of that instruction, nor does it set standards for evaluation. Educational Objective 23 follows a model of knowledge acquisition and demonstration of skills that suggests ethics is like other aspects of clinical training. The LCME's stipulation that ethics instruction should occur *before* patient interaction supports and reflects the usual form of ethics teaching, with didactic lectures and small-group discussions in the pre-clinical years and informal role-modelling and evaluation during the clinical years. The lack of standards for evaluation raises a number of questions: is ethics a set of knowledge, skills and techniques like biochemistry or an exercise intended to create proper habits of the heart? If ethics and professionalism are features of character that cannot be taught, should medical schools be using ethics exams (or perhaps personality tests) to select applicants?

Given the lack of clear guidelines, what are medical schools doing? To answer this question we looked to the American Association of Medical Colleges (AAMC) *Curriculum Directory*. We reviewed the directory from 1973 to 2007 and abstracted data on reported courses and content in ethics, humanities, social science, public health, community medicine and introduction to clinical medicine for 20 medical schools. The medical schools were chosen from the *US News and World Report* 2007 rankings as the Best Primary-Care medical schools and the Best Research medical schools. Of these 20 schools, eight reported courses or lectures in ethics as part of their overall curriculum summary, but all 20 reported a course that *may* have contained ethics content under a title such as, 'Doctoring', 'Physician, Patient and Society', 'Medical Humanities' or 'Human Context and Medical Practice'. Many also reported courses in history of medicine, community medicine, healthcare systems and doctor–patient relations which overlap with bioethics in the teaching of some of the social and interpersonal contexts of health and medicine. Nearly all of the courses reported in the AAMC directory are taught in the first two years of medical school, but the directory only makes suggestions regarding the details of ethics and humanities training. Columbia University, the University of Washington and the University of Pennsylvania, schools that use small, case-based discussion groups and approaches from literary analysis in years three and four, did not report these efforts in the overall AAMC curriculum survey.

Targeted surveys – looking at the content of medical ethics and professionalism education – and reviews of the syllabuses of ethics courses show little consistency in ethics curricula in the United States (DuBois and Burkemper 2002). A survey of syllabuses for medical-ethics courses conducted for the 1999–2000 school year showed the content areas of informed consent, healthcare delivery, confidentiality, quality of life, death and dying, euthanasia and patient–physician relationship were covered by more than half of the responding schools, with teaching on informed consent reported by 85 per cent. No content area, however, was universally reported and there were 1,191 distinct readings required or recommended, with no single reading used by more than ten schools. A recent survey of European medical schools also found that while ethics education was reported at all but one responding institution, there was wide variation in the extent, form and content of training (Claudot *et al.* 2007). A more recent survey of 125 US medical schools (to which 59 responded, a response rate of 47 per cent), confirmed that – in keeping with the LCME requirements – all schools require coursework in bioethics, with an average of 36 hours of instruction (sd = 23.6, range 9 to 125 hours). The survey confirms that most bioethics instruction is done in the first two years of medical school: on average 15.9 hours were taught in year one, 11.2 hours in year two, 6.5 hours in year three, and 2.0 hours in year four (Persad *et al.* 2008). The researchers also measured expertise of bioethics instructors, as indicated by number of publications in the bioethics literature; they discovered only 46 per cent had published at least one article, a worrisome finding suggesting that bioethics is not the primary area of those who teach it. A study of the bioethics curriculum at our own institution (see Box 11.1) showed somewhat uneven coverage of the 28 core topics and skills identified by the faculty. Most of the teaching was done in clinical rotations, enhancing its potential impact on practice, but this also placed teaching in areas such as advance care planning and refusal of care in the hands of faculty with little formal training in ethics.

Box 11.1 Evaluation of teaching in ethics and professionalism at the University of Michigan Medical School: a case study

> All care is teaching by role model. Good, bad, or indifferent. Most students identify with a resident. One resident hates drug abuse, does not like alcoholics. Students see that, and the attendings try, sometimes, to address resident attitude, but not always.
>
> (Attending Physician, University of Michigan)

In response to ongoing controversy about *what* and *how* to teach medical ethics in the four-year medical-student curriculum, University of Michigan bioethics faculty undertook an evaluation to identify:

1   What do bioethics faculty assess as the most important medical ethics and professionalism topics for medical-student education?
2   To what degree are students systematically exposed to teaching about those topics?

Phase 1. Defining key ethics topics

In Phase 1, the goal was to identify, 'What ethics and professionalism topics should be taught?' A bioethics expert panel was convened to develop a comprehensive list of potential topics. This yielded a master list of medical ethics and professionalism topics related to knowledge, attitudes, goals and skills. This list was then systematically assessed by faculty in the bioethics programme and those responsible for teaching ethics courses to medical students. Assessors were asked to rank each topic as: essential, strongly recommended or recommended, based on the criterion that a *graduating medical student should achieve competence in that topic before becoming a resident physician.* Twenty-eight topics were deemed essential (see Table 11.1).

Phase 2. Survey of course and clerkship directors

In Phase 2, a survey was sent to 50 course directors in an effort to determine if, when and how topics identified as core knowledge and skills were actually being

Table 11.1 Reported frequency of medical-student exposure to 28 'essential' ethics topics by course and clerkship directors

Topics well covered (n = 6)	Topics adequately covered (n = 9)	Topics marginally covered (n = 8)	Topics not routinely covered (n = 5)
Non-judgemental approach	Prudent use of resources	Impaired decision-making	Refusal of care
Protecting privacy and confidentiality	Professional balance	Decision to use hospice/palliation	Conflict of interest: incentives, pharmaceuticals
Involving patients in decision-making	Commitment to dying	Advance-care planning	Recognizing unethical behaviour in others
Honesty and forthrightness	Obtaining consent	Breaking bad news	
Accountability of students to patients, self and others	Accommodating sociocultural differences	Exceptions to protect patient confidentiality	Brain-death criteria
Assessment of decision-making capacity	Health-financing and influence on care	Medical errors and adverse events	Role/use of ethics committees
	Harassment	Boundary issues	
	Role models	Community service	
	Substance abuse		

taught, both in classroom and lab-based courses as well as in hospital-based clinical courses. Given the focus of the University of Michigan's competence-based curriculum, and the emphasis by accrediting bodies on demonstrating outcomes rather than simply exposure in the curriculum, each component was framed as a skill. The survey results ($n=25$) revealed the distribution of topic coverage as: six well covered, nine adequately covered, eight marginally covered and five not taught. This process also revealed the most active partners in ethics and professionalism teaching were courses and rotations in psychiatry, endocrinology, emergency medicine, doctor–patient relationships and 'family-centred experience' – a course in which students follow a family through their interactions with the healthcare system for the four years they are in medical school to see the impact of illness on work, school and family life. After the survey, qualitative interviews were conducted with six participants to assess how the ethics topics were being taught. These faculty members responded that there is little formal teaching about ethics, though through clinical rotations, students are routinely exposed to the topics creating an opportunity for teaching. Faculty confirmed that students tend to resist didactic 'talks' and emphasized their belief that ethics and professionalism (good and bad) are taught primarily by role-modelling.

Conclusions

Redirection of bioethics teaching out of the lecture hall and into small groups and clinical experiences increases the potential to teach ethics in an applied way and to demonstrate skills and techniques as well as knowledge. Faculty can define a corpus of medical ethics topics appropriate for systematic medical-student teaching and certain courses and rotations are particularly fertile for ethics teaching. Still, this shift puts a greater onus of teaching ethical skills on faculty and residents who typically have no training in bioethics. Role modelling, perceived as the main educational source for students, can include the good, the bad and the ugly. This project concluded that bioethicists and medical educators should work with course/ clerkship directors to develop specific ethics-teaching objectives, materials and evaluation appropriate to their clinical content.

Does bioethics education change the behaviour of physicians-in-training? The LCME requirement is premised on the notion that it does, but documenting that change has not been easy. Researchers continue to struggle with the development of measurements that can capture the effect of ethics education on what students know, and more importantly, how students behave. Not much has changed between 1986 – when James Rest published his influential text, *Moral Development: advances in research and theory* – and today. Social psychologists continue to wrestle with the problem of how to measure moral sensitivity, the first step in assessing the effectiveness of ethics education. Witness the conclusion of this 2007 review article:

> The purpose of this review was to summarize moral sensitivity assessment and to provide researchers with a *launching pad* for developing and validating instruments. The paucity of such tools and the lack of consensus in the

field have placed limitations on the extent to which moral sensitivity can be empirically investigated. Without valid measures of the construct, researchers cannot embark on investigations to uncover situational and individual differences that affect moral sensitivity or to determine the relation between moral sensitivity and related constructs.

(Jordan 2007: 354, emphasis added)

Medical educators have a more immediate problem: the need to find a way to assess (i.e. grade) a student's skill in bioethics. Because ethics education is expected to do so many different things, determining when those goals have been met is nearly impossible. Ethics training is supposed to improve students' professional bearing, bedside manner and ability to manage difficult clinical situations, as well as to convey or reinforce a range of other attitudes and skills. Assessing adherence to specific requirements such as patient confidentiality is relatively straightforward if teachers have the time and exposure to students in a range of settings that would allow them to comment. On the other hand, sensitivity, bedside manner and identification of ethical issues in clinical practice are much more subtle and subject to variation in assessments by different supervisors. These problems with student evaluation are not unique to ethics. Instead, they mirror the challenges of evaluating students' clinical skills. As is the case with clinical skills, ethics is sometimes taught only in the context of clinical subject matter where issues like consent and confidentiality are left to informal role-modelling; other programmes use formal methods of testing including written exams, oral exams, papers and structured clinical encounters. Still others regard '360-degree' evaluation by nurses, patients and peers as the best way to capture the nature and quality of trainee encounters outside of formal attending rounds (Liu *et al.* 2007).

Multiple-choice exam questions about criteria for competence to make medical decisions or justifiable reasons to violate patient confidentiality provide some information about knowledge acquired in bioethics courses, but they are at best blunt instruments. Efforts to standardize training in ethics, rather than leave it to haphazard role-modelling, parallel the creation since the 1960s of textbooks, courses and standardized patient encounters to assess medical students' skills in medical history-taking, physical examination and patient communication. In both cases, the dominant mode of assessment remains subjective and summative, either through narrative assessments or scores on a survey scale. Recent efforts to better assess both ethics and clinical skills use a checklist of behaviours to be observed in clinical encounters – or with 'standardized patients' (lay persons who play the role of a patient and who are trained to evaluate a medical student's examination skills) – to measure how well a student has mastered the knowledge and techniques required of a clinician (Stern 2006). These changes reflect greater attention to fairness and rationality in student assessment, the professionalization of medical educators over the past generation and widespread concerns that changes in the function and structure of teaching hospitals have reduced student contact with clinical teachers and continuity with patients (Ludmerer 1999).

Conclusion: making sociological sense of the rise of bioethics education

Sociology gains its analytic strength by looking at society and its institutions from the margins, from the outside. This perspective has generated brilliant insights about the way healthcare works – hospitals are a lot like prisons (Goffman 1961; Parsons 1951), social worth determines how patients are treated by doctors (Sudnow 1967), for surgeons in training technical mistakes are less serious than 'moral' mistakes (Bosk 2003) – but it has won us few fans in the arenas we study. In this case, we look at noble efforts to make future physicians more ethically aware. While we find these efforts commendable, as social scientists we necessarily look beyond 'official explanations' of how and why bioethics found its way into the medical curriculum. Persad and his colleagues (2008: 89) offer one such official, common-sense explanation of the emergence of bioethics when they claim, 'issues such as the growth of genetic testing, end-of-life decision-making for a burgeoning elderly population, confidentiality in the era of electronic medical records, and allocation of scarce medical resources make bioethics training clearly necessary for physicians'. As sociologists we find this explanation too thin; we seek more sociological, and perhaps less welcome, accounts of this turn in medical education.

Why bioethics now? Our short history of bioethics showed the rise of the field to be associated with the conjunction of the 'rights movement' and the new machines of medicine. Bioethics education in medical schools is part of this larger social change, a move from medical ethics – ethics managed by the medical profession – to bioethics, a specialty populated by physicians and 'strangers' (non-physicians). Three aspects of this move are sociologically interesting. First is consideration of the value of bioethics and bioethics education for medicine. In the 1980s and 1990s bioethics was gradually transformed from a 'watchdog' into a 'show-dog'; this product of the cultural and social changes of the 1960s was assimilated into the work of medicine, helping medical institutions to deflect societal challenges to its authority (Elliott 2001). Given its lack of demonstrable effectiveness and its less than felicitous placement in the early years of medical school, one may assume that bioethics instruction is also something of a show-dog, a cosmetic effort to demonstrate concern with the important ethical problems of medicine. More than two decades ago, Abbott (1983) made a similar, but somewhat softer argument about professional ethics. Using historical data, he showed that when those who entered the learned professions were drawn from the upper classes, there was no need for professional ethics – those admitted to professional training programmes were assumed to have a set of ethics (guided by the notion of 'disinterested service') controlling their behaviour. It was only when admission procedures became more democratic that professional ethics were needed – no longer did the uniform class background 'guarantee' ethical behaviour. According to Abbott, professional codes of ethics help secure and preserve the status of an occupation. Bioethics instruction can be seen as an effort to introduce a standard set of values to medical students from diverse backgrounds and to maintain the special status of the medical profession, serving simultaneously as public symbolism and professional socialization.

Second, bioethics education is one part of a larger change in the way medicine is taught. Curricular reforms over the past two decades have reduced the time spent in the anatomy lab peering into a microscope and doing physiology experiments. Those activities have been replaced by self-directed and informal learning, the use of computer-imaging and simulations, and other supplements to classroom instruction. In response to a number of internal and external critiques focusing on areas where graduating physicians are under-prepared (for example, newly minted doctors 'do not know how to examine the heart', 'don't talk to their patients' – though this may have more to do with the length of office visits – and 'do not have the knowledge required to recognize or resolve ethical challenges'), clinical skills are now being taught in the classroom rather than on the wards. This process of moving from ward to classroom, from informal to formal learning, highlights the extent to which these skills are seen as critical to good medical practice. Rather than students learning ethics by watching senior physicians at work in the wards, medical educators are now 'making the invisible visible' by direct instruction in these areas. Renewed emphasis on teaching these aspects of the 'art' of medicine – including physical examination, communication, doctor–patient relationships, ethics and professionalism – comes at a time when medicine seems ever more fragmented, technical and alienating to both patients and providers. While medical educators cannot alter the economics and structure of healthcare that leads to short-stay hospital care for childbirth and eight-minute office visits, they can respond to growing dissatisfaction by introducing a course on communication or ethics.

Third, the move to bioethics instruction can be seen as a move *away* from instruction in medicine and society grounded in the disciplines of anthropology, sociology, history, public health and community medicine. Fox points out that bioethics has pushed other, non-biomedical, course work out of the medical school curriculum:

> [B]ioethics has replaced psychiatry, the social (behavioral) sciences, and community medicine.... Psychiatry has become more biologically oriented and engrossed; both community medicine and the social sciences have disappeared from the organizational structure and the programs of many medical schools as attention to the social aspects and responsibilities of medicine has waned.
>
> (1999: 8)

Why now? Bioethics education is part of a movement that began as a challenge to medical authority, but has come to be co-opted by medicine. While it is true that theologians, philosophers, lawyers and social scientists have shaped the bioethical curriculum, bioethics occupies a marginal status within medical training. It has been more than three decades since bioethics was introduced to medical students and still there is no standard curriculum, widely agreed upon set of readings or reliable method of evaluating bioethics knowledge or skills. The individualistic emphasis of bioethics is much more congenial to medical practice than the societal perspective of the social science courses it replaced, easing its acceptance within clinical teaching. Sadly, the transmogrification of courses in medicine and society into bioethics courses means that medical students are required to think less about the social context of illness and the policy and political changes that can improve health across populations and more about whether Uncle Bob's 'Do Not Resuscitate' order should be honoured.

Note

1 We gratefully acknowledge Dr Susan Goold's assistance with the University of Michigan ethics assessment project. Dr De Vries' work on this paper was supported by a grant from the National Institutes of Health (US) National Library of Medicine (1G13LM008781–01).

References

Association of American Medical Colleges (AAMC) (1973–2000) *AAMC Curriculum Directory*, Washington, DC: Association of American Medical Colleges. Subsequent years online at http://services.aamc.org/currdir/section2/courses.cfm (accessed 28 March 2008).

Abbott, A. (1983) 'Professional ethics', *American Journal of Sociology*, 88: 855–85.

Bloom, S. W. (1988) 'Structure and ideology in medical education: an analysis of resistance to change', *Journal of Health and Social Behavior*, 29: 294–306.

Bosk, C. L. (2003) *Forgive and Remember: managing medical failure*, 2nd edn, Chicago, IL: University of Chicago Press.

Brainard, A. H. and Brislen, H. C. (2007) 'Viewpoint: learning professionalism: a view from the trenches', *Academic Medicine*, 82: 1010–14.

Charon, R. (2006) *Narrative Medicine: honoring the stories of illness*, Oxford and New York: Oxford University Press.

Christakis, D. A. and Feudtner, C. (1993) 'Ethics in a short white coat: the ethical dilemmas that medical students confront', *Academic Medicine*, 68: 249–54.

Christakis, N. A. (1995) 'The similarity and frequency of proposals to reform US medical education', *Journal of the American Medical Association*, 274: 706–11.

Claudot, F., Alla, F., Ducrocq, X. and Coudane, H. (2007) 'Teaching ethics in Europe', *Journal of Medical Ethics*, 33: 491–5.

Cocking, D. and Oakley, J. (2001) *Virtue Ethics and Professional Roles*, New York: Cambridge University Press.

Culver, C. M., Clouser, K. D., Gert, B., Brody, H., Fletcher, J., Jonsen, A., Kopelman, L., Lynn, J., Siegler, M. and Wikler, D. (1985) 'Basic curricular goals in medical ethics', *New England Journal of Medicine*, 312: 253–6.

Drane, J. F. (1988) *Becoming a Good Doctor: the place of virtue and character in medical ethics*, Kansas City, MO: Sheed and Ward.

DuBois, J. M. and Burkemper, J. (2002) 'Ethics education in US medical schools: a study of syllabi', *Academic Medicine*, 77: 432–7.

Elliott, C. (1999) *A Philosophical Disease: bioethics, culture, and identity*, New York: Routledge.

—— (2001) 'Throwing a bone to the watchdog', *Hastings Center Report*, 31: 9–12.

Feudtner, C. and Christakis, D. A. (1994) 'Making the rounds. The ethical development of medical students in the context of clinical rotations', *Hastings Center Report*, 24: 6–12.

Feudtner, C., Christakis, D. A. and Christakis, N. A. (1994) 'Do clinical clerks suffer ethical erosion? Students' perceptions of their ethical environment and personal development', *Academic Medicine*, 69: 670–9.

Fox, R. (1999) 'Is medical education asking too much of bioethics?' *Daedalus*, 128: 1–25.

Goffman, E. (1961) *Asylums: essays on the social situation of mental patients and other inmates*, Chicago, IL: Aldine.

Hafferty, F. W. (1998) 'Beyond curriculum reform: confronting medicine's hidden curriculum', *Academic Medicine*, 73: 403–7.

Hafferty, F. W. and Franks, R. (1994) 'The hidden curriculum, ethics teaching, and the structure of medical education', *Academic Medicine*, 69: 861–71.

Jonsen, A. R. (1998) *The Birth of Bioethics*, New York: Oxford University Press.

Jordan, J. (2007) 'Taking the first step toward a moral action: a review of moral sensitivity measurement across domains', *Journal of Genetic Psychology*, 168: 323–59.

Lerner, B. H. (2004) 'Beyond informed consent: did cancer patients challenge their physicians in the post-World War II era?', *Journal of the History of Medicine and Allied Sciences*, 59: 507–21.

Liaison Committee on Medical Education (LCME) (2007) *Functions and Structure of a Medical School: standards for accreditation of medical education programs leading to the MD degree*, June, online at www.lcme.org/functions2007jun.pdf (accessed 5 May 2008).

Liu, G. C., Harris, M. A., Keyton, S. A. and Frankel, R. M. (2007) 'Use of unstructured parent narratives to evaluate medical-student competencies in communication and professionalism', *Ambulatory Pediatrics*, 7: 207–13.

Ludmerer, K. (1999) *Time to Heal: American medical education from the turn of the century to the era of managed care*, Oxford: Oxford University Press.

Parsons, T. (1951) *The Social System*, Glencoe, IL: Free Press.

Percival, T. (1803) *Medical Ethics, or, A Code of Institutes and Precepts: adapted to the professional conduct of physicians and surgeons*, Manchester: S. Russell.

Persad, G. C., Elder, L., Sedig, L., Flores, L. and Emanuel, E. J. (2008) 'The current state of medical school education in bioethics, health law, and health economics', *Journal of Law, Medicine & Ethics*, 36: 89–94.

Rest, J. R. (1986) *Moral Development: advances in research and theory*, New York: Praeger.

Rhodes, R. (2001) 'Enriching the White Coat Ceremony with a module on professional responsibilities', *Academic Medicine*, 76: 504–5.

Rothman, D. J. (1991) *Strangers at the Bedside: a history of how law and bioethics transformed medical decision-making*, New York: Basic Books.

Russell, P. C. (2002) 'The White Coat Ceremony: turning trust into entitlement', *Teaching and Learning in Medicine*, 14: 56–9.

Stern, D. T. (ed.) (2006) *Measuring Medical Professionalism*, Oxford: Oxford University Press.

Sudnow, D. (1967) *Passing On*, Englewood Cliffs, NJ: Prentice Hall.

Veatch, R. M. (1973) 'National survey of the teaching of medical ethics in medical schools', in R. M. Veatch, W. Gaylin and C. Morgan (eds) (1973) *The Teaching of Medical Ethics*, Hastings on Hudson: Hastings Center.

—— (2002) 'White coat ceremonies: a second opinion', *Journal of Medical Ethics*, 28: 5–9.

Veatch, R. M. and Sollitto, S. (1976) 'Medical ethics teaching. Report of a National Medical School Survey', *Journal of the American Medical Association*, 235: 1030–3.

Wolpe, P. (1998) 'The triumph of autonomy in American bioethics: a sociological view', in R. DeVries and J. Subedi (eds) *Bioethics and Society: constructing the ethical enterprise*, Upper Saddle River, NJ: Prentice Hall.

12 Sociology in medical education

Graham Scambler

In the early days of medical sociology a distinction was usefully drawn between a sociology 'in' medicine and a sociology 'of' medicine. Its purpose was to highlight the different origins and conditions of emergence of the subdiscipline in different cultures and contexts. When medical sociology was introduced into fully fledged university departments of sociology, as often occurred in the US, it tended to take the orthodox form of a sociology 'of' medicine. In other words, practitioners with a grounding and apprenticeship in the parent discipline applied its tools – theories, concepts, methods and a critical or interrogative orientation – to issues of health and healing, *including the profession of medicine* (Bloom 2002). When, on the other hand, medical sociology found its feet courtesy of the patronage and sponsorship of interested physicians, as typically in Britain, then a sociology 'in' medicine resulted. Frequently self- rather than professionally trained, sociologists in the direct employ of physicians with their own research or policy agendas found their autonomy limited in the process, their critical edge either underdeveloped or gradually dissipated and lost. Sociologists 'in' medicine were handmaidens to medical professionals.

This distinction resonates here. Margot Jefferys (1997), a pivotal figure behind the introduction of sociology teaching into British medical schools, recalls that in 1969 the Royal Commission on Medical Education (the Todd Report) recommended that:

1   Sociology (and psychology) be taught to medical students.
2   The teachers be based in mainstream departments rather than in medical faculties.

Jefferys (1969) herself opposed point 2 on the grounds that the teachers needed to be (seen to be) fully immersed in the medical enterprise; and the fact that the prestigious London medical schools were largely independent bodies, if formally within the University of London, doubtless mitigated against this otherwise sensible proposal.

There is too a difference between a sociology 'in' and 'of' medical education. The chapter title signals discussion of the former, that is, of the variable and changing place and role of medical sociology in the education and training of physicians. Yet a sociohistorical narrative doing anything like justice to this – potentially quite mundane – topic must surely make full use of the tools of the parent discipline. So what follows is simultaneously an account of the insertion and development of sociology teaching in the medical curriculum, with the UK as the primary case study, *and* a sociological analysis of process and outcome.

The opening paragraphs are given over to a brief summary of the chronology, circumstances and characteristics of sociology's incursion into the medical curriculum in the UK; and the UK, notwithstanding the genesis of a medical sociology 'in' rather than 'of' medicine, proved something of a pioneer in this respect. This prolegomenon is succeeded by an excursus on the dynamics of change of medical curricula in general and sociological syllabuses in particular. London provides the context, and one of its – at the time of writing, five – medical schools the special point of focus. Although Aberdeen, under the leadership of Raymond Illsley (1980), was another principal focus for medical sociology in Britain at the time, it was Margot Jefferys in London, backed by Illsley and close colleagues like Meg Stacey, a convert to medical sociology at Warwick who was for a while a member of the General Medical Council (GMC), who became the driving force for the teaching of sociology to medical students. I draw liberally on my own personal experience of teaching medical students from 1975 onwards, of being what May and Clark (1980) called a 'cuckoo in the nest'. Bearing in mind the dangers of adopting an overly focused – city, national or non-comparative – perspective, the remainder of the chapter is committed to a sociological analysis of sociology in medical education.

Sociology and medical education

The origins of sociology, at least in its western professional disciplinary guise, are associated with mainland Europe, most notably through the pioneering triumvirate of Marx, Durkheim and Weber; and the writings of these three continue to bear on matters of health and healing. In many respects, however, it was in the US that sociology 'took off', not only in higher but also high-school education. The sociology of medicine was very much part of this American initiative, although Europe made its contribution to sociology in medicine. It is therefore somewhat surprising that 'sociology as applied to medicine' made its initial incursions into medical curricula in the UK. There is a difference between medical sociologists being 'around' – employed as collaborative researchers for example – and being recognized as core teachers of medical students and apprentice doctors. In terms of the latter, the period since the publication of the Todd Report in 1969 and the present can be divided into four reasonably distinct phases:

1   The *innovative* phase.
2   The *consolidation* phase.
3   The *rationalization* phase.
4   The *corporate* phase.

1 The innovative phase (1969–1983)

The post-Todd early 1970s saw a number of medical-sociology appointments to the largely autonomous Hospital Medical Schools (HMS) within the University of London (although some of the HMS opted to delay making appointments and to contract in their teaching). Many of the sociologists recruited were products of the MSc in Medical Sociology overseen by Margot Jefferys and George Brown, her co-director of the Unit of Medical Sociology at Bedford College (now Royal Holloway College), University of London. Others had strong associations: I did not take the MSc but my PhD was supervised by George Brown. After three years as a research officer studying the stigma attached to epilepsy in the Department of Neurology at St Bartholomew's HMS I was appointed to a half-time lectureship at Charing Cross HMS in 1975, courtesy of George Brown's active sponsorship. David Blane, also half-time, was already in post: he was medically qualified, held the Bedford College MSc, and had established a course mixing stand-up lectures and small-group discussions.

From the vantage point of the present, the innovation characteristic of these years seems even more remarkable. With an intake of 100 pre-clinical students, David Blane and I were able during their second years not only to cover the syllabus in conventional pedagogic fashion, but also to devise imaginative projects. One of these stands out and is instructive both in its scope and in the manner of its demise. Divided into groups of a dozen or so, each with its own tutor, the students were actively engaged in a credible research study of local illness behaviour. Overseen by David Blane and I, modes of sampling were debated; a questionnaire was designed; the students, in pairs, took the questionnaire round to households close to the hospital, stopping when four questionnaires had been completed; a coding frame was drawn up and the data processed; and finally the statistics lecturer collaborated in the analysis of the data, deploying simple descriptive statistics that students were required to master on his course. The result was a genuine quantitative study allowing sociology and statistics to be taught *in practice*. One finding I recall was that people's preference between non-appointment and appointment systems in General Practice was largely determined by the system they were most familiar with.

The termination of this project came about in a manner that anticipated post-innovative phases of medical-sociology teaching. Local General Practitioners (GPs) complained to the dean that their patients were being approached and 'interrogated' – not least about their use of and ideas about General Practice – without their approval or permission. We protested that an individual cannot, even ethically, be redefined and put out of reach, censored, as 'some GP's patient'; but we were informed that it was a sensitive issue and we must discontinue the project.

When I left to take a full-time post at Middlesex HMS in 1978, David Blane went on to devise an ingenious replacement project, again depending on medical-sociology tutors contracted in from outside. This involved students in researching their own family and kin backgrounds to draw up family trees, which in turn became resources for teaching and reflecting on all manner of issues of health and healing. It is worth noting at this point the emergence from the mid-1970s of an extraordinary group of peripatetic tutors in medical sociology whose expertise was available throughout the London HMS. This came to include Mel Bartley, Mary Boulton, Ann Bowling, Richard Compton, Jocelyn Cornwall, Judy Green, James Nazroo, Sarah Nettleton, Ruth Pinder, Annette Scambler, Clive Seale and Nikki Thorogood, to pick out just a handful.

These nomads lent their expertise also to Middlesex HMS. Flourishing in the shelter offered by the Head of the Department of Psychiatry, John Hinton, sociology was taught with psychology under the rubric of behavioural sciences. Moreover, the hours available were prodigious by the standards of the day: quadruple the 30 or so hours at Charing Cross HMS (although we prudently only used 60). David Tuckett, occupying a split-appointment with Bedford College, had pioneered the Middlesex medical-sociology course, as well as editing the first textbook, *Introduction to Medical Sociology*, in 1976. In 1978 I joined Ray Fitzpatrick, Tuckett's successor. If the teaching of behavioural sciences was not fully integrated, it was certainly a genuinely collaborative effort, including joint lectures and seminars. Very soon the sociology syllabus incorporated not only the standard didactic teaching but two sets of small-group seminars, run again by guest tutors, and visits to observe clinical encounters in General Practice. The assessment comprised two 2,500-word essays, reflecting the small-group work, and half a joint sociology/psychology three-hour examination paper. Courtesy of John Hinton, this was about as good as it was to get at Middlesex and most other HMS.

By this time each London HMS sent a representative to a University of London Special Advisory Committee in Sociology as Applied to Medicine (SACSAM). Chaired initially by Margot Jefferys, SACSAM gave a voice to otherwise isolated cuckoos in HMS nests. David Blane and I were once greeted by a Senior Professor of Physiology at Charing Cross HMS with the words: 'I can never see you two together without thinking of anarchy and bombs.' Although we were content to be treated as deviants by a colleague with a phobia for dirt who asked others to summon the lift because he refused to touch the button, this anecdote gives a flavour of the suspicion, and worse, that we sometimes occasioned among basic medical scientists and clinicians. Under such pressures SACSAM was a resource for solidarity and shared experiential learning and evolved into something akin to a pressure group.

It was under the umbrella of SACSAM that collective initiatives flourished in the innovative phase. An intercalated BSc was run for London medical students, normally taken between their two pre-clinical years and their three years of clinical firms. Compelling twice-over, through their selection to London HMS and their near-wilful determination to pursue an oddball discipline (some were actually pressurized by their parents to turn down Medical Research Council (MRC) scholarships to study sociology), these were special undergraduates. Talented, committed and engaged, I have yet to encounter their equals: I once had a six-hour seminar. The BSc lasted for 20 years, for some students a form of respite prior to entering the wards, for most a bout of education to punctuate a programme of professional training and socialization.

SACSAM collegiality was the source also of the first textbook on sociology as applied to medicine written especially for medical students. Donald Patrick and I became co-editors of *Sociology as Applied to Medicine*, published in 1982. The contributors were drawn from the London HMS, with David Blane, Ray Fitzpatrick, Sheila Hillier, David Locker, Myfanwy Morgan and Ellie Scrivens joining Donald Patrick and I; Margot Jefferys supplied the preface. Very much part of the London group, David Armstrong (1980) just beat us into press with a 'rival' single-authored volume. Concise, accessible and using a minimum of jargon, both books covered the basic syllabus and little more. The effect on student examinations was instant: cavalier guesswork was displaced by a less entertaining but largely uniform competence.

2 The consolidation phase (1983–1995)

There is a degree of arbitrariness in any attempt to delineate historical periods. The year 1983 has been selected because it marked the 'restructuring' of the Social Science Research Council (SSRC). Comprising social-science committees covering 14 disciplines ranging from anthropology to statistics, the SSRC had been formed in 1965. During the Thatcher years in general, and Keith Joseph's service as Education Minister in particular, a deep government antipathy towards the very idea of a science of society surfaced; the discipline of sociology bore the brunt. The transmutation of the SSRC into the Economic and Social Research Council (ESRC) in 1983 symbolized this hostility. Forced onto the back foot, sociologists had little choice but retrenchment. The post-Todd genesis and flourishing of medical-sociology courses and staffing in HMS stalled.

Most of the relatively well-established medical-sociology courses in the London HMS continued without undue threat. If there was little expansion in staffing or course ambition, most posts were retained, with SACSAM occasionally intervening to argue against the freezing of posts if a teacher left. Sociology teaching was, after all, a component of the education of doctors defined by the General Medical Council (GMC) post-Todd as non-optional. It was this GMC 'requirement' that underpinned SACSAM's major skirmish in the late 1980s and early 1990s. It was a skirmish that escalated to vice-chancellor level before fizzling out in obduracy and indecision.

By the time I was elected chair of SACSAM in 1989, my predecessor Sheila Hillier had prepared the ground. Using our representation on the committee overseeing medical education within the University of London, we had won support for exerting pressure on the medical school at Cambridge University to include medical sociology in its undergraduate curriculum, a step it had been reluctant to take. In the absence of a positive response, medical students from Cambridge were stopped from transferring to any of the London HMS to do their clinical training, hitherto a popular move. An epidemiologist representing

Cambridge insisted that their teaching already met the GMC requirement to address 'social factors' affecting health and healing. The London sticking point was Cambridge's refusal to introduce a medical-sociology course, taught and examined by sociologists, into the medical-student curriculum, a state of affairs long uniform across the London HMS. Cambridge did not budge. In the end the vice-chancellors of London and Cambridge met and decided that the stalemate, disrupting the training of growing numbers of Cambridge students, could not continue. We on SACSAM were apparently dismissed as 'a bunch of Ayatollahs' after the new ruler of Iran. From anarchists to theocrats! Although technically 'seen off', we took much encouragement from the support of our medical allies in London.

3 The rationalization phase (1995–2006)

The phase of consolidation, of fighting a rearguard action to retain the gains of the innovation phase, gradually gave way to an increasingly explicit phase of Weberian rationalization. In other words, pressures mounted for a standardized 'product', paying due attention to economies of scale. The dating of this transition is particularly difficult. At the Middlesex HMS, for example, the prospect of a merger with University College London (UCL) HMS gave rise to high emotions as early as the mid-1980s, the actual merger, experienced as a 'takeover', taking place in 1987. But 1995 has been selected here to mark the creation of Barts and The London School of Medicine and Dentistry under the aegis of Queen Mary College. In 1997 the Imperial School of Medicine was established, arising out of the merger of St Mary's HMS and Charing Cross HMS. This was followed in 1998 by the formation of the King's College School of Medicine and Dentistry as a result of the merger between King's College and the United Medical and Dental Schools of Guy's and St Thomas' HMS; and of the Royal Free and University College Medical School, a consequence of the mergers between UCL HMS and the Middlesex HMS in 1987 and the Royal Free HMS in 1998. Allowing for different periods of gestation, then, ten HMS in London had been reduced to four large multi-faculty London colleges, leaving only St George's HMS as an outlier in Tooting, South London.

Each merger of London HMS occasioned an overhaul of the undergraduate curriculum, and hence of the input of medical sociology. Thus when the Middlesex and UCL HMS came together in 1987 it was necessary to integrate two different courses rooted in different departments (Psychiatry in the former and Epidemiology and Public Health in the latter). With revenue at stake, educational arguments were tailored to political expediency. The result was the deconstruction of the old Middlesex mode of teaching in favour of more independent sociology and psychology courses. Because there was a strong Department of Psychology within UCL, the Middlesex psychology teachers were left high and dry; because there was no Department of Sociology, I remained fully engaged. The small-group teaching in sociology survived, but only because I persuaded the finance office to 'hide' the relevant monies (which thereafter remained static).

The additional merger with the Royal Free HMS in 1998 was more complex. This was partly because there were underlying political issues once more, but mostly because Charlotte Humphrey (sociology) and Jonathan Elford (epidemiology) had together built an ambitious and successful 'Population Studies' course, incorporating extensive small-group project work, leading to end-of-year presentations, again overseen by our expert circuit of external tutors. How could the impressive (quart-sized) Royal Free sociology-with-epidemiology course fit into the (pint-sized) UCL sociology-not-quite-with-psychology course? The answer, two curriculum-wide reviews later, was 'it couldn't'. By the turn of the century the compromise solution was clear.

The medical-sociology course had acquired a new set of properties. First, it was part of a 'Society and the Individual' programme, incorporating sociology, psychology and epidemiology, eventually settling into a first-year slot. Second, all small-group work had been lost, there being insufficient monies to either contract in tutors or provide rooms for an intake of approximately 350 students. The substitute was stand-up lectures to the whole year, plus episodes of private study or 'self-paced learning'. And third, the sole mode of assessment was a norm of two short-answer questions, subsumed in a general end-of-year examination, with model answers constraining more creative or independent-minded students. That the course was not examined by means of multiple-choice questions was entirely due to the efforts of Paul Higgs and Fiona Stevenson, by this time its convenors. The ideal form of assessment for many HMS was one that could be machine-marked.

4 The corporate phase (2006–)

If the argument based on economies of scale had largely been won by the close of the twentieth century, conspicuously so in London, the advent of the corporate phase can be dated from the introduction of university fees. Long eschewed by the Blair government, these eventually succeeded an atypical bout of rebellion inside as well as outside the Houses of Parliament in 2006. The corporate model seemed to evolve naturally enough in the four principal rationalized London HMS: Imperial School of Medicine; King's College School of Medicine and Dentistry; Barts and The London, Queen Mary's School of Medicine and Dentistry; and Royal Free and University College School of Medicine. St George's HMS as yet remains a stand-alone outpost of the University of London, although links with other universities have been mooted. At the time of writing Imperial College had already broken away from the University of London, and its three local multi-faculty rivals – King's College London, Queen Mary College, and University College London – are in many respects universities in their own right. Interestingly, none of these multi-faculty institutions has its own Department of Sociology. With the rationalization of the University of London has come devolution. The Subject Panel in Sociology Applied to Medicine which replaced SACSAM continued to meet at Senate House, but it had lost most of its teeth and has recently been wound up.

What marks the corporate phase is a process better understood via Marx than Weber. The London HMS have not only been amalgamated or rationalized into four large autonomous or semi-autonomous universities, but are now rivals, competing for status and customers in an international marketplace. Consonant with this, the management of the London 'big four' has become increasingly business-like. This shift in emphasis – which extends beyond medicine to embrace *all* faculties and departments – reflects an acceptance of America's top-rated, endowment-rich Harvard University as the global ideal. Ironically, however, British universities are opting for a micro-management of their staff exceeding that found in most of their US counterparts. Academics across disciplines are appraised for their cost-effectiveness, namely, their 'corporate worth' in terms of

1   Evolving national measures of research excellence.
2   Capacity to cover their own salaries.

Those who fall short on either criterion may be re-labelled as 'teachers' or invited to leave. Meanwhile senior appointments in fund-raising attain priority.

The impact of corporatization on medical-sociology teaching has varied, depending on assessments of individual corporate worth. The emphasis on (externally funded) research excellence over ability to teach has the potential to undermine the planning and delivery of courses. The need to pay attention to customer satisfaction is a mitigating factor. At the Royal Free and University College School of Medicine there has as yet been little change since the transition from the rationalization to the corporate phase. Paul Higgs, Fiona Stevenson and I, all acknowledged as 'research active', have survived our appraisals and can between us provide a 'rationalized' course. Like all our colleagues committed to teaching sociology to medical students, however, we must look over our shoulders. Sociologists employed in HMS are still anomalous cuckoos in the nest.

A sociology of medical education

Even in the lively innovative phase it is questionable to what extent London's medical students came to think sociologically, that is, to see beyond the world of events to their patterning and to the manner in which social structures like class, gender and ethnicity underpin this patterning. They were, however, exposed to projects and small-group work beyond the bounds of the didacticism of the lecture theatre: they could read for seminars, think out loud and enter a forum of discussion and debate. Essays and unseen written examinations made significant but manageable intellectual demands on students better versed in the natural and biological sciences than in the social sciences and humanities. If the majority came to appreciate the salience of 'social factors' for how people-cum-patients and health professionals behaved in and around illness, that was probably a reasonable return in the minds of their teachers.

David Armstrong (1979) listed his lecture topics at Guy's HMS in the mid-1970s as follows:

- Introduction – what is health?
- Why do people consult their doctors?
- Social structures and health.
- The social causes of disease.
- The nature of medical problems.
- Labelling.
- Disability and rehabilitation.
- Delivering healthcare.
- NHS – structure and function.
- Health policy.
- Evaluating healthcare.
- Health as a social value.

These lectures were backed up by the seminars and project work characteristic of the innovative phase. If medical sociology has grown exponentially since its first incursion into London HMS, adding a degree of sophistication of theory, concept and data analysis, David Armstrong's syllabus remains recognizable. The context in which lectures are given, however, has changed significantly during the consolidation, rationalization and corporate phases. The disappearance of seminar and project work is more effect than cause of this change.

The social change most pertinent to sociology in medical education can be approached via linked themes more familiar within mainstream sociology. A sociology 'of' is required to grasp the shifting fortunes of a sociology 'in' medical education. Five themes will be developed, together with appropriate illustrations as follows:

1 System colonization and sociology in medical education. The first theme utilizes Habermas's (1984, 1987) distinction between 'system' and 'life-world', framing his assertion that the modern era has witnessed the progressive 'colonization' of the latter by the former.
2 From system colonization to McDonaldization. This theme elaborates on this idea of colonization by exploring Ritzer's (1996) notion of the 'McDonaldization' of society and of academia.
3 Cultural relativity. This theme focuses on the extraordinarily rapid 'relativization' of culture between the innovative and corporate phases sketched above.
4 From education to the inculcation of skills. The fourth notes the changing nature of contemporary work and records the priority now accorded work skills over education.
5 The sociology of the taming of sociology in medicine. Finally, the risk of a 'taming' of medical sociology, not least in medical schools, is addressed.

1 System colonization and sociology in medical education

For Habermas, the system comprises the economy and the state, which act strategically or instrumentally, via the media of money and power respectively. This is inevitable in complex, highly differentiated and high-speed modern societies. Decisions can no longer wait upon public reason and affirmation – Habermas's communicative action – but must be taken on people's behalf, if 'behind their backs'. This only becomes problematic if agents of the economy and/or the state start acting beyond their remit and become unanswerable, even in principle, to their broader publics. This is when it becomes appropriate to write of the colonization of the (ordinary, everyday, public) lifeworld by the system.

The question of the extent to which any system colonization of the lifeworld has impacted on medical education in general, and constituent courses in medical sociology in particular, is an interesting one. My identification of rationalization and corporate phases since the mid-1990s is itself revealing. A significant and publicly unaccountable intrusion of state power into medical education is suggested by the first, while the second suggests a new salience for money, the 'steering medium' of the economy. Medical education, my terminology implies, has been significantly bureaucratized, then commodified, with a momentum beyond public deliberation or complaint. The modern (post-1858) British profession of medicine and its apparatus of education have of course evolved within parameters set by the state and economy, so processes of bureaucratization and commodification are not new. What the last decade has seen is a speeding up of systemic colonizing potentials.

There is a paradox here. The displacement of the rationalization by the corporate phase seems to accord state intervention causal as well as chronological priority. This is misleading. Extrapolating from an argument developed elsewhere – with reference to the reform of the National Health Service (NHS) rather than of university or medical education – it was the rapidly globalizing economy (from the mid-1970s) and consequent reinvigoration of relations of class that precipitated state intervention in the public sector (namely, an upsurge in relations of command) (Scambler 2002). The newly regulatory state emerged as the causal progenitor of a newly marketized state. This class/command dynamic has been the fundamental motor of the colonizing changes that have so marked medical education and the syllabuses and delivery of medical-sociology courses in HMS.

2 From system colonization to McDonaldization

Ritzer's (2001) thesis of the McDonaldization of academia overlaps with Habermas's notion of colonization. In a nutshell, Ritzer argues that the last generation has witnessed the institutionalized acceptance of new criteria of what counts intellectually and what should be rewarded by professional advancement: academic products, like those of McDonalds, have become more standardized. What this argument does is focus attention on:

1   The causes and consequences of the rationalization and corporate phases defined above.
2   The structural underpinnings of academic motivation.

The family of attributes that are now, according to Ritzer, required of American sociological research is of direct generic relevance to American and to British universities, including the London HMS. The first is *calculability* or an emphasis on things that can be quantified (what Sorokin long ago characterized as 'quantophrenia'); this encourages large grants to generate or re-analyse large datasets, leading to large numbers of uniform papers in major peer-reviewed journals. The second attribute is *predictability*: reading such papers mimics the consumption of standard products like 'Big Macs', a process reinforced by journal editors, referees and so on. Journal articles have to adopt a uniform format and be of a uniform length. This makes for a third attribute, *efficiency*, permitting sociologists simultaneously to contribute to and acquaint themselves with their fields. Underlying much of this is a reliance on *non-human technologies*, most notably electronic systems, a seemingly ineluctable shift lambasted also by Bourdieu and colleagues (1991). Ritzer offers his overall assessment of this quite fundamental and far-reaching re-focusing of academia and academics by referring to the *irrationality of this rational system*.

Ritzer readily accepts that American sociology has not been entirely McDonaldized, and this qualification applies no less to its British equivalent. A good case can be made, however, that sociologists in Britain, and perhaps especially those in HMS, are subject to more stringent and bureaucratic management than their American colleagues. In fact, Ritzer's is an uncomfortably apt interpretation of the colonization of medical sociology in medical schools. While teachers of medical sociology in London HMS have generally remained on permanent contracts, for historical reasons, researchers generally survive or build precarious careers on the basis of a series of short-term appointments. The teachers are encouraged, required or compelled (even permanent contracts are not what they were) to bid for increasingly competitive, commissioned funding to underwrite their posts and to enhance their status and income. Employers are satisfied and careers consolidated – if not exclusively, then above all else – by external monies raised and the accumulation of peer-reviewed articles in high-impact international journals in line with the latest national Research Assessment Exercise. Curricula vitae oriented to the past, as Sennett (2006) has so eloquently testified, mean less than present and future corporate potential. From such building blocks are global universities constructed. Echoing Ritzer once more, questionable, colonizing trends like those epitomized in his concept of McDonaldization are not incompatible with exemplary sociological work, or textbooks, or theory; they do, however, stand to make them more exceptional (Scambler 2006).

3 Cultural relativity

The advent of a so-called postmodern culture is generally dated from midway through the innovative phase, although there are earlier antecedents. Certainly there is a readily discernible difference between the medical students in London HMS *then* and *now*. What Lyotard (1972) called *grand* narratives have metamorphosed into *petit* narratives. The modern impulse towards a rational, universal consensus has yielded to a postmodern take-it-or-leave-it modality of 'choice': what were formerly contradictions have become alternative 'positionings'. Most London medical students are now self-confessed relativists, that is, they incline to the view that judgements of right and wrong, and even of truth and falsity, are largely culture-bound. A sociologist of medicine might reasonably infer that medical sociology courses in medical curricula have themselves become positionings. Although some judge that the bid for a postmodern medical sociology can now be deemed to have failed (Cockerham 2007), most medical sociologists, like other non-celebrity academics, have lost cultural authority. While they may not quite have become 'interpreters', they have lost their former status as 'experts' and are unlikely to recapture their roles as 'legislators' (Bauman 1987).

But there is another side to postmodern choice. The cultural relativity it reflects is functional for the rapid, irresistible spread of consumerism, leading commentators to refer to the 'consumer society'. Choice, even in identity formation, is exercised primarily through consumption. Our postmodern culture/consumer society has its structural origins in the reinvigoration of class power and its sway over government policy-making (see Harvey 2006). In Habermas's terminology, we are experiencing a colonizing thrust of the system over the lifeworld; and in Ritzer's, the hyper-commodification and hyper-bureaucratization epitomized in McDonaldization. Medical students too have become consumers, most tangibly in the corporate phase identified above, heralded by the introduction of university fees. At the time of writing medical students can expect to qualify with debts of around £37,000. They are paying good money, even if not yet an economic price, and have the consumer's right to transparency, quality control and redress when sold products they find deficient in some way. Of course they are not just consumers, and their teachers remain more than vendors of knowledge and practical skills, but the relationship between teachers and students has subtly changed.

4 From education to the inculcation of skills

These changes may not be wholly negative: there is thought to be more teacher accountability in the corporate than in the innovative phase for example. Students as consumers must be heard. Yet it is an odd bureaucratic form of accountability: teachers, and teachers' corporate employers, may take greater pains *to be seen to be* accountable than *to be* accountable: cast-iron paper trails are the order of the day, 'smoking guns' their potential undoing. Mere postmodern 'disinhibition' can be mistaken for democratic accomplishment (Scambler 2002). This has led Habermas (1989) to define postmodern culture as a form of neo-conservatism: after all, for the cultural relativist there can be no rationally compelling argument for rejecting the status quo of the day.

It is a commonplace of social-scientific analysis that the rationalization and corporate phases have led to a significant 'neo-liberalization' of British universities, including their medical schools (Callinicos 2006). As the appropriately named Law and Work (2008: 137) note, 'academic labour is becoming increasingly defined by market relations and the managerial conditions under which it operates as paid wage labour'. Students too must be prepared for the workforce. Ironically medical students have long received more of a hands-on, skills- as well as knowledge-based training for work than an education: one charge levied against sociology since the experimental days of the 1970s has been that it is too far removed from the praxis of the workplace. The notion that education is intrinsically worthwhile, once a cornerstone of educational philosophy and the training of teachers in primary and secondary as well as tertiary education, is harder to defend as a *petit* than a *grand* narrative.

In such times medical-sociology teachers in the London HMS and elsewhere might be expected to come under sharper pressure from their customers as well as their employers, the more so given the rationalization and corporatization of their courses discussed earlier. That medical and other students and their families and sponsors have become consumers or customers has given them too a strategic impulse. The fact that medical students, like many of their university-educated, professional-apprentice peers, have always made day-to-day decisions using strategic as well as communicative reasoning should not disguise the renewed force of this impulse. And strategic reason, it will be recalled, exercised reflexively or otherwise, is oriented to outcome not consensus, to grades and jobs rather than the acknowledgement of meretricious performance.

5 The sociology of the taming of sociology in medicine

The preceding paragraphs imply hazard rather than opportunity (Scambler 2006). I have argued elsewhere that the processes delineated in this chapter do indeed represent a significant threat to the subdiscipline of medical sociology in Britain (Scambler 1996). Arguably, however, sociologists employed in HMS have always and of necessity trimmed their sails. If they have sought to go beyond merely asserting the salience of 'social factors' for health and healing, exhorting students to consider the ways in which social structures shape events and behaviours for example, they have done so for the most part with circumspection. Starting in the innovative and extending into the consolidation phase, this seemed a matter of self-preservation, with employers and colleagues in the life and clinical sciences often finding sociological interrogations of healthcare systems, medicine and professional practice beyond the pale. Later, in the rationalization and corporate phases, and now almost part of the furniture, medical sociologists in London HMS, like many of their academic consociates, have become caught up in broader but more insistent employer demands for cost-effectiveness.

The 'taming' of those of us who teach medical students has been indirect and circuitous. The dwindling of a critical sociological focus on health and medicine has had knock-on effects in terms of research completed and therefore resources for teaching. Professional and policy sociology have a greater elective affinity with the demonstrable cost-effectiveness required by the recent surge in system colonization, McDonaldization and the neo-liberal work ethos than critical and public sociology (Burawoy 2005).

Concluding comments

References here to theorists like Habermas, and to propositions asserting the systemic colonization of the lifeworld, McDonaldization, the neo-liberalization of universities and the taming of the discipline, may suggest the use of too many sledgehammers to crack too few nuts. However, wider social changes often provide the causal backcloth to phenomena like revised curricula and modes of teaching and assessment. This chapter has used a case study of the genesis of medical sociology courses in the London HMS to illustrate externally induced change over a generation. Arguably London has special salience in this context, even internationally. Although sociology was most decisively institutionalized in schools and universities in the US, for example, it was in Britain, in London in particular, that, at the behest of the General Medical Council, it came to form an established part of medical education. This narrative of sociology's introduction into London HMS has a number of symbolic aspects: first, it might be said to represent a 'path' now being trodden elsewhere in Britain and in other countries; second, events in London HMS over the last 30 or 40 years might be expected to find an echo regionally, nationally and internationally given the global reach and spread of the neo-liberalism epitomized in the Washington Consensus; and third, the path followed in London HMS might be characterized in terms of threat rather than opportunity.

What this chapter has shown is that in London HMS, after early phases of innovation and consolidation, phases of rationalization and corporatization have secured telling changes. What will future audits of these changes reveal? Teachers may have become more productive in the light of controversial bureaucratic indices, but they have lost independence and a measure of freedom to ask research questions for which there is no external funding on offer. Students have become paying customers, are less educationally and more vocationally oriented, and seek bureaucratic and, increasingly, legal redress if they do not receive value for money. As far as the teaching of medical sociology to medical students is concerned, the quality and subtlety of student output has declined across many London HMS. This is a function not of any deterioration in student or teacher talent, or even in *what* students are taught, but rather of *how* they are taught in environments in which students and teachers alike are adapting, more precisely 'being adapted', to the external constraints of Durkheimian 'social facts' in a rapidly changing social world.

The sociology 'of' medicine (latterly of health and illness) has a rich history, especially in the US. Moreover sociologists have long worked in HMS in the US, Britain and elsewhere, typically in professional or policy sociology: these have been practitioners 'in' medicine. The calculated decision to establish medical-sociology courses in London HMS, complementing basic medical-science teaching, gave the sociology 'of' medicine an educational rather than vocational niche in the socialization of British doctors. Those of us appointed to this task are hanging in there.

References

Armstrong, D. (1979) 'Medical sociology', *Medical Teacher*, 1: 25–30.
—— (1980) *An Outline of Sociology Applied to Medicine*, Bristol: Butterworth-Heinemann.
Bauman, Z. (1987) *Legislators and Interpreters: on modernity, postmodernity and intellectuals*, Cambridge: Cambridge University Press.
Bloom, S. (2002) *The Word as Scalpel: a history of medical sociology*, Oxford: Oxford University Press.
Bourdieu, P., Chamboredon, J.-C. and Passeron, J.-C. (1991) *The Craft of Sociology: epistemological preliminaries*, New York: Walter de Gruyter.
Burawoy, M. (2005) 'For public sociology', *American Sociological Review*, 70: 4–28.
Callinicos, A. (2006) *Universities in a Neoliberal World*, London: Bookmarks Publications.
Cockerham, W. (2007) 'A note on the fate of postmodern theory and its failure to meet the basic requirements for success in medical sociology', *Social Theory and Health*, 5: 285–96.
Habermas, J. (1984) *Theory of Communicative Action. Volume 1: reason and the rationalization of society*, London: Heinemann.
—— (1987) *Theory of Communicative Action. Volume 2: lifeworld and system: a critique of functionalist reason*, Cambridge: Polity Press.
—— (1989) *The New Conservatism*, Cambridge: Polity Press.
Harvey, D. (2006) *Spaces of Global Capitalism: towards a theory of uneven geographical development*, London: Verso.
Illsley, R. (1980) *Professional or Public Health? Sociology in health and medicine*, London: Nuffield Provincial Hospitals Trust.
Jefferys, M. (1969) 'Sociology and medicine: separation or symbiosis?', *Lancet*, i: 1111–16.
—— (1997) 'Social medicine and medical sociology 1950–1970: the testimony of a partisan participant', in D. Porter (ed.) *Social Medicine and Medical Sociology in the Twentieth Century*, Amsterdam: Rodopi.
Law, A. and Work, H. (2008) 'Ambiguities and resistance: academic labour and the commodification of higher education', in G. Mooney and A. Law (eds) *New Labour/Hard Labour: restructuring and resistance inside the welfare industry*, Bristol: Policy Press.
Lyotard, J.-F. (1972) *The Postmodern Condition*, Manchester: Manchester University Press.
May, D. and Clark, I. (1980) 'Cuckoo in the nest: some comments on the role of sociology in the undergraduate medical curriculum', *Medical Education*, 14: 105–12.
Patrick, D. and Scambler, G. (eds) (1982) *Sociology as Applied to Medicine*, London: Baillière Tindall.

Ritzer, G. (1996) *The McDonaldization of Society*, 2nd edn, Thousand Oaks, CA: Pine Forge Press.

—— (2001) 'The McDonaldization of American sociology: a metasociological analysis', in G. Ritzer (ed.) *Explorations in Social Theory: from metatheorizing to rationalization*, London: Sage.

Royal Commission on Medical Education (1968) *Royal Commission on Medical Education 1965–68: report* (the Todd Report), London: HMSO.

Scambler, G. (1996) 'The "project of modernity" and the parameters for a critical sociology: an argument with illustrations from medical sociology', *Sociology*, 30: 567–81.

—— (2002) *Health and Social Change: a critical theory*, Buckingham: Open University Press.

—— (2006) 'Medical sociology: past, present and future', in G. Scambler (ed.) *Medical Sociology* (four volumes), London: Routledge.

Sennett, R. (2006) *The Culture of the New Capitalism*, New Haven, CI: Yale University Press.

Tuckett, D. (ed.) (1976) *Introduction to Medical Sociology*, London: Tavistock.

13 Epistemology, medical science and problem-based learning

Introducing an epistemological dimension into the medical-school curriculum

Margot L. Lyon

Introduction

Debates about medical education are closely bound to issues of the quality and adequacy of training. At base, such debates are also inevitably about the foundations of medical knowledge and how such knowledge might best be embodied in training. The shift to a problem-based learning (PBL) model in the curriculum of a majority of medical schools, with its emphasis on student-driven, context-dependent learning, has heightened awareness of what is at stake. Concerns about the knowledge implications of this model are forcing the deeper engagement by medical educators with fundamental questions about the nature of the profession of medicine today and what it may become in the future.

Problem-based learning's emphasis on student-directed, problem-solving methods versus the transmission of information through more conventional didactic techniques has meant fewer hours – and fewer staff – devoted to lecturing and laboratory-based teaching components (Jones *et al.* 2001). The teaching of the basic sciences is now largely embedded, albeit in varying degrees depending on the school, in the problem-based learning context itself. The reduction of time devoted to anatomy, particularly the move away from dissection, as well as reduced teaching of embryology and histology, is seen by many to have undermined not only the competencies required for understanding pathophysiological processes but for many aspects of practice as well.[1] This in turn has led to accusations of the 'dumbing down' of the medical school curriculum.

Included in the typical PBL curriculum are components oriented toward the skills seen as necessary for a more patient-centred model of practice, sometimes labelled as a 'know how' rather than 'know all' approach (Jones *et al.* 2001: 699). What is perceived as an increasing dominance of these more procedural skills has led to what is seen as an imbalance between 'hard' and 'soft' sciences. The 'hard' sciences are seen as having been displaced by so-called 'soft' components such as the psychosocial dimensions of care, ethics, health promotion and communication skills (Cribb and Bignold 1999: 202), and also newer 'buzz' areas such as 'cultural competence'. The soft components are often lumped together and represented as belonging exclusively to the behavioural or social sciences, or to the humanities. Variations on the opposition of hard versus soft science include the opposition between basic and clinical sciences, medical science versus medical practice, or even between the scientific components of practice and what are sometimes represented as its 'touchy-feely' dimensions.

However, framing the debate in terms of an opposition between hard and soft science in fact obscures or masks more fundamental conceptual issues that need to be openly addressed. Constructing these domains as in opposition to one another implies an ontological difference between them and thus their potential exclusivity. It suggests that the hard or 'real' science components are concerned with one type of phenomena, and so opposed to the soft or 'not' science components that either masquerade as science, or are somehow not subject to scientific enquiry. Yet clearly both domains – including their interconnections – must be subjected to scientific analysis.

While clinical training of course entails the acquisition of diverse practical techniques, skills and information relevant to acquiring the necessary capacity for professional practice, the clinical components of a curriculum in their wider sense are logically grounded in – and should embrace – the full scope of current scientific knowledge. In a real sense they are the embodiments of that knowledge. And that scientific knowledge properly encompasses all dimensions of life including social phenomena. The distinction between science and praxis thus has limited value. It does not open a way toward a deeper understanding of the interpenetration of science in both domains. To ignore the conceptual foundations for the integration of basic and clinical sciences is to risk reinforcing the body–mind dualism that characterizes so much of medical thinking.

One way to cut through the hard versus soft, basic versus clinical science division is to consider how such distinctions in themselves reflect a particular epistemological stance, one that can cloud our view of the importance of a deeper engagement with science. Epistemology is a relatively unexamined dimension of medical education but one that may assist in revealing and clarifying core problems within it. This chapter seeks to consider some core epistemological issues that arise from the ways in which medical education is organized. In the process, I shall suggest how these issues may at least be made more explicit, in the hope that it may contribute to future curricular design as well as to students' ability to better come to grips with the ever-changing field of medical science.

The following section provides a brief overview of the key characteristics of problem-based learning, its stated advantages, and major points of critique. The chapter then addresses the epistemological dimension of medical education and how the addition of an 'epistemological layer' into PBL curricula may assist in generating student awareness of the structure, foundations and limits of medical knowledge.

Problem-based learning and its critics

Introduction

Problem-based learning is now the core of curricula in many medical schools throughout the world. It was first developed as a teaching tool in the fields of medicine and engineering as a means to assist students in the application of learned knowledge to real problems. Involving small groups of students working together, PBL is a form of active learning. The emphasis is on problem-solving through the use of specific cases or scenarios designed to stimulate student interest and to structure the learning process. Scenarios can take the form of paper-based case descriptions, articles from scientific journals or from the press, laboratory data, video clips, real or simulated patients, or a combination of these and other materials. Working through the cases can be said to loosely mimic processes of diagnosis and formulation of treatment plans.

Case scenarios in a PBL-based curriculum are of course written with particular learning goals in mind, and their structure and content are meant to guide the study process so as to meet those specific learning objectives (Wood 2003: 329). Yet, once presented with the case materials, it is primarily the students themselves who must formulate the key learning tasks for each case. Although under the guidance of a tutor, students are expected to work together to ascertain what types of knowledge they need to acquire to understand all dimensions of the case. Group members are expected to engage in independent reading and research using a variety of relevant resources, and then meet to share, discuss and critique what they have learned within a group context.[2]

The 'key cases' approach that is at the heart of PBL is seen as breaking down the barrier between pre-clinical and clinical education, while enabling the delivery of a core curriculum for common study by all students (Wood 2003: 328). This context-based learning model has also been represented as assisting in the integration between science and praxis. It is argued that the medical sciences are learned in relation to their relevance to, and manifestation in, actual pathological processes in real populations. Therefore theoretically PBL should make possible a deeper engagement with science through seeing it not as independent sets of facts, but as revealed in complex bodily and social processes. Yet to its critics it does not seem to have fulfilled this promise.

Although the small-group teaching format fundamental to PBL is sometimes said to be rather more labour intensive than, for example, large-group lectures, in fact it has its own economies. It draws less heavily on research-based academic staff in the various medical-school departments and specialties to provide lecture and laboratory teaching. Once the PBL curriculum is designed, goals defined and the scenarios constructed, this ordered set of teaching materials and assessment plans provides a sort of potted curriculum which can be quite cost-effective. Supplemental components of the curriculum are now frequently drawn from the increasingly available and comprehensive online and software-based learning tools, including programs to assist in the study of the basic sciences.

This acts to further minimize the curriculum components that must be presented through more didactic-style teaching in labs and lecture halls. It would seem that PBL-based curricula are seen as particularly useful in new medical schools at smaller, more resource-poor institutions where the relevant science departments or faculties may not be well established.

In practice, of course, there is considerable variation in the approaches taken within a PBL format. In most schools, PBL generally occupies a place at the centre of a wider curriculum which includes some amount of additional teaching in the basic sciences, clinical-practice skills, professional development, and so on. Many schools retain or have reintroduced separate coursework in anatomy and pathology and other areas, either as required or elective components of the curriculum.

Stated advantages of problem-based learning

The PBL curriculum structure is considered to have a number of advantages. Presenting case scenarios as problems is designed to enhance student motivation through the excitement of discovery. Cases provide a meaningful context for learning and so are thought to encourage the active engagement with and processing of knowledge, thus facilitating not only understanding but retention. The integration of knowledge and practice required by the key-cases approach is also seen as a solution to information overload, a problem much exacerbated by technological advances and rapid changes in medical knowledge.

The active learning process is also said to facilitate *deep learning* (for example, Wood 2003: 330). Students are said to 'interact with the learning material more than in an information-gathering or theoretical approach. Concepts are related to everyday experience and evidence is related to conclusions. These are features of the deep approach to learning' (Davis and Harden 1999: 133).

As problem-based learning is *student-centred*, that is, the learning process itself is student-driven rather than faculty-driven, students are encouraged to take responsibility for their own learning. The aim here is said to be the development of the skills necessary for self-directed learning. These are seen as essential in preparing the student for the continuation of learning through their lifetime: 'The speed of developments and of innovation in patient care and in healthcare delivery requires all health professionals to make a commitment to keeping up to date through lifelong learning' (Davis and Harden 1999: 133).

PBL thus is meant to instil generic competencies such as problem-solving, communication and team-working skills. But although students start with individual examples, the goal in learning is to be able to use the specifics of these cases to arrive at general principles, which can then presumably be applied in other, differing contexts. Its promotion of active engagement with knowledge is seen as fostering clinical reasoning and decision-making abilities. Its integrative character is held to assist in the organization of knowledge and even concept formation.

Critiques of PBL and curricular change

The central place now given to problem-based learning in medical-school curricula has also evoked intense criticism. The basis for critique of main concern here is the place given to the study of the basic sciences. Though often presented as a solution to information overload, the reliance on PBL has also been seen as symptomatic of 'underload' as more traditional components of training are pushed into the background.

Student-driven, context-based learning techniques are seen as resulting in superficial or incomplete learning of scientific facts and principles – learning that is ultimately inadequate for the demands of clinical practice. In the United Kingdom, for example, the *British Medical Journal* publishing group initiated a campaign to encourage debate about the soundness of current training in academic medicine (Clark and Smith 2003; Tugwell 2004). In Australia the rather recent turn toward PBL by both established and new medical schools triggered a series of exchanges regarding the place of hard science in the curriculum in the *Medical Journal of Australia* (*MJA*). For some schools, the curricular change accompanied a shift to a post-graduate training model. A 2003 editorial in the *MJA* pointed out that '[m]edical students in the UK and Australia have called for more, not less, hard science', and urged wider consultation with the profession and the accumulation of hard evidence on the relative benefits of the different components of the curricula (Van Der Weyden 2003: 601). Such concerns have led many medical schools to attempt to adjust and fine-tune PBL curricula or to create hybrid programmes in order to reintroduce more rigorous training in the basic sciences.

As crucial as the debate about the diminution of science training is, as has been suggested above, the setting up of a dichotomy between science and other curricular components obscures deeper issues about the nature of medical science as a whole. These issues permeate teaching in both the basic sciences and clinical skills.

Sobel and Levine, writing on the undermining of the value of science in medicine, argue that the social transformation of medicine has altered both medical education and medical practice, and in so doing has led to the 'disqualification of physician-scientists' (2001: 713). The authors take the example of current uses of evidence-based medicine (EBM) to illustrate what they term the de-emphasis of 'traditional scientific reasoning predicated on an understanding of physiology and pathophysiology' (ibid.). The 'unintended consequence of evidence-based medicine is excessive reliance on a tool box of processes such as appraisal skills, meta-analyses, and practice guidelines' (ibid.: 714). Their critique parallels others such as that of Talbot (2004), who sees a reduction of medical-science training to a competency model. Such changes in the nature of medicine are 'driving the primary care physician to forsake consideration of scientifically established principles, rely on algorithms mandated by healthcare economists, triage patients, and mouth a litany of new objectives including market share, throughput, and productivity' (Sobel and Levine 2001: 715). And, despite the development of new curricula, many 'fail to adequately incorporate the seminal developments in genetics, molecular biology, and technology that offer so much promise' (ibid.: 715–16).

The epistemological dimension in medical education

The ultimate consequence of the lack of scientific rigour in current curricula for Sobel and Levine is the 'minimization of the value of critical thinking' (ibid.: 714). They insist that '[m]edical schools must empower their graduates with skills in critical thinking and expertise in integrating advances in basic science into clinical practice if physicians are to retain any leadership role in the health-care system's hierarchy'. In light of continual exponential developments in technology, they argue against 'a reductionist, cookbook approach to training physicians', stating that residents 'must know also how to think critically and assimilate advances in science pertinent to their patients'. Further, '[m]outhing of the results of the "latest" (not necessarily the best designed) clinical trial', they say, 'cannot substitute for a broader epistemology' (ibid.: 716).

Epistemology by definition is concerned with the investigation of the nature of knowledge and the grounds on which a body of knowledge can be justified as 'fact'. Thus, it considers the processes through which knowledge claims in any given domain come to be developed and justified. A broader epistemology can only be nurtured through education, not just training. From the perspective of Sobel and Levine what students require is 'knowledge of "classics" in medical science and the logical fabric of mechanistic research and its contribution to clinical judgment' (ibid.).

Epistemology and critical thinking

But what is the connection between epistemology and critical thinking? A crucial matter is that education must be sufficient to foster not only the ability to reflect upon the structure of medical knowledge, but also its limitations. The explosion of information in many areas of medicine has increased the importance of an awareness of how knowledge is produced and the bases of its claims for legitimacy. This is central not only for establishing uniform diagnostic criteria, consistent definitions and nomenclatures, and for the systematic manipulation of medical data (Lindahl 1990: 1); it is even more crucial in coping with the epistemological uncertainty that characterizes medicine today (Fox 2000). Fox, who first wrote about training for medical uncertainty in 1957, has outlined in a later work how major changes in medicine have created new 'modalities of uncertainty'. Not merely scientific and technological, these changes are also 'cognitive and ethical, conceptual and empirical, methodological and procedural, and social and cultural in nature' (2000: 422).

The lack of attention in medical education to the epistemological foundations of medical knowledge and practice has been noted by many (for example, De Cuzzani and Lie 1991; Lindahl 1990; Pena *et al.* 2002; see also Wulff 2001).

However, in the medical-education literature it is more common to see reference to the need for research on the existing epistemological beliefs of students, that is, the taken-for-granted understandings that students bring to the study of medicine. Roex and Degryse point out that despite major changes in the medical-school curriculum, 'insights into students' epistemological beliefs have yet to find their way into the curriculum' (2007: 616; see also Knight and Mattick 2006).

Less common is comment on the degree to which the medical curriculum directly engages with epistemological dimensions of medical science and its practice. Much of curriculum content regarding the practice of medicine is in fact 'hidden', not made manifest, and yet it is from this 'hidden curriculum' that 'students learn what a doctor is' (Cribb and Bignold 1999: 205; see also Hafferty 1998, and Hafferty and Castellani, Chapter 2 this volume). The same can be said for curriculum content regarding the nature of medicine itself. The invisibility of epistemological concerns has been commented on by Phillips, who recounts that through all the years of her medical training and practice, including teaching at two universities, she never heard anyone explicitly refer to the notion of the body-as-machine – a central metaphor of biomedicine – or use the term ideology (Phillips 1997: 499). She argues that although 'newer educational formats such as problem-based learning offer an opportunity to acknowledge and discuss the presumptions of medicine, their design and content can and do work to reinforce rather than challenge values' (Phillips 1997: 499).

Starting from the fact that all 'scientific knowledge subsumes a set of epistemological, logical and ethical foundations', Pena *et al.* (2002) studied resident physicians' knowledge. As physicians must acquire and use basic scientific principles 'to explain, diagnose, and manage complex medical problems', the ability to identify and integrate these principles 'should be necessary for improved application, teaching and learning of medical practice' (Pena *et al.* 2002: 1). Yet data from a survey of resident physicians' understandings of the meaning of epistemology showed that 67 per cent had no idea what epistemology is, and only 24 per cent were able to provide a definition of scientific theory.

Similarly, a study by two medical ethicists at the University of Oslo showed how a lack of understanding of the limitations of medical knowledge can have significant implications for decision-making in clinical intervention (De Cuzzani and Lie 1991: 87–8). Using the example of a particular intervention in cardiological disease, they show how it is 'not only a *lack* of knowledge about the pathophysiology of the disease that led to the adoption of inappropriate therapies, but also a lack of awareness of the *limitations* of such knowledge for clinical intervention' (De Cuzzani and Lie 1991: 87–8). They point out the need for better understanding of how knowledge gained from the basic sciences is used, and how it is grounded in the need to understand the knowledge-acquisition process itself. They state: '[w]e would like to suggest that more attention should be directed to an examination of the epistemological presuppositions of medical knowledge if we want to solve the ethical problems which arise from an application of this knowledge' (De Cuzzani and Lie 1991: 89).

Such issues, in turn, have a bearing on how professionalism is to be defined and nurtured. In an article reflecting on theories of the acquisition of medical professionalism, Hilton and Southgate discuss what they see as six domains of professional behaviour. One of these is the capacity for reflection and self awareness, which they compare with the Aristotelian concept of 'practical wisdom' (*phronesis*) (2007: 270): 'This is the application of judgment to address complex problems and conflicting interests' (ibid.: 267). They state that '[k]nowledge, skills and competences are necessary, but not sufficient ... what is required is good quality or effective reflection, which in turn requires the developed meta-skills' (ibid.: 271).

The structure of medical knowledge

The capacity for reflection and an awareness of the limitations of medical knowledge are therefore fundamental to critical thinking. The development of these skills in turn entails an awareness of the categories of thought that are at the foundation of any given system of knowledge. Critical reflection is thus about how knowledge and meaning are made. Students need to be made aware of how 'all knowledge is constructed by the learner', says Graffam, who sees critical reflection as a crucial component of processes of active learning (2007: 39).

However, in the active, self-directed learning context that is characteristic of PBL, the onus is on students to determine learning objectives, that is, the directions of enquiry, appropriate sources to be consulted, and so on. Without some prior sense of the structure of knowledge across differing disciplines, as well as the ability to organize, manage and integrate that knowledge, students may simply reproduce in the new learning context their own past limitations in knowledge and understanding. '[P]eople construct knowledge based on previously held beliefs and experiences', as Graffam notes (2007: 39). Students with narrow or limited backgrounds may find it difficult to engage with deeper levels of learning. If student learning experiences and information resources are lacking in depth and rigour, then the scaffolding necessary for building knowledge is weakened, impairing the ability to reflect on its meaning, as well as on its limitations. Critical reflection cannot extend much beyond the understandings the student either already has or those he or she can acquire through sufficient learning. It is no surprise that in some disciplines of medicine there is a move toward faculty-driven learning where senior faculty act as expert mentors, rather than having students determine appropriate goals and strategies for learning (see, for example, Trappler 2006). True critical reflection thus requires understanding of larger questions of context, and thus the place of one's perspective in a broader epistemological frame.

Poorly designed case scenarios may contribute to this tendency to replicate conventional ways of thinking. In addition, cases may be written or tutored in such a way as to reproduce gender and ethnic stereotypes. Examining PBL cases in use at one university, Phillips clearly shows how problem-based learning 'can and does effectively and implicitly reinforce traditional values and stereotypes' (1997: 497).

Proper scenario design is a complex process, particularly if it is to move students into a deeper interrogation of the material. To create maximum impact and have maximum learning potential an ideal scenario needs to be *ill-structured*, that is, one that does not have a single solution pathway, and that changes as more information is obtained (see, for example, Dolmanns *et al.* 2005: 734–5). Problems must be truly open-ended such that students cannot know if they have made the correct decision, so generating controversy and forcing the consideration of an expanding domain of questions. They must require information that is not initially available and that is of sufficient complexity to require collaboration with others, including working across disciplines (Stanford University CTL Newsletter 2001: 3).[3] In dramatized form, a sufficiently ill-structured scenario might be said to resemble a plot sequence from the American TV serial *House*. The fictional Dr Gregory House and his team repeatedly think they are able to make a diagnosis only to be presented each time with new information or new symptoms that negate the prior solution and force a rethink of the case. Uncertainties and conflicts that arise in student debate about the case should help bring to the fore and make apparent their taken-for-granted assumptions. It is in this process that 'epistemological beliefs typically come to the surface', say Roex and Degryse (2007: 617). And it is here that they need to be challenged.

Therefore the question of at what level knowledge is being engaged in case-based learning is an important one. In what ways are students thinking about – and learning to think about – what they are learning? Is it of sufficient breadth and depth to provide that 'broader epistemology' that Sobel and Levine say is needed? They argue that this is a knowledge that comes from a deeper engagement with medical science, a medical science whose scope, it should be added, includes an understanding of its historical, scientific and social foundations.

The introduction of an epistemological dimension into a problem-based learning curriculum: a practical example

PBL as a locus of opportunity

How might a meta-cognitive dimension be introduced to the curriculum, one that can make the learner more aware of the construction of scientific knowledge? Although not a solution to the perceived lack of rigour in scientific training, it is worth considering if such a component could be developed. The PBL framework in fact presents an opportunity for the introduction of this dimension. The very integrative character of context-based learning can facilitate the introduction of this additional 'layer' in teaching, one that is directly relevant to, and yet sits 'outside' the immediate case material. Through it, students can be made aware of epistemological issues – though the term itself need not even be used – and thus become more acutely aware of the structure of medical knowledge and its limitations.

Properly conceived and executed, the additional component could be used to challenge students to reflect upon the larger, usually unquestioned context in which medicine resides. This can be a particularly effective device at the first-year level[4] when students are beginning to differentiate between types and levels of information, and degrees of inclusiveness-exclusiveness of categories. It is here that there exists the possibility of introducing material that can foster a self-conscious awareness and questioning of the origins, construction, organization and veracity of categories and models that they are learning.

The remaining sections of this chapter outline a concrete example of curricular materials intended to introduce an epistemological layer into medical teaching.

A sample curriculum

An attempt to deepen engagement with such issues within medical education can be illustrated by a set of materials that I authored for a recently established, postgraduate-entry medical-degree programme in Australia.[5] Entitled 'The Social Foundations of Medicine' (SFM), the content attempts to address the wider social theoretical dimensions of medicine, yet also constitutes an integral component of the curriculum (Lyon 2003a, 2003b).[6] My aim was to develop a series of dynamic modules that could engage simultaneously with medicine as science and as praxis, and so play an integrative role in the medical-education curriculum as a whole.

The design of the course involved the selection of materials that would facilitate development of students' awareness of the assumptive bases of medical knowledge, and also of their own taken-for-granted ideas and beliefs about health, sickness and healing. 'The Social Foundations of Medicine' thus provides an arena in which to raise questions about the nature of medicine and to provide insight into how biomedicine is shaped by the material, historical, social and cultural contexts in which it is located.

The modules work primarily through contrasting perspectives whereby the juxtaposition of two readings and/or other materials brings into question or 'de-naturalizes' a particular set of ideas or beliefs about some aspect of medicine. This momentary de-centring of viewpoint seeks to prompt students to think about the origins, construction, organization and veracity of medical knowledge. The modules do not so much speak directly *about* epistemology per se, but rather aim to *reveal* something about the epistemological foundations of medicine by engaging directly with the nature and structure of that knowledge.

The questioning – at the very outset – of the epistemological bases of what is being learned is therefore a worthwhile step in itself. A programme such as SFM provides for the introduction of an additional level of learning into the curriculum, but does so in a way that links directly to case scenarios and other teaching components in the curriculum.

Structure and organization of the 'Social Foundations of Medicine' and its place in the curriculum

As noted, 'The Social Foundations of Medicine' was written to function as an integral part of a four-year, post-graduate training programme. The first two years of the curriculum are organized around four main areas or 'themes': Medical Sciences (45%), Clinical Skills (30%), Professionalism and Leadership (15%) and Population Health (10%).[7] Content is variously delivered through large-group lectures, small tutor-led groups, seminars, demonstrations, laboratory sessions, clinical-skill practice sessions including those undertaken in a hospital setting and so on. At the centre of the curriculum structure, and around which theme the teaching revolves, are the problem-based learning cases. 'The Social Foundations of Medicine' component, however, is conceived of as a 'framework' that transects the four themes, and is intended to play a supportive and integrative role in the medical programme overall. Although as a framework it is technically independent of the four themes, SFM is a required component of the curriculum and therefore assessable, with questions on the material included in exams as part of overall assessment.

SFM lecture topics were chosen so as to link with the clinical material in the various case scenarios, as well as with other aspects of the teaching programme. Approximately 17 in-class hours are allotted to SFM teaching distributed throughout the two main 'Blocks' that comprise the first-year curriculum.[8] In Year Two further but fewer sessions are conducted. The focus in SFM teaching in Years Three and Four is on assisting students to make use of perspectives gained in the first two years as they undertake their various rotations.

Each module topic is designed to encourage reflection on different aspects of medical knowledge and practice. For each session students are provided a brief study guide which includes reference to its aims and a synopsis of content. Readings, generally two, are provided. All materials are available in an online format to be read online or printed off. As readings by non-medical professionals tend to be given little authority by students, an attempt was made to use sources by scientists and professionals working in medical fields, and where relevant to point out to students the career trajectory of the author or their standing in the field of medicine.

The study guide for each session includes a question of one or more parts to be answered by students, generally in learning-diary format. The questions are short and are designed to direct attention to the most relevant and important aspects of the material and so assist in efficient time use. Students are to read not for detail but rather for the particular perspectives or concepts being addressed in the readings. They are asked to reflect on these and to consider their potential relevance to other curricular components. It is important to point out that this structure is flexible. It is a simple matter to change or substitute readings to better intersect with other parts of the curriculum, to include more timely topics, or to better capture shifting student interests.

Course-content examples

By way of illustration, I shall outline some examples of module topics and readings. Emphasis will be given to the nine modules taught as part of the Foundation Block of the first-year curriculum.

The first six of these provide students with an introduction to major conceptual issues that arise in the study of biomedicine. As already indicated, the aim is to encourage students to reflect on wider contexts of their study of health, sickness and healing, as well as on the structure and content of the categories of knowledge presented to them in the course of their training. These modules address, for example, the nature of biomedicine, biomedicine's implicit, so-called 'hidden' values, the social and historical development of nosological categories, the idea of the embodiment of sickness and distress, the foundations of efficacy, and the 'therapeutic process'. Subsequent modules, numbers seven and eight, address sickness and social inequality, followed by a ninth module on contested views of what constitutes clinical death.

In combination or singly, the texts assigned aim to help develop a self-directed and self-conscious awareness of these fundamental issues in medical knowledge and practice, and the subsequent enhancement of critical thinking. In the first module concerning the nature of biomedicine, for example, students read short excerpts on striking differences in the everyday practices of scientific biomedicine in France, Germany, Great Britain and the United States (Payer 1988). Though popularly written, the differences, when pointed out, momentarily de-familiarize something normally assumed to be a single entity, thus serving to suggest that what we see as medical science is always informed by the societal contexts in which it is practised. A second reading then provides a more explicit framework for articulating how the biomedical model in our society functions both as a scientific model, and as a folk model (Rhodes 1990). Such readings do not at any time deny or discount the importance of the scientific foundations of biomedicine; their introduction at this point aims to give students a model for understanding and appropriate terminology for the articulation of the wider dimensions of medicine as both knowledge and praxis.

In the follow-up module on hidden values in biomedicine, readings by two medical scientists are used to develop a further grasp of the implicit dualisms in biomedicine. One addresses medicine's dominant emphasis on the body as machine and the inevitable clinical implications of mind–body distinctions (Kirmayer 1988). The second uses the title chapter of Cassell's (1991a) 'The nature of suffering', which shows how suffering is related both to physical symptoms and personhood, thus providing further development of the implications of a mind–body duality for patients.

Module three takes up the construction of disease categories. Using an article on the origins and changes over time in the classification of psychological disorders in the *Diagnostic and Statistical Manual of the American Psychiatric Association* (DSM), it introduces the idea that what we see as given nosological categories – in this case for psychological illness – have been profoundly influenced by historical and social forces (Gaines 1992). It is paired with another chapter by Cassell entitled, 'Ideas in conflict: the rise and fall of new views of disease' (1991b), providing discussion of how our models or theories of disease affect what we see and what we do, and how an awareness of this can move us to think beyond them to be open to other dimensions in the understanding of sickness. Further, understanding the history of the development of disease categories provides a good foundation for later discussion of potential future sites of medicalization.

Module four considers how social and economic forces are embodied in the experience, manifestations and representations of sickness, pairing a reading on perceptions of an illness category, *debilidad*, common among Hispanic populations (Oths 1999), and an historical overview of chronic fatigue syndrome in the West (Aronowitz 1992).

Modules five and six ask students to consider diverse dimensions of the question of the nature of healing. Module five, for example, introduces debates about the nature of placebo/nocebo phenomena, and how placebo phenomena may be considered a component of all healing. Module six introduces the notion of the 'therapeutic process' in biomedicine as a complex, multidimensioned topic, and asks how its differing aspects might be explored, for example, which dimensions of the medical encounter might be said to have therapeutic 'effects'. Such a topic can also encompass a consideration of how authority relations in any given society (including our own) tend to be reflected or reproduced in the structuring of medical encounters.

The programme continues with two modules that address suffering and social inequality, using the examples of diseases of nutritional deficiency and infectious diseases. The first of these addresses the relationship of social and political inequality to the distribution of disease and suffering, drawing on a reading by Paul Farmer (1998), who calls for 'a critical epistemology of emerging infectious diseases'. The second, using the example of AIDS, explores how a population's understandings of and reactions to sickness are shaped by the political, economic and cultural contexts in which they arise. Case material is drawn from both Haiti (Farmer 1999) and South Africa (Leclerc-Madlala 1997). The importance of including curriculum content on diseases of the developing world, particularly in the training of primary care doctors, has been flagged by many and evokes high student interest.

The Foundation Block finishes with a module on death in conjunction with the case scenario involving the unexplained death of a young person. A reading by a medical anthropologist (Lock 1997) raises the question of the origins and development of biomedical definitions of what constitutes clinical death. Comparing changing constructions of death in America and Japan, it also examines the implications of such differences for attitudes toward transplant technologies. A very different reading on the natural processes of dying is excerpted from Nuland's *How We Die: reflections on life's final chapter* (1993). The problematization of just how death is to be defined in biomedicine is later built upon in the second semester in a module on the history of the development of organ-transplant technologies and the commodification of human body parts. Such critical material helps to underpin the learning process for students who will some day have to address patient questions regarding brain death and organ donation.[9]

Other topics addressed in later modules in the first year are phenomenological accounts of chronic illness and disability, the gendering and legitimation and delegitimation of certain illness presentations, differing sociocultural perspectives on the medical encounter and the conception of medicalization and related notions such as 'disease mongering'. In the latter case, in conjunction with a case scenario on sleep apnoea, the module explores the history of the increasing interest in defining 'normal' patterns of sleep and wakefulness. A reading which details the huge diversity in sleep patterns across different societies is used (Worthman and Melby 2003). This is then paired with website descriptions of seemingly science-fictionesque research into the effects of acute and chronic sleep deprivation on fighter pilots and their prevention, one of the biological sciences research projects of the Defense Sciences Office (DSO) within DARPA (Defense Advanced Research Projects Agency) of the United States Department of Defense.[10]

In any of these topic areas, choices of readings can be taken from a range of scientific fields and medical subspecialties, as well as from social sciences and history. Further, the number of thought-provoking yet popular books on medical topics continues to grow which, together with works from medical classics, makes for a formidable list. Careful selection of web-based resources including list-serves, medical blogs and particular online science publications and medical websites, and so on, can provide further easily accessed material that can be harnessed for teaching.

For student groups unable or unwilling to engage with such material, sources that emphasize the import of the psychosocial domain for biological systems can be used, for example, literature in the fields of psychoneuroimmunology or placebo phenomena. Important also are recent developments in the neurosciences that are bringing about a new convergence of the biological and social sciences and making possible research aimed at understanding the simultaneity of biological and social being.

Conclusion

It should be clear from the above that a set of modules such as SFM can be easily located within a problem-based learning curriculum. The questions raised and the concepts introduced should then help to put the curricular content in perspective, and function in the integration of its various components.

Although the addition of such a teaching programme to a typical problem-based learning curriculum does not necessarily impact on the level or quality of science training in the medical curriculum as a whole, one can argue that it may contribute to a deeper engagement with science. Such modules, properly conceived and taught, can help to reveal to students the structure of the knowledge systems with which they are grappling, the assumptions on which they are based, and their potential limitations. In turn, this awareness should assist in the development of better thinking and reasoning skills, and perhaps the ability for a more efficacious application of knowledge in practice.

These other ways of knowing are thus also part of the process of learning the skills that are necessary for the development of professional competence. If one of the purposes of this volume is to 'suggest future directions for the sociological study of medical education and for medical education itself', I would argue that the question of how to encourage the awareness of, and reflection on, the depth and breadth of developments in science, as well as their limitations, is a crucial step. Addressing how this may be imparted is a step in the development of professional judgement and critical thinking.

Notes

1 For example, the lack of gross dissection has led to a situation whereby surgical residents learn anatomy while doing surgery, leading to criticisms such as that made by Beahrs (quoted in Cahill *et al.* 2000: 70): 'Lack of anatomic knowledge too often leads to disaster. To learn basic anatomic information by trial and error at the expense of a patient undergoing an elective or emergency operation is morally wrong.'

2 The nature and principles of problem-based learning in medical education are well covered in the literature. Guides and overviews are readily available, e.g. Dolmanns *et al.* (2005), Davis and Harden (1999) and Wood (2003).

3 The newsletter article draws on material from Allen *et al.* (1996) and Gallagher (1997).

4 Comments here refer to the first year of a post-graduate entry programme. The possibility of integrating SFM into an undergraduate programme would depend on the structure of the curriculum, and would probably be better brought in during the second or third years.

5 The Australian National University Medical School commenced teaching in 2004. Located in the national capital of Canberra, it is one of several recently established medical schools in Australia.

6 The examples presented here concern 'The Social Foundations of Medicine' curriculum component only. I do not attempt to discuss, and make no claims about, the curriculum as a whole nor the place of basic science teaching within it.

7 Medical Program Curriculum Information can be accessed at http://medicalschool. anu.edu.au/curriculum/themes.asp.

8 Block One ('DNA to Death') comprises the 'Foundation Block' with PBL cases roughly organized around the life cycle. Block Two focuses on anatomical systems with emphasis in the first year on cardio-respiratory and renal medicine, and endocrine and reproductive health. SFM occupies nine sessions in Block One and eight sessions in Block Two.

9 A study to assess medical-student knowledge in Ohio showed that medical students had less knowledge about brain death than a random sample of non-medically trained adults (Essman and Thornton 2006).

10 See, for example, www.darpa.mil/dso/thrusts/bio/index.htm.

References

Allen, D. E., Duch, B. J. and Groh, S. E. (1996) 'The power of problem-based learning in teaching introductory science courses', in L. Wilkerson and W. H. Gijselaers (eds) *Bringing Problem-based Learning to Higher Education: theory and practice*, San Francisco, CA: Jossey-Bass.

Aronowitz, R. A. (1992) 'From myalgic encephalitis to yuppie flu: a history of chronic fatigue syndrome', in C. E. Rosenberg and J. Golden (eds) *Framing Disease: studies in cultural history*, New Brunswick, NJ: Rutgers University Press.

Beahrs, O. H. (1991) 'Gross anatomy in medicine', *Clinical Anatomy*, 4: 310–12.

Cahill, D. R., Leonard, R. J. and Marks Jr, S. C. (2000) 'A comment on recent teaching of human anatomy in the United States', *Surgical and Radiologic Anatomy*, 22: 69–71.

Cassell, E. J. (1991a) 'The nature of suffering', in *The Nature of Suffering and the Goals of Medicine*, New York: Oxford University Press.

—— (1991b) 'Ideas in conflict: the rise and fall of new views of disease', in *The Nature of Suffering and the Goals of Medicine*, New York: Oxford University Press.

Clark, J. and Smith, R. (2003) 'BMJ publishing group to launch an international campaign to promote academic medicine', *British Medical Journal*, 327: 1001–2.

Cribb, A. and Bignold, S. (1999) 'Towards the reflexive medical school: the hidden curriculum and medical education research', *Studies in Higher Education*, 24: 195–209.

Davis, M. H. and Harden, R. M. (1999) 'AMEE Medical Education Guide No. 15: problem-based learning: a practical guide', *Medical Teacher*, 21: 130–40.

De Cuzzani, P. and Lie, R. K. (1991) 'The importance of epistemology for clinical practice', *Theoretical Medicine*, 12: 87–90.

Dolmanns, D. H. J. M., De Grave, W., Wolfhagen, I. H. A. P. and van der Vleuten, C. P. M. (2005) 'Problem-based learning: future challenges for educational practice and research', *Medical Education*, 39: 732–41.

Essman, C. and Thornton, J. (2006) 'Assessing medical student knowledge, attitudes, and behaviors regarding organ donation', *Transplantation Proceedings*, 38: 2745–50.

Farmer, P. (1998) 'Social inequalities and emerging infectious diseases', in P. J. Brown (ed.) *Understanding and Applying Medical Anthropology*, Mountain View, CA: Mayfield.

—— (1999) 'Sending sickness: sorcery, politics, and changing concepts of AIDS in rural Haiti' *Infections and Inequalities: the modern plagues*, Berkeley: University of California Press.

Fox, R. C. (1957) 'Training for uncertainty', in R. K. Merton, G. G. Reader and P. L. Kendall (eds) *The Student-Physician: introductory studies in the sociology of medical education*, Cambridge, MA: Harvard University Press.

—— (2000) 'Medical uncertainty revisited', in G. Albrecht, R. Fitzpatrick and S. Scrimshaw (eds) *Handbook of Social Studies in Health and Medicine*, London: Sage.

Gaines, A. D. (1992) 'From DSM-I to II-R: voices of self, mastery and the other: a cultural constructivist reading of US psychiatric classifications', *Social Science and Medicine*, 35: 3–24.

Gallagher, A. A. (1997) 'Problem-based learning: where did it come from, what does it do, and where is it going?', *Journal for the Education of the Gifted*, 20: 332–62.

Graffam, B. (2007) 'Active learning in medical education: strategies for beginning implementation', *Medical Teacher*, 29: 38–42.

Hafferty, F. W. (1998) 'Beyond curriculum reform: confronting medicine's hidden curriculum', *Academic Medicine*, 73: 403–7.

Hilton, S. and Southgate, L. (2007) 'Professionalism in medical education', *Teaching and Teacher Education*, 23: 265–79.

Jones, R., Higgs, R., de Angelis, C. and Prideaux, D. (2001) 'Changing face of medical curricula', *Lancet*, 357: 699–703.

Kirmayer, L. J. (1988) 'Mind and body as metaphors: hidden values in biomedicine', in M. Lock and D. R. Gordon (eds) *Biomedicine Examined*, Dordrecht: Kluwer Academic Publishers.

Knight, L. V. and Mattick, K. (2006) 'When I first came here, I thought medicine was black and white: making sense of medical students' ways of knowing', *Social Science and Medicine*, 63: 1084–96.

Leclerc-Madlala, S. (1997) 'Infect one, infect all: Zulu youth response to the AIDS epidemic in South Africa', *Medical Anthropology*, 17: 363–80.

Lindahl, B. I. B. (1990) 'Editorial', *Theoretical Medicine*, 11: 1–3.

Lock, M. (1997) 'Displacing suffering: the reconstruction of death in North America and Japan', in A. Kleinman, V. Das and M. Lock (eds) *Social Suffering*, Berkeley: University of California Press.

Lyon, M. L. (2003a) 'The Social Foundations of Medicine'. Curriculum materials prepared for Australian National University Medical School, Canberra, Australia.

—— (2003b) 'A guide to the introduction of epistemological issues into the medical curriculum: syllabus and course readings', Manuscript.

Nuland, S. B. (1993) 'Three score and ten', *How We Die: reflections on life's final chapter*, New York: Vintage Books.

Oths, K. S. (1999) '*Debilidad*: A biocultural assessment of an embodied Andean illness', *Medical Anthropology Quarterly*, 13: 286–315.

Payer, L. (1988) *Medicine and Culture*, New York: Penguin.

Pena, A., Paco, O. and Peralta, C. (2002) 'Epistemological beliefs and knowledge among physicians: a questionnaire survey', *Medical Education Online*, 7: 1–9.

Phillips, S. (1997) 'Problem-based learning in medicine: new curriculum, old stereotypes', *Social Science and Medicine*, 45: 497–99.

Rhodes, L. A. (1990) 'Studying biomedicine as a cultural system', in T. M. Johnson and C. F. Sargent (eds) *Medical Anthropology: contemporary theory and method*, New York: Praeger.

Roex, A. and Degryse, J. (2007) 'Introducing the concept of epistemological beliefs into medical education: the hot-air balloon metaphor', *Academic Medicine*, 82: 616–20.

Sobel, B. E. and Levine, M. A. (2001) 'Medical education, evidence-based medicine, and the disqualification of physician-scientists', *Experimental Biology and Medicine*, 226: 713–16.

Stanford University (2001) 'Problem-based learning. Speaking of teaching', *Center for Teaching and Learning (CTL) Newsletter*, 11: 1–7.

Talbot, M. (2004) 'Monkey see, monkey do: a critique of the competency model in graduate medical education', *Medical Education*, 38: 587–92.

Trappler, B. (2006) 'Integrated problem-based learning in the neuroscience curriculum – the SUNY Downstate experience', *BMC Medical Education*, 6: 47.

Tugwell, P. (2004) 'The campaign to revitalise academic medicine kicks off', *Medical Journal of Australia*, 180: 372–3.

Van Der Weyden, M. B. (2003) 'Medical education and hard science: from the editor's desk', *Medical Journal of Australia*, 180: 601.

Wood, D. F. (2003) 'ABC of learning and teaching in medicine: problem-based learning', *British Medical Journal*, 326: 328–30.

Worthman, C. and Melby, M. (2003) 'Toward a comparative developmental ecology of human sleep', in M. A. Carskadon (ed.) *Adolescent Sleep Patterns: biological, social and psychological influences*, Cambridge: Cambridge University Press.

Wulff, H. R. (2001) 'Editorial: a return to biological thinking in medicine', *Medicine, Health Care and Philosophy*, 4: 1–3.

Part III

Medical education in national contexts

14 Medical education and the American healthcare system

William C. Cockerham

American medical schools rank among the best in the world. Typically these schools have quality research facilities, advanced technology and well-trained faculties. They all have high standards of admission and their graduates are readily accepted into the medical profession and by the public at large upon meeting the requisite qualifications for their area of practice. However, the medical profession has experienced radical changes over the past decades as society itself has changed, and many of these changes have affected medical education or – in some instances – medical schools themselves have served as a pipeline to change.

The United States has the most expensive healthcare delivery system in the world. This system is a conglomerate of health practitioners, agencies and institutions, all of which operate on a more-or-less independent basis under a fee-for-service arrangement. In this financing scheme, patients are responsible for paying for the services rendered. Physicians are relatively well paid and hospitals charge high fees. Given the high cost of care, health insurance is a necessity for individuals and families. The insurance system consists of both private and public components, with employer-based insurance the foundation of the private sector and government-sponsored Medicare (for the elderly) and Medicaid (for the poor) comprising the public sector. However, some 16 per cent of the population is uninsured and underserved with respect to their health needs. While much of the healthcare provided is of high quality, the uninsured are least likely to have access to it.

The purpose of this chapter is to examine the relationship between medical education and the healthcare delivery system in the US. At the outset, it should be noted that changes taking place in American society have caused this relationship to be unsettled. That is, society, not the medical profession, has had the primary causal role with respect to changes in the organization of clinical practice and medical education. This is why classical theorists in sociology like Durkheim, Simmel and Weber did not regard medicine as a basic social institution. They apparently recognized that medicine did not mould the fundamental nature and structure of society in the same way as the economy, politics and religion. Rather, it was the case that the nature and structure of society shaped medical practice instead of the reverse. When society changes, medicine adapts and these adaptations often make their way into medical education.

Therefore, as Cooke *et al.* (2006: 1339) observe: American 'medical educa-tion seems to be in a perpetual state of unrest'. Not only do Cooke *et al.* find 'messy' real-world issues difficult to teach in medical schools, but they observe that the values of the profession are increasingly difficult for students to learn, the delivery of care has become vastly more complicated and the expectations of the public higher. At the same time, there has been a decline in the status and autonomy of physicians as healthcare corporations, insurance companies and government entities exercise more control over clinical practice, and allied health professions and occupations are making inroads on their once all-powerful professional dominance. Moreover, the large number of medically uninsured in American society represents an unmet challenge that neither medicine nor the federal government has solved. Physicians prefer not to treat patients who have no health insurance and such patients avoid doctors in order to evade their fees. But accidents and disease bring these two parties involuntarily together, causing unsettled circumstances in which one group or the other is likely to be penalized.

The story of medical education and the American healthcare delivery system is clearly one of change over time. This chapter begins by briefly reviewing medical education during the so-called 'golden age of doctoring' that began in the 1950s, followed by the introduction of managed care in the 1990s, and con-cluding with a discussion of current directions.

The golden age of doctoring

The term 'the golden age of doctoring' was introduced by John McKinlay (1999) to describe the state of the American medical profession at the mid-twentieth century during the height of its power, prestige and public trust. This was the period in which Eliot Freidson (1970a, 1970b) formulated his influential 'profes-sional dominance' thesis in sociology to account for an unprecedented level of professional control by physicians over the delivery of healthcare in the US that no longer exists. It was also a period of escalating prices and overcharging for services to a degree previously unachieved in the history of American medicine. As Donald Light (2000) describes it, there was a proliferation of unnecessary tests, hospitalizations, prescriptions and surgical operations, along with provider-structured insurance that paid for practically everything without question, poor investments in technology or facilities, and neglect of the poor – all in the name of professional autonomy. Light (2004: 15) refers to the 'golden age of medi-cine' as the 'age of gold' for the medical profession.

According to the British historian Roy Porter (1997), health had become one of the major growth industries in America. It encompassed not only physicians, but also hospitals, health-insurance companies, pharmaceutical corporations and manufacturers of costly diagnostic technology, laboratory instruments and thera-peutic devices, as well as vast numbers of other medical personnel, receptionists, clerks, lawyers, accountants and various other supporting occupations. By 1966, health expenditures were approaching 15 per cent of the GDP. Porter determined that health costs were largely unchecked as insurance companies paid whatever the market would bear, physician incomes were seven times higher than the national average, and hospitals in competition for patients added costly technology that was often duplicated in nearby facilities.

Medical education in the golden age of doctoring

As for medical education during the 'golden age of doctoring', essentially all medical schools had adopted the recommendations in Abraham Flexner's famous report in 1910 to establish full-time faculties, laboratory facilities and hospital access for students, and high standards for student admissions and faculty qualifications. This also included locating medical schools in universities to provide graduate level instruction and the integration of teaching with research within these schools. Medical historian Kenneth Ludmerer (1999) observed that from the beginning, modern American medical schools had a three-fold mission of:

1 Education.
2 Research.
3 Patient care.

However, these activities were never in balance. At different times, one or the other was more important. Ludmerer finds that the educational role dominated medical education until 1945 and the end of the Second World War, research until 1965, and patient care in the years thereafter.

During the 'golden age of doctoring', medical schools shifted emphasis from their teaching mission to research as large amounts of federal and private monies flooded into medical schools to fund searches for cures or improved treatments for a wide spectrum of diseases. According to Samuel Bloom (1988), medical education's humanistic mission of teaching and patient care was a screen for its research mission that was the major focus of the medical school during this period. As Ludmerer (1999: xxii) points out, 'all medical schools shared the wealth, and at virtually every school, the research enterprise grew to a size that before ... [the Second World War] would have been considered unimaginable'.

Ludmerer further notes that medical schools were staffed by faculties who made research a high priority in the belief that in order to educate students more effectively, determine standards of patient care and improve that care, it was necessary to be engaged in research. 'The ascendancy of American medical research', states Ludmerer (1999: 139), 'occurred as part of the more generalized expansion of science and higher education in the United States produced after the war by federal spending.' This effort was accelerated by the establishment of the National Institute of Health (NIH), organized in 1948 to conduct research in its own facilities, as well as to fund research at medical schools, universities, hospitals and elsewhere through a nationwide programme of grants and contracts. Ludmerer (1999: 141) depicts the growth in funding during the first 20 years of the NIH as 'staggering' and describes the 1950s and 1960s as a 'golden era' for medical research in the US as well, with vast amounts of money pouring into medical-school labs and other research sites.

The emphasis on research appeared to have strong public support in a period of economic prosperity and industrial growth, in which scientific investigation was emerging as a major function in the nation's leading universities. This emphasis paralleled the expanding modernization taking place in the wider society on a massive scale – as newly designed automobiles, newly invented televisions and other consumer goods such as improved clothing, dish washers, dryers and refrigerators became readily available. Advances in medicine at this time included open-heart surgery, kidney and heart transplants, the discovery of the double helical structure of DNA, the establishment of the link between smoking and lung cancer and improvements in antibiotics.

However, Ludmerer points out that the success of biomedical research was not problem-free for medical education. Research scientists could no longer be produced by medical schools as a simple byproduct of training for an MD (the basic medical degree), since the latter typically had little or no training in research methods, statistics and theory. Although medical schools often adjusted their curriculum to provide at least an introduction to biostatistics and research methodology, biomedical research increasingly demanded sophisticated and advanced methodologies beyond the usual medical school experience. According to Cooke *et al.*:

> Gifted clinical investigators tended to be equally gifted as clinicians and clinical teachers. After 1960, however, as medical research became increasingly molecular in orientation, patients were bypassed in most cutting-edge investigations, and immersion in the laboratory became necessary for the most prestigious scientific projects. Clinical teachers found it increasingly difficult to be first-tier researchers, and fewer and fewer investigators could bring the depth of clinical knowledge and experience to teaching that they once had.
>
> (2006: 1340)

Consequently, a division between the research and clinical-teaching faculty in medical schools began to appear, despite efforts to maintain a balance between the two groups. 'Biomedical research', states Ludmerer (1999: 151), 'acquired an independent quality, no longer requiring the presence and stimulation of medical students'. Research faculty increasingly used basic science graduate students, research fellows and post-doctoral students in their laboratories instead of undergraduate medical students. Some research-oriented students interrupted their medical studies to work in labs relevant to their interests in order to learn more sophisticated research techniques and establish their initial credentials as researchers. Others sought residencies with research opportunities or acquired research positions after residencies and the training that went with them.

However, beginning in 1965 with the advent of Medicare and Medicaid, clinical practice ultimately evolved to supplant research as a medical school's most important source of income. 'If research had once been the master', Ludmerer (1999: 221) observes, 'that role at most medical schools was increasingly assumed by patient care – to the increasing subordination of both research and teaching'. Faculty practices staffed by the clinical faculty at medical schools became nearly universal in response to the rising demand for healthcare. This demand came initially from newly insured Medicaid and Medicare patients and later from patients with private insurance who were attracted to the quality of the doctors and the institutions. This situation evolved when monies from federal grants declined as the growth of the NIH slowed and other national priorities attracted government revenues. Connections to universities weakened as medical schools became integrated into local and regional healthcare-delivery systems as major providers in these care networks.

Demands on faculty time, first with the research emphasis and later with increasing patient loads, reduced the time many professors spent with medical students. Generating profits for the institution through patient care became the priority, not the lecture hall. Bloom citing Lewis Thomas (1987), notes that the:

> professors are elsewhere, trying to allocate their time between writing out their research requests (someone has estimated that 30 per cent of a medical school faculty's waking hours must be spent composing grant applications), doing or at least supervising the research in their laboratories, [and] seeing their patients (the sustenance of a contemporary clinical department has become significantly dependent on the income brought in by the faculty's collective private practice).
>
> (1988: 303)

This situation did not mean that the physicians graduating from American medical schools were poorly trained. To the contrary, Ludmerer (1999: xxiii) finds that even though education by the 1980s was rarely a high institutional priority, 'the quality of medical education obtainable in the United States remained superb'. This was because medical schools depended less on passive learning through lectures and instead emphasized self-learning through problem-solving in case-based, small-group discussions and computer-based independent learning modules that the highly self-directed medical students seemed to prefer. Typically these students preferred practical information that could help them solve clinical problems and pass examinations, rather than theoretical knowledge presented in a lecture format. As Ludmerer explains:

> all medical learning was ultimately self-learning. Throughout the [twentieth] century, the high quality of American medical education depended far less on the formal curriculum than it did on attracting motivated, capable students and providing them unfettered opportunities to learn. Essential to this learning environment were good laboratories and libraries, an ample and diverse supply of patients, and stimulating teachers and colleagues. Most important of all was the fact that medical education was conducted in

settings where learners were provided sufficient time with patients so that patients could be studied and understood.

(1999: xxiii)

The 1950s and 1960s were a period when sociologists began joining medical faculties to teach behavioural science in the first (basic science year) of medical school. Their presence signified recognition by the medical profession that many health problems were due to unhealthy social behaviour and living conditions. The initial studies of medical education by sociologists were conducted at this time in American medical schools and primarily focused on the socialization of medical students into the medical profession. The first extensive study appeared in the book, *The Student-Physician* (1957), edited by Robert Merton, George Reader and Patricia Kendall, with Renée Fox's chapter ranking as a major contribution. Fox (1957) determined that students at Cornell Medical School acquired two basic traits as a result of their medical training: the ability to be emotionally detached from patients and to tolerate uncertainty. The students came to realize they could not learn everything about medicine, that limitations in medical knowledge existed that affected the faculty as well, and that they had to learn to distinguish between personal ignorance and the limits of available knowledge.

In the 1980s, however, evidence-based medicine (EBM) developed in the UK and was introduced in American medical schools to reduce uncertainty among students and improve their diagnostic skills. EBM uses clinical practice guidelines that provide step-by-step instructions that students can refer to in making a diagnosis and determining a course of treatment (Timmermans and Kolker 2004). These instructions are based on established diagnostic and therapeutic procedures corroborated by research and clinical trials. EBM does not remove all uncertainty, but improves judgement in situations where outcomes are generally known and helps where uncertainty still persists in existing medical knowledge (Timmermans and Angell 2001).

The best-known study is that of Howard Becker and his colleagues, reported in their book *Boys in White* (1961), containing observations of the socialization process at the University of Kansas Medical School. Becker *et al.* found that the students developed a strong appreciation for clinical experience and a sense of responsibility for their patients. They also learned to be emotionally detached from patients and to view disease and death as medical problems, not emotional ones. The students had entered medical school openly idealistic about helping people but became somewhat cynical and more concerned with navigating successfully through the training. Idealism allegedly returned on graduation as the students again became interested in service to humanity. Neither the Becker *et al.* nor the Merton *et al.* studies were critical of the US healthcare-delivery system or of the medical profession itself. These early studies were conducted during the so-called 'golden age' of medicine when doctors were all-powerful and medical sociologists were dependent on them for research opportunities. Consequently, the initial focus was on medical students who were relatively powerless. It was not until the late 1970s that sociological critiques of the health-care system and the medical profession started to become common as social inequities in health continued and in some cases worsened, while physician power waned (see Cockerham 2010).

What is often overlooked, as Frederic Hafferty (2007) points out, is that both the Merton *et al.* and the Becker *et al.* studies had an agenda. They were less about medical training and more about advancing a particular theoretical perspective in sociology – structural-functionalism in the case of Merton and his associates as opposed to symbolic interaction for Becker and his colleagues. Another focus of the Becker *et al.* study was on the methodological techniques of participant observation.

There has been little comprehensive research on the medical-school experience over the years. The few subsequent studies have usually focused on particular aspects, such as student protests (Bloom 1973), learning to be unemotional with patients (Coombs 1978; Haas and Shaffir 1977) and dealing with feelings about death (Hafferty 1991). The Merton and Becker studies thus remain the most frequently cited works even though they were conducted in the mid-twentieth century. Hafferty (2007) says this is a glaring commentary on the current lack of well-designed and comprehensive sociological research on medical education. But further research on this topic was undermined by Freidson's (1970a, 1970b) claim that the work environment in medicine was a stronger determinant of physician attitudes than prior socialization in medical school. That is, the demands of residency training following graduation from medical school more strongly embedded professional attitudes in novice physicians. Also the major sociological studies of medical students took place in the infancy of medical sociology, but as the subdiscipline matured and gained access to populations of working physicians, interest in medical students declined. 'The sociological study of medicine', observes Hafferty (2007: 2930), 'began to shift away from a more micro focus on professionalism and identity transformation to a more macro focus on organizational dynamics and structural change'. The era of large-scale studies of medical education was over as sociology transferred its concentration to the practising physician and the major changes taking place in the medical profession at large.

The changing environment of medical practice

Yet as the 'golden age of doctoring' was promoting an 'age of gold' for medicine and professional dominance was in its ascendancy, Light (2000) and Light and Hafferty (1993) accurately observed that countervailing powers were accumulating that soon shattered the status quo. The medical profession was but one of many powerful groups in society – government, big business, patients as consumers, and large health-insurance companies – that were also stakeholders in healthcare delivery. The medical profession's control over its market began to falter as these countervailing powers established strong positions of their own, primarily in reaction to the escalating costs of care. The profession's monopoly began dissolving as it reached its highest point. As Light (2000: 204) points out: 'Dominance slowly produces imbalances, excesses, and neglects that offend or threaten other countervailing powers and alienate the larger public.' And this is exactly what happened.

Change came from several directions outside medicine. The rising costs of healthcare resulted in increased public demands for government intervention and the government responded. Medicaid and Medicare health-insurance pro-grammes were created by federal legislation in 1965 to meet the needs of the poor and the elderly, respectively. Other legislation in the 1970s established Pro-fessional Standards Review Organizations (PSROs) to evaluate the quality of care given to Medicare and Medicaid patients, followed by authorization of Diagnostic Related Groups (DRGs) in the early 1980s. DRGs were a schedule of fees placing limits on how much the government would pay for specific services rendered to patients by doctors and hospitals.

However, as the poor gained health-insurance coverage, the crisis passed to the middle class that was finding it increasingly difficult to adjust to rising charges for care and higher insurance premiums. Fee schedules similar to DRGs were soon adopted by private health-insurance companies, along with such companies some-times requiring second medical opinions for recommended but highly expensive procedures. Third-party payers, namely the government and private insurance companies, had intervened in the doctor–patient relationship to limit physician fees, review the quality of care and in some instances require their approval. And, in doing so, they limited physician autonomy. Additionally, support, through plan-ning grants and loan guarantees, was provided by the government to encourage the development of health-maintenance organizations (HMOs) as a new form of group practice emphasizing preventive care. HMOs are a form of managed care in which patients pay a set fee on a per-capita basis every month and in return are entitled to whatever healthcare they require. HMOs were intended to prevent health problems through regular physician visits or to discover them in early stages so they could be treated less expensively. HMOs soon spread across the nation along with pre-ferred provider organizations (PPOs) in which groups of physicians contracted with employers to provide discounted health services for their employees.

Another limitation on medical practice came from large private health-care corporations purchasing or building chains of hospitals, nursing homes, emergency-care centres, medical-supply companies and other facilities. The interest of these corporations was not in treating patients with government insur-ance, but attracting patients with private health insurance that would cover the higher costs of profit-making hospitals in providing quality facilities and care. In corporate-owned hospitals and care centres, however, physicians were employees and subject to corporate standards of performance, monitoring and scrutiny of mistakes. Corporate hospitals typically do not have a teaching role in undergraduate medical education. This role is generally filled by university and community hospitals.

There were also changes in the public's attitudes toward medicine. Given the American Medical Association's (AMA) strong objections to healthcare reforms like Medicaid and Medicare and any other measure that threatened the incomes and prerogatives of physicians, the public came to view the medical profession as more interested in financial well-being than public welfare. In 1984, the AMA had even unsuccessfully sued the federal government for its cost-containment measures for Medicare, claiming the government did not have the authority to impose limits on physicians' fees and such action interfered with their right to contract for services. The emphasis on financial gain undermined public confidence in the medical profession more than any other single issue at this time (Cockerham 2010).

Not surprisingly, there were changes in the patient–physician relationship as well, with educated patients opting for more of a provider–consumer relationship in which the patient as consumer sought more equality in decision-making about the patient's health. As Eric Cassell (1986) explained, the scientific knowledge of medicine became increasingly available to lay persons – a process accelerated by the ubiquity of the internet. Knowledgeable patients were better able to review their symptoms and probable outcomes with their doctors and were more cognizant of the effects of particular drugs and medical procedures. Thus the internet has changed the doctor–patient relationship by empowering patients with information and giving them a greater role in decision-making about their health. 'Because physicians are no longer the primary gatekeepers of medical information', states Pam Rajendran (2006: 804), 'shared decision-making is now emerging as the hallmark of the patient–physician relationship.'

Yet, as Cassell (1986: 195) also observes, something else 'happened to displace physicians from their previous pre-eminent status, something powerful enough to allow patients to express the common belief that "doctors aren't Gods"'. This shift began during the 1960s, which were a time of radical change between individuals and their respect for authority in the United States. 'In fact', states Cassell (1986: 195), 'the fall of doctors from absolute authority on matters of health occurred at a time when all authority found itself challenged.' The anti-Vietnam War, Civil Rights, and the women's movement all contributed to a greater sense of individualism that questioned the motives of higher authority and rejected its arbitrary exercise.

The result of all these changes was a decline in the autonomy of physicians to control their work and a slippage in their professional status. While people would think highly of their own individual doctor, the public was suspicious of the motives of the medical profession in general and the AMA in particular with respect to the public's welfare (Cassell 1986). George Ritzer and David Walczak (1988) referred to this process as one of deprofessionalization. Ritzer and Walczak (1988: 6) defined deprofessionalization as 'a decline in power which results in a decline in the degree to which professions possess, or are perceived to possess, a constellation of characteristics denoting a profession'. Deprofessionalization does not mean a profession loses its professional standards; rather, it refers to a decline of a profession's control over its clients.

Drawing on Max Weber's (1978) concept of rationality, Ritzer and Walczak maintain that the rise of the profit orientation in medicine identified a trend away from substantive rationality (stressing ideal values like serving the patient) toward the dominance of formal rationality (stressing efficiency) in medical practice aimed at greater financial profits. The decline of the substantive element signalled a loss of public support and an invitation to countervailing powers to enter into an unregulated market that the medical profession had previously kept for itself. A quest for a share of the medical market by healthcare corporations and the public's demand for cost controls led to greater external control over the work of physicians by the government and business corporations. 'The basic thrust of professionalism', state Hafferty and Light (1995: 138), 'is toward a loss and not a continuation or strengthening of medicine's control over its own work.'

The managed-care era

As the 'golden age of doctoring' was ending with the external imposition of cost controls, the present era of managed care was rising. This era emerged in 1994 when Bill Clinton was elected President and included the provision of national health insurance as part of his political agenda. The measure failed in Congress after the initially high level of public support eroded in the face of an intense public-relations campaign by opponents and strong opposition by the small-business lobby who objected to the high costs to be borne by the employers they represented. However, the Clinton plan had stimulated movement toward the massive reorganization of American healthcare into a delivery system in which managed care is now the dominant approach.

About 62 per cent of all Americans are enrolled in managed-care pro-grammes. As noted, the term 'managed care' refers to healthcare organizations, such as HMOs and PPOs, that manage or control the cost of healthcare by moni-toring how doctors treat specific illnesses and injuries, limit referrals to special-ists, require authorization prior to hospitalization and second medical opinions prior to expensive procedures, among other measures. Physicians are obligated to practise in accordance with the regulations and fee structure set by the managed-care plan that employs them.

Managed care also changes the doctor–patient relationship by inserting a third party – the case manager – into the decision-making process. The case manager represents the bill payer, usually an insurance company, who certifies that the care to be rendered is both effective and cost-effective. The case manager addi-tionally authorizes hospitalization. Another feature is capitation or per-capita financing that consists of a fixed sum paid monthly by an individual and his or her employer that guarantees care to the person and the person's immediate family for little or no additional cost. Healthcare providers must provide the necessary care and are not paid for any additional services. This measure dis-courages inefficient and unnecessary treatment.

However, managed care not only appeared in the private sector in response to anticipated government controls under the proposed Clinton reforms, but also in accordance with changing market conditions. The medical market was under considerable pressure from the government, insurance companies and the public to control costs and managed care was considered the most effective means for doing so. Managed-care organizations were created because of the crisis of excess spending by physician-dominated healthcare-delivery systems and a new system was needed to control these costs. Managed care was the answer.

Managed care also affected medical schools. With respect to teaching, Ludmerer (1999: 378) observed more emphasis on cost-cutting decision-making, preventive care, appropriate use of diagnostic tests and effective communication with patients. Another major change occurred in faculty practice. Managed care became the major vehicle for adjusting to the realities of the new medical market, generating revenues for the schools and providing a basis for the continued expansion of faculty practice. 'By the late 1990s', says Ludmerer (1999: 381), 'the level of private practice by full-time faculty dwarfed that which anyone would have dared predict a mere 10 to 15 years before.'

Many medical schools evolved into academic healthcare systems; some became major regional-care providers. Beginning initially with a medical school and a teaching hospital, full-fledged healthcare complexes emerged that included research centres and laboratories, rehabilitation facilities and schools of nursing, dentistry, optometry, pharmacy, public health and allied health professions, along with various types of clinics and specialized hospitals (such as children's hospitals, veterans' hospitals and eye hospitals). Some academic health centres might contain as many as seven or more different hospitals.

The clinical income of medical schools increased as healthcare rendered by faculties expanded. Much of this expansion was necessary because the managed-care model reduced profit margins, threatening to lower the operating budgets of the schools, so expanded faculty patient care emerged as the primary means of generating the needed revenue. Faculty practice also allowed academic health centres to subsidize their teaching and research missions; it was therefore of critical importance to medical schools on several levels. By 2000, 50 per cent of an average medical school's budget was derived from clinical revenues and 35 per cent from external research grants (Griner and Danoff 2000). Today, dependence on revenues from faculty practice is likely to be even greater in many medical schools. On the downside, Ludmerer finds the emergence of a less academic atmosphere in medical schools now that the primary role of a majority of faculty is to treat patients instead of to conduct research or teach students. Teaching clearly has the lowest priority. 'No medical school was strong enough', states Ludmerer (1999: 375), 'to fully resist the "proprietarization" process' in which the faculty earned their income primarily through the patient care they provided.

Current directions

Although there are different types of practice settings, managed care remains the dominant style of practice in many clinics and hospitals associated with medical schools. It has been found to reduce the cost of care, although that advantage is showing signs of eroding as patients opt for direct access to specialists and more expensive services. Whereas managed care is not very popular among medical students, faculty members and practising physicians, it is the dominant mode of care and future physicians find they need to adapt to it (Harter and Kirby 2004; Simon *et al.* 1999). Current challenges for medical schools include how to conduct education in clinical settings without interrupting the flow of patients, pressure on clinicians and researchers to increase revenues to offset rising costs and budgetary shortfalls, and limited monetary allocation for teaching.

While teaching occupies the lowest rung of the patient care, research and education mission triad, American medical schools nevertheless strive to provide a quality education. Students are trained in basic science principles linked to clinical scenarios in the first two years which are revisited in the last two years in clinically integrated case approaches to instruction in clinical clerkships, electives and residency preparatory courses. Students are also exposed to patients early in their education and learn from them as well, while working on their interview and communication skills. As previously noted, many schools now have fewer lectures and more case-based small-group sessions with faculty preceptors, along with computer-based, independent, self-study learning modules. The goal for the student is to learn to evaluate data critically and to consistently arrive at the correct decision, even in complex situations.

The overall intent of such programmes is to provide a less passive, lecture-based medical education and instead orient the student toward active problem-solving, being part of a team that may include multiple specialists, nurses, pharmacists, therapists and others, and thinking like a practising physician. Compared to the past, the doctor is unlikely to be a solo practitioner and more likely to be a leader of a team of healthcare professionals. Additionally, many American medical schools require their students to complete faculty-supervised research projects in a laboratory, clinic or community setting in order to promote the development of physician-scientists.

Consequently, medical schools are adapting to changes in medical practice that, in turn, have origins in a changing society. From a sociological perspective, medical schools can be viewed as recipients rather than catalysts of change. However, such institutions nonetheless act as conduits to changes that are taking place in the medical profession and the wider society. The best example of this process is the increase in gender and racial diversity of medical students that is having a profound current and future effect on the physician population. In 1960, some 5 per cent of all medical-school graduates were women – a percentage that had remained virtually unchanged since 1910. But in the mid-1960s, stimulated by the women's movement and anti-discrimination legislation, increasing numbers of women began applying to medical schools and were getting accepted. Prior to this period, medical doctors were predominately white males.

By 1970, some 9.2 per cent of medical-school graduates were female and this figure increased to nearly 31 per cent in the mid-1980s. The most recent figures for 2006 show women now comprise 49 per cent of all medical students. There has also been an increase in the percentage of racial-minority students from 3 per cent in 1969 to 37 per cent in 2006. The gender and racial composition of physicians in the US has therefore changed profoundly in the last 60 years and medical schools have been the pipeline through which this change has emerged. These changes reflect other changes in medical practice with women and minorities now more likely to be treated by a physician who is more like them, with a closer understanding of their life situation and role demands. Although men and women doctors have been found to possess similar diagnostic and therapeutic skills, they appear to have different communication styles, with women proving more empathic and egalitarian in their relationships with patients, more respectful of their concerns and more responsive to their psychosocial difficulties (Martin *et al.* 1988).

Elianne Riska (2005) has asked whether medicine will remain a masculine-dominated profession, given the increasing number of women entering its ranks. This is an important question because female-dominated professions tend to have lower status and lower salaries. In time this may be the case, but at present this change is unlikely. Men still fill the vast majority of leadership positions in medicine. There is also a conspicuous segregation of medical work by gender in the US, Great Britain, Scandinavia and elsewhere. Women doctors tend to choose specialties consistent with the female role like paediatrics and geriatrics. Male physicians, conversely, are more likely to opt for male-dominated fields like surgery and internal medicine. Women enter these fields, but in far fewer numbers. Over time, however, women are more and more likely to move into leadership positions and enter all specialties in greater numbers. When this happens, whether or not a particular doctor is a man or a woman may not be especially meaningful. Like the 'golden age of doctoring', the era of white-male dominance is passing into history.

When it comes to social change and the medical profession, change typically impacts first on the profession and then extends to its schools. Medical schools, in turn, are part of the change process as they train students to practise in line with the new realities and reflect the gender and racial/ethnic adjustments taking place in the wider society. The changes taking place are indeed unsettling and yet the quality of training remains high, even though the era in which teaching was the primary mission of medical schools is now long past.

References

Becker, H. S., Greer, B., Hughes, E. C. and Strauss, A. (1961) *Boys in White: student culture in medical school*, Chicago, IL: University of Chicago Press.

Bloom, S. W. (1973) *Power and Dissent in the Medical School*, New York: Free Press.

—— (1988) 'Structure and ideology in medical education: an analysis of resistance to change', *Journal of Health and Social Behavior*, 29: 294–306.

Cassell, E. J. (1986) 'The changing concept of the ideal physician', *Daedalus*, Spring: 186–208.

Cockerham, W. C. (2010) *Medical Sociology*, 11th edn, Upper Saddle River, NJ: Pearson Prentice Hall.

Cooke, M., Irby, D. M., Sullivan, W. and Ludmerer, K. M. (2006) 'American medical education 100 years after the Flexner Report', *New England Journal of Medicine*, 355: 1339–44.

Coombs, R. H. (1978) *Mastering Medicine: professional socialization in medical school*, New York: Free Press.

Fox, R. (1957) 'Training for uncertainty', in R. K. Merton, G. Reader and P. L. Kendall (eds) *The Student-Physician: introductory studies in the sociology of medical education*, Cambridge, MA: Harvard University Press.

Freidson, E. (1970a) *Professional Dominance*, Chicago, IL: Aldine.

—— (1970b) *Profession of Medicine*, New York: Dodd, Mead.

Griner, P. F. and Danoff, D. (2000) 'Sustaining change in medical education', *Journal of the American Medical Association*, 283: 2429–31.

Haas, J. and Shaffir, W. (1977) 'The professionalization of medical students: developing competence and a cloak of competence', *Symbolic Interaction*, 1: 71–88.

Hafferty, F. W. (1991) *Into the Valley: death and the socialization of medical students*, New Haven, CT: Yale University Press.

—— (2007) 'Medical school socialization', in G. Ritzer (ed.) *The Blackwell Encyclopedia of Sociology, Vol. VI*, Oxford: Blackwell.

Hafferty, F. W. and Light, D. W. (1995) 'Professional dynamics and the changing nature of medical work', *Journal of Health and Social Behavior*, 36 (Extra Issue): 132–53.

Harter, L. M. and Kirby, E. L. (2004) 'Socializing medical students in an era of managed care: the ideological significance of standardized and virtual patients', *Communication Studies*, 55: 48–67.

Light, D. W. (2000) 'The medical profession and organizational change: from professional dominance to countervailing power', in C. Bird, P. Conrad and A. Fremont (eds) *Handbook of Medical Sociology*, 5th edn, Upper Saddle River, NJ: Prentice Hall.

—— (2004) 'Introduction: ironies of success – a new history of the American health care system', *Journal of Health and Social Behavior*, 45 (Extra Issue): 1–24.

Light, D. W. and Hafferty, F. W. (eds) (1993) *The Changing Medical Profession: an international perspective*, New York: Oxford University Press.

Ludmerer, K. M. (1999) *Time to Heal: American medical education from the turn of the century to the era of managed care*, Oxford: Oxford University Press.

McKinlay, J. B. (1999) 'The end of the golden age of doctoring', *New England Research Institutes Newsletter*, [Summer]: 1, 3.

Martin, S. C., Arnold, R. M. and Parker, R. M. (1988) 'Gender and medical socialization', *Journal of Health and Social Behavior*, 29: 333–43.

Merton, R. K., Reader, G. and Kendall, P. L. (eds) (1957) *The Student Physician: introductory studies in the sociology of medical education*, Cambridge, MA: Harvard University Press.

Porter, R. (1997) *The Greatest Benefit to Mankind: a medical history of humanity*, New York: Norton.

Rajendran, P. R. (2006) 'The internet: ushering in a new era of medicine', *Journal of the American Medical Association*, 285: 804.

Riska, E. (2005) 'Health professions and occupations', in W. Cockerham (ed.) *The Blackwell Companion to Medical Sociology*, Oxford: Blackwell.

Ritzer, G. and Walczak, D. (1988) 'Rationalization and the deprofessionalization of physicians', *Social Forces*, 67: 1–22.

Simon, S. R., Sullivan, A. M., Pan, R. J., Connelly, M. T., Peters, A. S., Clark-Chiarelli, N., Singer, J. D., Inui, T. S. and Block, S. D. (1999) 'Views of managed care: a survey of medical students, residents, faculty, and deans in the United States', *New England Journal of Medicine*, 340: 928–36.

Thomas, L. (1987) 'What doctors don't know', *New York Review of Books*, 24 September: 6–11.

Timmermans, S. and Angell, A. (2001) 'Evidence-based medicine, clinical uncertainty, and learning to doctor', *Journal of Health and Social Behavior*, 42: 342–59.

Timmermans, S. and Kolker, E. (2004) 'Evidence-based medicine and the reconfiguration of medical knowledge', *Journal of Health and Social Behavior*, 45 (Extra Issue): 177–93.

Weber, M. (1978) *Economy and Society, Vol. 2*, Berkeley: University of California Press.

15 *Tomorrow's Doctors*, a changing profession

Reformation in the UK medical-education system

Oonagh Corrigan and Ian Pinchen[1]

Introduction

Since it was first published in 1993, *Tomorrow's Doctors* (General Medical Council), the General Medical Council's guidance has had a radical impact on undergraduate medical training in the UK.[2] Insisting for the first time that all medical schools explicitly follow its advice, the General Medical Council (GMC) demanded that universities introduce sweeping changes in undergraduate medical education. Emphasis has been placed on a more rounded education and while clinical and basic sciences are still seen as crucial aspects of the curriculum, increasingly the accent is on their integration with other forms of learning. The importance of developing good communication skills, understanding the legal and ethical aspects of medicine and the acquisition of knowledge about the social and cultural environment in which health experience is embedded and medicine is practised in the UK are achieving greater prominence. All this is part of a drive to produce practitioners who are better prepared to meet the challenges of the future. The new curriculum is less concerned with learning biological facts, a practice which has increasingly been seen as leaving students ill-prepared for the complexities and uncertainties of medical practice; instead, growing emphasis is being placed on learning about the clinical realities faced by practising doctors. This has implications for both the content of medical education and the methodologies through which future learning takes place. Human sciences, medical humanities, ethics and skills training are increasingly occupying space alongside traditional curriculum subjects while modes of delivery are gradually shifting from a tradition of 'rote' learning to student-led processes with the notion of 'reflective practice' at the core.

Tomorrow's Doctors also contains guidance on the delivery of the curriculum, advice on the use of new technologies to deliver teaching and learning experiences, balancing large- and small-group sessions and providing student training in conjunction with other healthcare workers in multiprofessional settings. A central tenet of these recommendations is a more overtly patient-centred orientation, one that understands patients' needs and 'respects the rights of patients to be fully involved in decisions about their care' (GMC 2003: 9). As this chapter will demonstrate, *Tomorrow's Doctors* and further changes introduced for the education and on-going training of doctors in the UK have been prompted by a number of major criticisms of healthcare and medical treatments over recent decades. These include: a growing critique of professionalism and medical practice within the academic world; criticisms from policy analysts and policy-makers of the efficiency and effectiveness of medical interventions; anxieties expressed by some members of the general public; and a number of recent incidents which have found their way into the media spotlight. Many of the current reforms required by *Tomorrow's Doctors* are directed at improving patient care, in the broadest sense, at (re)securing public trust in the medical profession and at refashioning medical practice in the context of changing demands for healthcare provision and concerns about rising levels of public spending in general and on health in particular.

As well as generating changes in basic medical education, concern about patients and the public, in particular issues related to maintaining public trust, have also played a central role in instigating new reforms in medical education at the post-graduate level. The two years that immediately follow undergraduate training in the UK have been subject to controversial developments. Furthermore, emphasis has been placed on improving the quality of training, and 'Modernising Medical Careers' (MMC) (NHS 2008), a government programme of reform has been established with the aim of 'improving medical education' and providing 'a transparent and efficient career path for doctors' (NHS 2008: 310). Moreover, for the first time in the history of UK medical education the training of doctors and their registration is not the sole province of the medical profession and medical schools. Drawing on contemporary sociological work on medical professionalism, this chapter will explore changes within the UK undergraduate curriculum and new post-graduate reforms in training and registration.

Medical professionalism: the decline of medical dominance and the erosion of trust?

Traditionally, in the social sciences, the professions have been understood through 'trait theory' (Carr-Saunders and Wilson 1964 (1933)), literally the identification of a series of traits and characteristic practices which favourably distinguished professionals from other sorts of workers. Traits included, most importantly: the ownership of a specialized body of knowledge that gives the owner a range of associated, valuable skills; an altruistic orientation towards those served by the profession; and a code of ethics through which to define and monitor that service.

The claim to ownership of a specific body of esoteric knowledge paves the way for professions to present themselves as experts in a given field of activity. In doing so they are able to exclude other occupations from certain areas of practice and the rise of medicine in the nineteenth century gradually marginalized other forms of healing. The natural corollary of this claim was that only those in possession of the esoteric knowledge could determine who should enter into training for the profession and how they should be trained. This effectively allowed the profession a complete monopoly over the conditions of its work. At the same time, however, the 'promise' of altruism and a set of ethical codes, monitored by the profession itself, in the case of medicine, through the GMC, suggested the resultant monopoly of practice would not be abused for personal gain.

Trait theory was largely based on an uncritical acceptance of the professions' own accounts of their work and medicine was often used as the ideal-type model. By the mid-twentieth century it had become embedded into the functionalist sociology of Talcott Parsons (1951) who viewed the altruism of the professions as a desirable bridge between the cold rationality of market relationships in the public sphere and the affective relations of the private realm. In the case of medicine, this view fitted well with Parsons' famous description of the 'sick role' where the doctor's assumed skills in healing illness combined with the functional requirement of managing sickness as a form of deviance, itself a potentially disruptive force that might destabilize the wider social order. For several decades in the middle of the twentieth century, a period when the profession of medicine was consolidating its position in most western societies as the 'natural' mechanism for defining and treating health and illness, trait theory went largely unchallenged. This process was aided in the UK through increasing statutory recognition of medicine, particularly in 1948, with the establishment of the National Health Service (NHS) (Klein 2006). Hunter (2006: 4) suggests that Aneurin Bevan (the Minister of Health responsible for the establishment of the UK National Health Service) viewed the NHS as an administrative system for doctors and nurses 'freely to use in accordance with their training for the benefit of the people of the country'. Healthcare provision between 1948 and the early 1960s was not without some significant problems but these tended to be viewed as technical difficulties in the context of building and consolidating a new service rather than a problem of medicine and the professionals who practised it (Klein 2006). This was not to last and by the 1970s medicine itself began to face a range of challenges from a number of quarters. While there is not space here to explore them in detail, they are important insofar as they served to question the complacency over trait theory and laid the foundations from which new theories of the professions would emerge. Furthermore, this scrutiny began to provide the basis and sometimes the ammunition for a policy attack on what gradually came to be seen as the privileges of doctors and the problem of medical practice. This has led to major changes in the way medicine has been managed over recent decades and has increasingly had a major impact, directly and indirectly, on the nature of medical education.

The 'trait theory' view of medicine, as a product of modernity, rested on a number of assumptions, particularly the infallibility of science as an explanatory paradigm, that have increasingly come to be seen as problematic. Medicine was built upon the newly established biological sciences that by the nineteenth century were coming to be seen as providing a set of objective 'truths' about the natural world and the human body in particular. Various discoveries, notably the emergence of germ theory, led to the doctrine of 'specific aetiology' (Nettleton 2006), the view that illnesses were caused by specific, identifiable organisms or pathogens which scientific investigation could reveal. All doctors had to do was inspect the patient's body, diagnose and treat the presenting condition. If treatment was not yet available research would eventually deliver it. Medicine and its cures were seen mostly as a matter of scientific progress. By the 1970s such confidence was beginning to evaporate. Research from within the world of medicine itself began to suggest that improvements in the nation's health over a period of 100 years or more had little to do with the rise of medicine (McKeown 1976 in Davey *et al.* 1995). Furthermore, Cochrane (1971 in Davey *et al.* 1995) argued that despite claims of scientific rigour, in reality many medical treatments were untested and unproven. His response to this revelation was to call for more robust research and evaluation with the randomized control trial (RCT) at the pinnacle of a range of methodologies, paving the way for what has come to be known as evidence-based practice.

Outside medicine a chorus of other voices added to the refrain. A comprehensive study by Illich (1977) suggested that one in five medical interventions actually caused iatrogenic (treatment-induced) illnesses of varying severity and that the paternalistic nature of medical practice created dependency among the general population. One of the problems of the doctrine of specific aetiology was that the patient, as a person (as subject), became increasingly irrelevant to the practice of medicine (Jewson 1976). Normal biomedical practice was individualistic and built around the one-to-one encounter between doctor and patient, a relationship imbued with an almost spiritual reverence in the accounts of functionalism and trait theory, and indeed in doctors' own accounts of their work. However, micro-sociological studies into doctor–patient relationships increasingly showed that patients often felt dissatisfied with the medical encounter and that doctors had very little understanding of their needs or of the social world in which their experiences of health and illnesses were embedded. Rather than the cosy paternalistic relationship assumed by trait theory, the doctor–patient encounter was revealed to be a hotbed of potential misunderstanding and conflict.

Finally, during this same period, research from a public-health and political-economy perspective began to raise questions about whether current medical practice, well delivered or not, was the appropriate mechanism to address a nation's health. National research on inequalities in health (Whitehead *et al.* 1992) suggested that social class, gender and ethnicity may be more important determinants of people's health experiences than the individualistic focus of biomedicine. In response to the recognition of this at the international level a growing body of opinion was beginning to advocate policies of prevention and public health. This trend was most fully expressed in the World Health Organization Conference of 1978 and the publication that followed, *Health for All by the Year 2000* (WHO 1978) which called for countries to restructure health services around public-health and primary-healthcare measures and to turn away from high-cost, high-technology hospital systems – systems upon which most national health services of the western world were based and which had doctors and biomedicine at their core. Although its goals were ultimately difficult to achieve, the programme highlighted growing doubts about the direction of healthcare provision with curative biomedicine at its centre.

Out of this climate, new, more critical theories of the professions have emerged that play down the idea of altruism and emphasize the role of doctors in serving sectional interests. For example, Marxist writers draw attention to the links between medicine and the interests of capitalism. The American sociologist Navarro (1977) suggests that doctors and biomedicine, with their individualistic focus on disease, disguise the way in which capitalism causes illness through polluting industrial processes, oppressive working conditions and low pay. In addition, Marxists argue that in treating people's ailments, doctors provide a service to capitalism by maintaining the health of the workforce in the interests of the capitalist productive process. The profession's reward for this is the high wages and prestige that medicine offers. Doyal and Pennell (1979), in the UK, have emphasized the link between medicine and the pharmaceutical industries, arguing that the biomedical professions serve the needs of this industry rather than those of their patients. Similarly, in the US, such developments have been documented by Paul Starr (1982) who showed how insurance companies and drug companies had gained control over the prescribing practices of General Practitioners who were no longer able to exercise autonomous professional judgements in the care of their patients. Instead, they were given profit targets that worked in the interests of the companies. This brought to an end 'the golden age of medicine' (Starr 1982).

Other perspectives focus on the medical profession as a self-serving elite that uses the idea of professionalism as an occupational strategy to pursue its own needs. In particular, the seminal work of Eliot Freidson (1970) has become the subject of recent discussion. Professions, according to Freidson, are organized occupations that seek to control the conditions of their own work. Freidson viewed the medical profession as the epitome of this. Professions exercise their control by developing and defining a relevant body of knowledge and by educating, testing and credentializing practitioners; in doing so, they maintain exclusive jurisdiction over some areas of the labour market. For Freidson, the distinguishing feature of the medical profession, one that differentiates it from others, has been its dominance over its sphere of work. Dominance is maintained as the medical profession is able to exercise autonomy over work undertaken by its members, it controls and manages the work of others in the healthcare field, evokes deference from patients and the wider public and exercises institutional power, maintaining cultural and legal authority over its jurisdiction. Legal authority is of particular importance and Freidson argues that it was the ability of the medical profession to persuade successive governments to support it (for example, through legal recognition of the AMA in the United States and the GMC in the UK) that secured for it its dominant position. Historically, doctors have presented themselves as having to fight for autonomy of practice in the interests of their patients against state intervention, but Freidson argues that doctors only achieved the pre-eminence they have through government patronage and support. Legal recognition by government allowed the medical profession to colonize health and define it as its own area of jurisdiction in the face of competing claims from other healers. Freidson argued that the individual autonomy exercised by doctors is such that it resists efforts to monitor the quality of their work, thereby avoiding political and societal accountability and maintaining autonomy at the collective level.

More recent debates on medical professionalism, however, have focused on a number of significant changes in medical practice during the past three decades and many commentators are now suggesting that medical autonomy is under threat. Harrison and Ahmad (2000) argue that in the UK medical autonomy has declined at the micro, macro and meso levels. Freidson (Freidson 1988 and 1994) too revised his original thesis in the face of the rising consumer movement in the US and the growing corporatization of healthcare. In the UK, from the 1980s onwards, the NHS has been increasingly subjected to a combination of managerial interventions and quasi-market forces in an attempt to rein in public spending and make the impact of doctors' work more transparent. In light of such developments, Freidson drew a distinction between the social and economic conditions of medical provision on the one hand and the conditions of technical practice on the other, arguing that governments control the former and doctors the latter. However, Johnson (1995) suggests these distinctions began to blur as it was recognized that doctors' technical decisions in themselves have major cost implications. Such changes have led to the thesis that a process of 'proletarianization' (McKinlay and Marceau 2002) or deprofessionalization has taken place.

While Freidson maintained that medicine had retained its dominance insofar as it continued to control subordinate health workers and retained the power of licensure, it is clear that doctors are not being accorded quite as much deference by patients or the general population as in the past. Various scandals in medical practice have prompted media-fuelled public critiques and dented the cultural credibility of the profession. Bury and Gabe (2004) argue that media representations of doctors and medicine have become more ambivalent in recent decades. Programmes such as the TV documentary *The Cooke Report* of 1988, which exposed the inappropriate use of tranquillizers, *Operation Hospital* in 1991, which explored the problems of managing a large hospital and even the soap opera *Casualty*, with its mixed representations of the professions, suggest the media no longer either present the doctor as a professional held in the highest esteem or take the benefits of medicine for granted. In 1997 the BBC *Panorama* programme (Taylor 1997) drew attention to the 'Costly Cure' of poorly judged and widely varying levels of radiotherapy treatment for cancer patients across the UK, and the more recent scandals which led to the Bristol Royal Infirmary Inquiry and the Shipman Inquiry discussed below have all contributed to an apparent decline of faith in doctors and medicine. The various public failures and crises of medicine can be seen, at some level, to have eroded trust and confidence in the ability and integrity of those who practise it. However, the medical profession has since developed a number of reflexive strategies aimed at preventing similar future risks that might continue to undermine public trust.

Clearly, the changing fortunes of the medical profession and the way government and the public view it has implications for the control, structure and content of medical education and over recent decades, as the following section shows, changes have indeed been taking place. A reduction in confidence in the profession's ability to conduct its affairs in the public interest might be expected to lead to external intervention while continued faith in the profession would leave professional control untouched. Whether the recent changes in medical education represent the continued decline in medical dominance or an attempt to reassert it is unclear. Research in this area is currently relatively underdeveloped. As Donald Light argues there needs to be a new sociology of medical education, one that studies it as a social institution focusing on the organizational aspects and power dimensions: 'At issue is the relationship of medical education as a social institution to the health care system and to the training experience of future physicians who will take care of patients' (Light 1988: 307).

Key players in medical education

Medical education in the UK is forged by a number of key players: the Royal Colleges; university medical schools; the GMC; the British Medical Association (BMA); national and international medical-education professional bodies and associations such as the Association for Medical Education in Europe (AMEE), the Association for the Study of Medical Education (ASME) and the Academy of Medical Educators; doctors; the NHS; and the government, as well as patients and the public. Evidently not all are equal and in his account of the historical outline of the GMC, Sir Donald Irvine, President of the GMC from 1995 to January 2002, claims that the Royal Colleges and medical schools are the real 'power brokers' (Irvine 2006: 204). Nevertheless, given that the GMC has been the body responsible for registration and licensure as well as advising on basic undergraduate medical education and professional discipline, it would appear, at least on the surface, to be a powerful arm of the medical profession. Irvine, however, claims that during much of its history the GMC has been a reactionary body that has not wielded much power, having been predominantly 'anchored in the regulatory backwater to which the leaders of the profession had consigned it' (Irvine 2006: 205).

While the reforms introduced by the GMC, contained within *Tomorrow's Doctors*, are quite radical, many of these recommendations reflect earlier changes in medical education outside the UK. Perhaps the most significant reform was in the response to the now famous North American report by Abraham Flexner (Flexner 1910) based on a survey of the curricula and education of medical schools. Published in 1910, it noted huge disparities in the quality of medical education and proposed standardizing the quality of all medical schools to that of America's best schools. It is thought to be the most important event in the history of American and Canadian medical education and gave rise to modern medical education (Beck 2004). Other important developments such as the self-directed, problem-based learning (PBL) approach pioneered at McMaster University in Canada were developed in the late 1960s. This approach has since been adopted by a number of countries and is present in some form or another in most UK medical schools. The 'new pathway project', another novel initiative introduced at Harvard Medical School in the late 1980s, was premised on a more integrated science-based approach in medical education (Weatherall 2006). Meanwhile, in the UK, the 1980 'Recommendations on Basic Medical Education' was published by the GMC after a major review by its statutory Education Committee and was regarded as being highly innovative (Walton 2006). These specified, for the first time, the knowledge, skills and attitudes to be acquired by medical students, emphasizing the crucial importance of communication skills in the training of doctors. The importance of psychology and sociology was stressed, as was the value of early clinical exposure for medical students at the time when they were learning the basic medical sciences as a foundation for clinical and medical practice. These recommendations brought the Council into conflict with the Universities of Oxford and Cambridge, who did not agree that the behavioural sciences should play a part in the pre-clinical curriculum, but eventually they conceded '...and also, with some reluctance, introduced early clinical exposure along somewhat limited lines' (Walton 2006: 1148).

While general developments had a major impact on the teaching and delivery of medical education in the western world more widely, prior to the introduction of the GMC's recommendations in 1993, the UK was seen as largely conservative with regard to the delivery of medical education, which had undergone little change since the period following the Second World War (Irvine 2006). The pattern which had been retained in most medical schools was of a first-year course where students studied chemistry, zoology and botany followed by two years dissecting the whole body and being taught physiology, biochemistry and sometimes psychology and related subjects with a final course starting with pathology and bacteriology and proceeding eventually to clinical training on the wards. In absorbing many of the criticisms and developments outlined above, *Tomorrow's Doctors* has sought to shift the balance in the curriculum to include more emphasis on the ability to understand 'the working, organisational and economic framework in which medicine is practised in the UK' (GMC 2003: 15), and 'the social and cultural environment in which medicine is practised' (GMC 2003: 17). Unsurprisingly, in comparison with what went before, the GMC's recommendations for training were seen as a radical departure from the past and, while welcomed by many, there were those within the profession who were then, and have since remained, opposed to and sceptical about the reforms and the new role being played by the GMC more generally.

The GMC, first established in 1858 as a statutory body, was and remains today, financed by the profession itself. It was, however, established to ensure that the public could trust any doctor who was registered with it, and while not preventing other kinds of healing practitioners it established professional boundaries by ensuring that no others could be classified as 'registered medical practitioners' (Stacey 1991). As such the GMC plays a crucial role in maintaining the professional boundaries of medicine through access to accredited education. Its original 24 members represented the Royal Colleges, the universities and General Practitioners. Following the Medical Education Act in 1886 the Council was granted powers to insist that candidates were required to pass examinations in medicine, surgery and midwifery in order to be eligible for registration. Although the Council had powers to discipline errant doctors, 'the President was concerned that the Council "should not seem overanxious to be at work since the spreading abroad of the shortcomings of any erring members of our honourable profession is a proceeding to be carefully restrained within precise limits"' (Irvine 2006: 204). This feature of non-interference by the GMC allowed the medical profession to establish its dominance and to carry on its business unfettered, and according to Irvine (2006), this position was maintained until the early 1990s. At the same time of course this raises questions about the balance between altruism and self-interest central to recent debates about professionalism.

Revolution and reform

Tensions emerged between the GMC and doctors and the Royal Colleges during the 1960s. Between 1968 and 1973, the unity of the profession and the legitimacy of the GMC were almost lost (Stacey 1991). In a climate where wider structural changes in the NHS, the emergence of new Royal Colleges and the demands placed on junior doctors were all having an impact on the practice of medicine, 'the GMC appeared out of touch with the profession' (Irvine 2006: 205). Further tension arose between the GMC and the wider profession and although the GMC's *Recommendations on Basic Medical Education* (General Medical Council 1967) had been accepted by the Royal Commission on Medical Education and subsequently partially implemented by some medical schools, tension arose as the GMC wanted more money from the medical profession to offset rising operating costs. Furthermore, the Royal Colleges were frustrated by the GMC's lack of initiative in tackling poor GP practice and errant GPs, so when the Council introduced a levy retention fee, most doctors decided not to pay. The GMC lost control and the government temporarily intervened. This led to the 1978 Medical Act, which doubled the size of the Council and gave a majority to elected, rather than appointed or nominated, members (Irvine 2006; Stacey 1991). The GMC's remit was to register doctors, regulate basic medical education, coordinate all stages of medical education, deal with doctors' fitness to practice and give advice on professional standards and ethics. In the interim an inquiry that had been instigated by the BMA and Royal Colleges noted among its many conclusions that even in the area of basic medical education, where the GMC was seen to be more proficient, the Council had failed to insist that its recommendations were adhered to. It was to be another 15 years before the GMC introduced *Tomorrow's Doctors* and made its guidance mandatory.

Despite the 1978 reformation of the Council and the mandatory system of elected membership, the BMA tried to influence GMC members (Irvine 2006). However, the government strengthened the Council by introducing lay activists and academics as members in order to ensure that the Council was influenced by thinking from outside the profession. There were also a number of other sources of pressure from both inside and outside medicine that urged the GMC to become more effective. For example, in his 1980 radio broadcast Reith Lecture address, 'Unmasking Medicine' (British Broadcasting Corporation 1980), medical lawyer and ethicist Ian Kennedy argued for improved professional standards and better teaching on communication and ethics. The pressure for reform did not disappear and in 1989 Richard Smith, editor of the *British Medical Journal*, published a series of articles criticizing the GMC. Also Meg Stacey, a medical sociologist and lay member of the GMC who had served on the Council for nine years between 1976 and 1984 was highly critical of the GMC's activities, arguing that doctors needed to do more to protect patients (Stacey 1992). As Stacey (1991) noted, the 1978 reforms were profession-led and addressed problems identified by medical people. Among other things, they reduced the proportion of lay members although their absolute numbers increased, as did those of all other groups. The GMC was seen as failing in its duties and it was only in the 1990s that the Council started to act like a normal regulator (Stacey 1991).

Patients and citizens

In the late 1990s, two major cases exposed serious failures of the medical profession to control standards in professional practice and to monitor and discipline errant doctors. In the case of the Bristol heart-surgery scandal, between 1991 and 1995, some 30 to 35 children undergoing heart surgery at Bristol Royal Infirmary died who would probably have survived if treated elsewhere. The Bristol Inquiry report (Bristol Royal Infirmary Inquiry 2001) claimed there was a flawed system of care at the hospital with poor teamwork between professionals, with 'too much power in too few hands'. Surgeons lacked the insight to see that they were failing and continued to operate (Dyer 2001: 181). The report went further than simply blaming the action of individuals, claiming that there were inadequacies at every point of the process – from referral to diagnosis, surgery and intensive care – and that these flaws and failures existed within the wider NHS. Furthermore, the failure to pay attention to the original whistleblower, a consultant anaesthetist at the hospital who had been forced to leave his position after reporting the actions of the surgeons and was subsequently unable to get another post, was, the report said, an indication of the lack of openness and what was described as a 'club culture'. 'The style of management had a punitive element, and the environment did not make speaking out or openness safe or acceptable' (Dyer 2001: 181). This episode drew attention to wide variations in medical practice, once more raised questions about the efficiency and effectiveness of treatment and demonstrated the importance of doctors keeping their learning up-to-date. Moreover, while traditional assumptions about professionalism took for granted the altruistic disposition of the doctor, these events increasingly demonstrated that 'professionalism' has to be learned and made explicit. It could no longer be assumed and needed to be included in the curriculum as a key component of medical training.

In January 2000 Harold Shipman, a former GP, was convicted of murdering more than 200 of his patients. There was immense media attention and public concern about how he had maintained his position as a GP for so long and about the efficiency of existing systems for checking mortality patterns. Furthermore, as Shipman had previously been convicted in 1976 for committing forgery and fraud for prescribing drugs for his own drug addiction to pethidine, there was concern that the GMC had failed at that point to withdraw his licence to practice. These medical scandals were seen at the time by the public and the profession as shocking and worrying insofar as they exposed what Irvine describes as a cultural gap between medicine and society. Historically the culture of British medicine was strong on science, technology and clinical practice but 'inward-looking, paternalistic, secretive and self protective in its social attitudes' (Irvine 2006: 202). The media attention and public outcry was a serious indictment of the profession's ability to effectively self-regulate. Patient loss of trust in the profession was considered to be a major problem. However, the events in retrospect appeared to prompt a wake-up call to the profession and the GMC responded at last, acting with the authority a regulator should. From this time the GMC began to be viewed more positively as it responded to a more obvious patient-consumerist voice in the wake of public and media attention that followed the Bristol heart-surgery and Harold Shipman cases. The GMC's response to the doctors who had performed poorly in their surgical competency and had misinformed patients as in the Bristol heart-surgery deaths was viewed as positive and the Council was, in the end, commended on how it conducted its inquiry. Richard Smith went as far as to claim in the *British Medical Journal* that a new social contract between doctors and the public was emerging:

> The contract is renegotiated not by bald men in suits in back rooms but rather by the public expressing its disquiet in a myriad of forms – through, for example, parliament, the media and patients' organisations – and by the profession recognising the disquiet and responding.
>
> (1998: 1622)

In their 1998 guidance, *Good Medical Practice* (General Medical Council 1998) the Council set new standards that doctors would be expected to meet, stating that failure to meet them could result in them being removed from the registry. Drawing on the Royal College of General Practitioners who had a 20-year history of operating a national, standard-based, assessment-driven system of quality assurance in continuing medical education, the GMC's Standards Committee set a standards-based model of medical licensure. These standards highlighted the importance of patient care, and the protection and promotion of the health of patients and the public as the foundation of good medical practice. The standards had the effect of uniting the profession around a set of generic duties and attributes that both they and the public thought were important aspects of a 'good doctor' (Irvine 2006).

Reform continued and in 1999 the GMC decided that a system of revalidation would need to be introduced and that all doctors in active practice should have their performance regularly evaluated to show that their skills are up-to-date and that they are fit to practise. In 2003 a new smaller GMC with 40 per cent lay membership was established. However, as Irvine observed, the 'battle between reformers and conservatists was bitter' (Irvine 2006: 208). The 'battle' was one between the GPs and Royal Colleges who both backed the GMC's reforms and the BMA hospital specialists and public-health committees who opposed the form of revalidation the GMC intended. In his 2006 article on the history of the GMC, Irvine lamented that the 'GMC backed down under pressure' and he accused them of 'reverting back to their old practices of protecting the interests of doctors' (ibid). He argued, rather damningly, that the culture of the medical profession had not really changed and was still strong on individualism and weak on teamwork. Irvine was not the only critic of the GMC's failures, and during the early years of the new millennium the government continued, in a more determined manner, their challenge to the role of the GMC.

Clinical governance

Concerned that patients and the public needed to maintain trust in the medical profession following the Shipman Inquiry, the government's Chief Medical Officer was asked to undertake a broad review of medical regulation. The ensuing report, *Good Doctors, Safer Patients* (Hewitt 2006) gave advice on measures to strengthen the arrangements in place for the protection of patients. The report contained 44 recommendations, including devolving some of the powers of the GMC to a local level, changing its structure and function, and creating a new framework for revalidation. This was followed in 2007 with the publication of a government White Paper (Hewitt 2007). In the paper's Foreword the government's Health Secretary, Patricia Hewitt states:

> For any consideration of the regulation of health professionals, the preservation of that trust has to be the starting point. Professional regulation must create a framework that maintains the justified confidence of patients in those who care for them as the bedrock of safe and effective clinical practice and the foundation for effective relationships between patients and health professionals.
>
> (2007: 1)

Although not specifically addressing educational aspects, the White Paper set out a programme of reform to the UK's system for the regulation of health professionals. The paper claimed that the regulators needed to be independent of government, and include the professionals themselves, employers, educators and all the other interest groups involved in healthcare. It made clear that recertification will be based on standards and assessment methods, defined by the relevant medical Royal Colleges and faculties, with the approval of the GMC. In July 2008 the government's Chief Medical Officer announced that a new five-year revalidation process would start to be implemented. The process involves two strands:

> ...relicensing (confirming that doctors practise in accordance with the General Medical Council's generic standards) and recertification (confirming that doctors on the specialist and GP registers conform with standards appropriate for their specialty of medicine).
>
> (Department of Health 2008: 7)

Prior to this, the Chief Medical Officer's report *Unfinished Business* (Donaldson 2002) recommended reform for the training of Senior House Officers (those in the early years of post-graduate clinical training) and set out plans for a new two-year 'Foundation Programme', followed by a number of broad-based specialist training programmes running through to consultant level or General Practice. 'Modernising Medical Careers' (MMC), a programme of radical change, was launched in February 2003. Introduced by the four UK Government health departments, this new system for the training of newly qualified doctors was rolled out in 2005. This involved a shorter period of training to consultant level than previously. The Foundation Programme represented a fundamental change for the Senior House Officer grade. In August 2005 all medical graduates undertook this new, integrated, planned programme of general training. The GMC was made responsible for the first year of the programme and published new guidelines, *The New Doctor* (GMC 2007a), setting out the standards providers must meet and the outcomes that Foundation Programme doctors must demonstrate before they could move to full registration. Although the first year was similar to the previous system (the pre-registration year) in their second year, doctors were to be given further generic skills training in a mixture of specialties. For the first time a curriculum was produced defining a series of clinical competencies which must be achieved. However, while the GMC guidance set standards for the first year, an independent regulatory body called PMETB (Postgraduate Medical Education and Training Board), established in 2005, was given responsibility for the second year of the Foundation Programme. PMETB is an independent regulatory body accountable to Parliament, designed to administer a system for doctors' applications to specialist and GP registers beyond their two-year postgraduate training. PMETB sets the overarching standards within which selection for specialist training must operate.

However, the first year of operation of the new MMC system resulted in some serious problems. An IT system and a badly designed application form led to a mismatch in allocating the best qualified doctors to vacant posts. Following the chaos that ensued and the hostile reaction to events by the medical profession,

Sir John Tooke, Dean of the Peninsula College of Medicine and Dentistry, was asked to chair an inquiry into the MMC programme and to provide recommendations for improvement. In his report, Tooke made eight key recommendations, including the suggestion that PMETB should be merged with the GMC to facilitate a common approach and the linkage of accreditation with registration (Tooke 2008). Another major recommendation put forward by Tooke was that a new body – NHS Medical Education England (NHS: MEE) – should be established. Tooke proposed that NHS: MEE would be accountable to the Department of Health's Senior Responsible Officer for medical education and would be guided by an advisory board with professional, service, academic, BMA and trainee representation, which Tooke claimed would be able to articulate the principles of post-graduate training and implement them successfully. The report also contained a warning that training could suffer when the European Working Time Directive comes fully into force in 2009 and was concerned to ensure that the limit on doctors' working hours will not mean that there is insufficient time to train them to the skill levels needed.

The debate rages on. The Department of Health in England published an official response to Tooke's inquiry into the MMC reforms and has agreed to implement many of the recommendations. A Government report, *A High Quality Workforce* (Darzi *et al.* 2008), published in June 2008, endorses many of Tooke's recommendations, including the creation of the new body, NHS: MEE, to oversee post-graduate medical training. Tooke also called for post-graduate medical education to be integrated into university medical schools, through the trialling of new 'graduate schools' which would take on some of the NHS deaneries' current work, including handling applications by junior doctors to specialist training and overseeing career development of trainee clinical academics and managers (Tooke 2008).

Conclusion

It is clear from this brief outline of the key changes to medical education in the UK that doctors' education, training, revalidation and the systems in place to administer this, have undergone a radical transformation with change still ongoing. Patients, government and the public have in various ways become stakeholders in the training of doctors. If in the past the medical profession acted on behalf of and for the medical profession alone this position has now become untenable. Nevertheless, while greater emphasis is being placed on the social aspects of medicine delivery as outlined in *Tomorrow's Doctors*, and more recently in reports by Tooke and Darzi *et al.*, there remains a tension between the so-called 'soft sciences' and the increasing drive within biomedicine towards advancing scientific and technological developments. Medical careers are likely to be influenced by the high status accorded to doctors undertaking scientific biomedical research. While medical education constructs medicine as both art and science, the concept of medicine as a science with the drive towards evidenced-based medicine and massive investments in new technological advances such as genetics, helps to maintain professional dominance in society.

Patients', government and the public response to key (media-driven) events have played a significant role in the changes implemented in medical education, particularly since the Bristol heart-surgery and Harold Shipman cases. The events in the UK are not divorced from wider changes in medical education such as those in North America and Europe. However, they have taken their own particular trajectory in the UK and have been shaped not least by the key role played by a public-owned National Health Service. Nevertheless, it would be a mistake to see recent changes as representing a major decline in professional autonomy and power. Indeed, the failure of the new MMC programme to deliver the changes has returned some power to the profession. The report by Tooke represents a very significant move within the profession to regain the balance of power. Furthermore, the GMC has come under attack again for not implementing changes following its own recommendations during the Shipman Inquiry:

> At a meeting convened at the Royal Society of Medicine in London to discuss trust between doctors and patients after the Shipman case, Janet Smith, chairwoman of the Shipman Inquiry, said that the case had 'disclosed a raft of flaws in professional governance' and that 'inaction cannot be defended'.
>
> (Richards 2006: 1111)

Eminent speakers attending the conference argued that there had been a demise of community health councils' and patients' forums which had weakened the patients' voice, and that patients' representation on the GMC needed to be strengthened and their interests protected to the same extent as those of the medical profession (ibid).

The GMC has responded to these criticisms and the government's proposals for revalidation. Its plans include methods to identify for further investigation, and remediation where appropriate, doctors whose practice is impaired, or may be impaired, where local systems are weak or non-existent (GMC 2007b). The GMC admits that among other things, revalidation requires a more structured, systematic approach to continuing professional development in support of doctors' professionalism.

It is also interesting to note that the issue of professionalism is being reconfigured by the profession itself. As a further example of institutional reflexivity, the medical profession is debating the fundamentals of what it means to be a 'good doctor'. In recognition that 'social and political factors' and certain events which have undermined public trust have 'challenged characteristics that were once seen as hallmarks of medicine', the Royal College of Physicians (2005) has produced a report, *Doctors in Society: medical professionalism in a changing world* (Royal College of Physicians 2005: Foreword). Its report follows the International Medical Professionalism Project launched in 1999 (a European-

and American-based project) resulting in a new charter on medical professionalism focusing on the ethical tenets and responsibilities of the profession. The Royal College of Physicians' report defines medical professionalism as 'a set of values, behaviours, and relationships that underpins the trust the public has in doctors' (Royal College of Physicians 2005: 14). In doing so, it has abandoned previous aspects of professionalism, in particular the notions of 'mastery, autonomy, and privilege, and self regulation' (ibid.: 16). More emphasis is placed on the patient and doctor–patient interaction. The thrust of the report though appears to be about (re)securing public and patient trust in the profession: 'Securing trust is the most important purpose of medical professionalism. Trust – and so professionalism – operates at two levels: in the doctor providing care (individual professionalism) and in the system where care is given (institutional professionalism)' (ibid.: 15).

It could be suggested that medicine's concern with the concept of professionalism is an attempt not simply to respond to public concern and to rebuild trust but also to take control over the definition of a good doctor and to bring this back under the aegis of the profession itself rather than leaving it in the hands of government or policy-makers. Also, in relationship to institutional professionalism, the report calls for an end to what the authors describe as 'internal tribalism' and suggests that leadership skills and managerial competence are developed as these are increasingly important facets of the profession. The report recommends that the GMC revises *Tomorrow's Doctors* '…to strengthen leadership and managerial skills as key competencies of professional practice' (ibid.: 27). The recent Department of Health report which is part of a key NHS review (Darzi *et al.* 2008) further emphasizes the need for clinicians to take senior leadership and management posts.

Furthermore, although in this chapter we have focused primarily on the structural and political landscape of medical education in the UK, as Bleakley and Bligh (2008) argue, while there has been a good deal of rhetoric surrounding patient-centred education in medical schools, in practice this has been situated within a broad professionalism framework which tends to refocus on the role-modelling of the physician rather than encouraging collaborative working relationships between students and patients.

Freidson, in his revised professionalism thesis, claims that the erosion of professional autonomy and the legal, economic and political pressures it is now experiencing, have been brought about because of the failure of the profession to regulate itself in the public interest (Freidson 1988). It is clear that there is some truth in this and that this is reflected by changes in the way medicine is regulated and the way the structure and content of medical education has been reconfigured. Nevertheless, these changes may not signify a linear decline in medical power and autonomy. Johnson (1995) argues that the relationship between the state and the professions has always been more fluid than many analysts think. Professions are an integral part of the process of governmentality and in the process of being recognized by the state and given jurisdiction over an area of social life, according to Johnson, they effectively become a part of it. However, those jurisdictions themselves are fluid and can shift according to the changing priorities of a particular government. In recent decades, problems of public spending, medical failures, media attention and public dissatisfaction have all contributed to a reconfiguration of professional power; doctors are increasingly held to account for their performance and this is reflected in the changing structure and content of medical education. However, this has happened in such a way that doctors and their representative organizations still lie at the very centre of the debates.

Notes

1 We would like to thank our colleagues John Bligh, Julian Archer and Julie Brice for their helpful comments on an earlier draft.
2 Following informal visits to medical schools between autumn 1998 and 2001, the GMC reviewed progress and considered the strengths and weaknesses of its guidance. Taking account of developments in educational theory and research and professional practice, it introduced an updated version of *Tomorrow's Doctors* in 2003. The main principles remain much the same as the 1993 version.

References

Beck, A. H. (2004) 'The Flexner Report and the standardization of American medical education', *Journal of the American Medical Association*, 291: 2139–40.

Bleakley, A. and Bligh, J. (2008) 'Students learning from patients: let's get real in medical education', *Advances in Health Sciences Education*, 13: 89–107.

Bristol Royal Infirmary Inquiry (2001) *Learning from Bristol: the report of the public inquiry into children's heart surgery at the Bristol Royal Infirmary, 1984–1995*, London: Stationery Office.

British Broadcasting Corporation (1980) 'Reith Lecture: Unmasking Medicine', online at www.bbc.co.uk/radio4/reith/reith_history.shtm (accessed 4 June 2006).

Bury, M. and Gabe, J. (eds) (2004) *The Sociology of Health and Illness: a reader*, London: Routledge.

Carr-Saunders, A. M. and Wilson, P. A. (1933) (1964) *The Professions*, London: Frank Cass and Co.

Cochrane, A. L. (1995) 'Efficiency and effectiveness', in B. Davey, A. Gray and C. Seale (eds) *Health and Disease: a reader*, Buckingham: Open University Press.

Darzi, A., Keen, A. and Nicholson, D. (2008) *A High Quality Workforce: NHS next stage review*, London: Department of Health.

Davey, B., Gray, A. and Seale, C. (eds) (1995) *Health and Disease: a reader*, Buckingham: Open University Press.

Department of Health (2008) *Medical Revalidation – Principles and Next Steps: the report of the Chief Medical Officer for England's Working Group*, London: The Crown.

Donaldson, L. (2002) *Unfinished Business: proposals for reform of the Senior House Officer grade. Consultation Paper*, London: The Crown.

Doyal, L. and Pennell, I. (1979) *The Political Economy of Health*, London: Pluto Press.

Dyer, C. (2001) 'Bristol inquiry', *British Medical Journal*, 323: 181.

Flexner, A. (1910) *Medical Education in the United States and Canada: bulletin number four*, New York: Carnegie Foundation for the Advancement of Teaching.

Freidson, E. (1970) *Profession of Medicine: a study of the sociology of applied knowledge*, New York: Dodd, Mead.

—— (1988) *Profession of Medicine: a study of the sociology of applied knowledge, with a new Afterword*, Chicago, IL: University of Chicago Press.

—— (1994) *Professionalism Reborn: theory, prophecy and policy*, Cambridge: Polity Press.

Gallen, D. and Peile, E. (2004) 'A firm foundation for senior house officers', *British Medical Journal*, 328: 1390–1.

General Medical Council (GMC) (1967) *Recommendations on Basic Medical Education*, London: General Medical Council.

—— (1993) *Tomorrow's Doctors*, London: General Medical Council.

—— (1998) *Good Medical Practice*, London: General Medical Council.

—— (2003) *Tomorrow's Doctors*, London: General Medical Council.

—— (2007a) *The New Doctor*, London: General Medical Council.

—— (2007b) *Regulating Doctors: ensuring good medical practice*, online at www. gmc-uk.org/about/council/papers/2007_12/4d%20-%20Taking%20Forward%20 the%20White%20Paper_%20Revalidation.pdf (accessed 4th June 2008).

Harrison, S. and Ahmad, W. I. U. (2000) 'Medical autonomy and the UK state 1975 to 2025', *Sociology*, 34: 129–46.

Hewitt, P. (2006) *Good Doctors, Safer Patients: proposals to strengthen the system to assure and improve the performance of doctors and to protect the safety of patients. A Report by the Chief Medical Officer*, London: The Crown.

—— (2007) *Trust, Assurance and Safety: the regulation of health professionals in the 21st century. Government White Paper*, London: The Crown and Stationery Office.

Hunter, D. J. (2006) 'From tribalism to corporatism: the managerial challenge to medical dominance', in D. Kelleher, J. Gabe and G. Williams (eds) *Challenging Medicine*, 2nd edn, London: Routledge.

Illich, I. (1977) *Medical Nemesis*, New York: Bantam Books.

Irvine, D. (2006) 'A short history of the General Medical Council', *Medical Education*, 40: 202–11.

Jewson, N. D. (1976) 'The disappearance of the sick man from medical cosmology, 1780–1870', *Sociology*, 10: 225–44.

Johnson, T. (1995) 'Governmentality and the institutionalisation of expertise', in T. Johnson, G. Larkin and M. Saks (eds) *Health Professions and the State in Europe*, London: Routledge.

Klein, R. (2006) *The New Politics of the NHS: from creation to reinvention*, 5th edn, London: Radcliffe.

Light, D. (1988) 'Toward a new sociology of medical education', *Journal of Health and Social Behavior*, 29: 307–22.

McKeown, T. (1995) 'The medical contribution', in B. Davey, A. Gray and C. Seale (eds) *Health and Disease: a reader*, Buckingham: Open University Press.

McKinlay, J. and Marceau, L. (2002) 'The end of the golden age of doctoring', *International Journal of Health Services*, 32: 379–416.

National Health Service (NHS) (2008) *Modernising Medical Careers*, online at www. mmc.nhs.uk/default.aspx?page=280 (accessed June 2008).

Navarro, V. (1977) *Medicine under Capitalism*, London: Croom Helm.

Nettleton, S. (2006) *The Sociology of Health and Illness*, 2nd edn, Cambridge: Polity Press.

Parsons, T. (1951) *The Social System*, London: Routledge and Kegan Paul.

Richards, T. (2006) 'Chairwoman of Shipman inquiry protests at lack of action', *British Medical Journal*, 332: 1111.

Royal College of Physicians (2005) *Doctors in Society: medical professionalism in a changing world*, London: Royal College of Physicians.

Smith, R. (1998) 'Renegotiating medicine's contract with patients', *British Medical Journal*, 316: 1622–3.

Stacey, M. (1991) 'Operating in the public interest?', *Health Matters*, 9: 12–14, online at www.healthmatters.org.uk/issue9/publicoperator (accessed July 2008).

—— (1992) *Regulating British Medicine: the General Medical Council*, Chichester: Wiley.

Starr, P. (1982) *The Social Transformation of American Medicine*, New York: Basic Books.

Taylor, D. (1997) 'A costly cure', *Panorama*, UK: BBC 1.

Tooke, J. (2008) *Aspiring to Excellence: final report of the independent inquiry into Modernising Medical Careers*, London: MMC Inquiry.

Walton, J. (2006) 'Medical education and the role of the General Medical Council', *Medical Education*, 40: 1148–9.

Weatherall, D. J. (2006) 'Science in the undergraduate curriculum during the 20th century', *Medical Education*, 40: 195–201.

Whitehead, M., Townsend, P. and Davidson, N. (1992) *The Black Report and the Health Divide*, London: Penguin.

World Health Organization (1978) *Health for All by the Year 2000*, Geneva: WHO.

16 The challenges to achieving self-sufficiency in Canadian medical education

Ivy Lynn Bourgeault and Jennifer Aylward

The issue of self-sufficiency in human resources for health has become increasingly salient in many countries, particularly in light of concerns about looming shortages and the global consequences of the increased reliance on internationally educated health professionals. The Harvard-based Joint Learning Initiative (2004) report, for example, explicitly recommends reducing the 'pull' forces of health professionals in source countries through the emphasis on aiming for educational self-sufficiency on the part of destination countries. It argues that it would be wise for wealthy countries to strive for self-sufficiency because reliance on immigration is short-sighted, inequitable and risky; self-sufficiency is both sound and fair (JLI 2004: 106). These calls were echoed by the World Health Organization (WHO) (2006) and the World Health Assembly (WHA) (2006). In the 2006 World Health Report, the WHO recommends self-sufficiency through recommendations directed at increased domestic production, improved recruitment and retention, and enhanced political and technical workforce strategic planning. Paralleling this, the fifty-ninth World Health Assembly, recognizing the importance of achieving the goals of self-sufficiency in health workforce development, passed a resolution in May 2006 for the rapid scale-up of health workforce production (WHA 2006: 2).

The self-sufficiency debate that has emerged particularly within the medical profession reveals some especially interesting themes and complex contextual influences. Nearly every country claims to have a shortage of physicians, though in relative terms this is felt most acutely in low- and middle-income countries (WHO 2006). The ability to 'solve' these shortages with international medical graduates (hereafter referred to as IMGs) is a unique feature to high-income, western countries. Countries like Canada, the US, the UK and Australia, for example, rely on IMGs in the range of 23 to nearly 30 per cent of their overall medical workforces. The ethical issues raised by this extensive reliance on IMGs are part of the overall call for high-income countries to become more self-sufficient in medical education and training. This chapter aims to shed light upon the concept of self-sufficiency with a particular focus on the context of medical education in Canada.

The data on which this chapter is based form part of a larger study comparing policy in regards to internationally educated health professionals in Canada, the

US, the UK and Australia. For each of the four countries, data have been collected through:

1   The acquisition of key public-domain policy documents from the various professional and stakeholder groups.
2   Interviews with key informants involved in or influenced by the policy decision-making process.

These data have been analysed using the constant comparative technique of qualitative policy analysis which draws upon thematic content analysis as its basis.

We present here the key themes that have emerged from this analysis related to the issue of self-sufficiency. We describe who is raising the issue and why; we then address the ethical implications associated with achieving self-sufficiency, the difficulty in defining self-sufficiency and the limits to this being achieved. Briefly, what we find is that the issue of self-sufficiency has been raised primarily by representatives of professional associations and medical educators as a response to the increasing practice of international recruitment. Arguments supporting self-sufficiency are also bolstered by the growing awareness of the ethical issues associated with the healthcare brain drain from developing countries that can least afford to lose precious health human-resources. To provide the necessary context for this discussion, we begin with some background information on the structure of Canadian medical education, recent changes in the process of becoming a doctor in Canada and the related issue of medical shortages and health human-resource planning.

The structure and evolution of medical education in Canada

The basic structure of medical education in Canada is similar to other high-income countries. It involves two main components: undergraduate medical education and post-graduate training in a residency programme. There are 17 medical schools across Canada, each affiliated with a university-based health-science centre. The language of instruction for 14 of these medical schools is English, while for the remaining three it is French. Financial support is provided to each school from provincial governments; however, both undergraduate and post-graduate medical-education programmes are managed by the universities themselves (Reudy and Gray 1998).

Until the mid-1990s, the common path for most medical-school graduates was to undertake rotating internships which in some cases was followed by specialty training. Upon completing the rotating internship, medical graduates could enter more permanent practice in primary care. What this system offered was a core of younger physicians looking for community experience before establishing a practice or moving onto specialty training (Reudy and Gray 1998). By 1993, all provinces increased the post-graduate training requirements from one year of a rotating internship to two years in a programme in family medicine accredited by the College of Family Physicians of Canada (CFPC), or the completion of specialty training to certification by the Royal College of Physicians and Surgeons of Canada (RCPSC)[1] which could take from four to six years (Reudy and Gray 1998). Students, therefore, no longer have the choice of completing a rotating internship as a means to gaining licensure.

Since the elimination of the rotating internship, residency-training programs are the sole path of training for a career in primary care in Canada (Reudy and Gray 1998: 1048–9). Residency or specialty training is provided by each of the medical schools in Canada with the curriculum evaluated either by the CFPC or the RCPSC. Following graduation, medical-school graduates apply for a residency training position via the Canadian Resident Matching Service (CaRMS).[2] The process is largely dictated by the choices put forth by the applicants. Prior to 2006, the 14 English-language medical schools participated in the matching process, while the remaining three French-language schools in Quebec had their own training positions that were offered to their students. All medical schools are now part of the CaRMS process. Students submit their applications to the CaRMS, and they are reviewed by the selection committee. Subsequently, a list of potential interviewees is developed and these students undergo interviews with the residency programme directors. Following the interview process, students and directors submit their match lists to CaRMS. The preliminary round of the match process is only available to Canadian medical-school graduates. Following this round, the remaining residency positions are made available for a second round, which is accessible to those who were not matched in the first round, physicians returning to practice and international medical graduates (Reudy and Gray 1998).[3] It has been noted by many stakeholders that because the number of residency positions is limited, medical students selecting a residency position may feel that there will be little opportunity to alter their career path once in training (Task Force Two 2003: 50).

In addition to these changes in residency positions, there have also been changes to undergraduate medical education, enrolment in particular. The number of students enrolled in undergraduate medical-education programmes had declined by more than 10 per cent since the late 1980s, following concerns raised over a potential oversupply of physicians in Canada (discussed more fully below) (Reudy and Gray 1998: 1047). More recently, however, there has been a significant upswing in medical-school enrolments since 2000 in response to a physician human-resource task force (Task Force One). First-year enrolments now exceed the peak of enrolments seen in the early 1980s (Chan 2002). This rise in intake levels can be partially attributed to the opening of the Northern Ontario School of Medicine in September 2005 – the first medical school to be opened since 1969. The school was not only established to increase medical-school enrolment in general, it focused specifically on increasing the number of practising physicians in rural and northern communities (Padmos 2008).

The other change in medical education is in regards to its rising costs since the early 1990s. Prior to this time, the overall costs of medical education were reasonable, particularly in comparison to the US. Since the 1990s, however, there have been dramatic increases in tuition fees largely as a result of deregulation. Added to this, the costs of credentialling and examinations, malpractice insurance and licensing fees, and obtaining an appropriate residency training position have all become more costly. The debt loads of Canadian medical students at graduation are now much greater (Reudy and Gray 1998: 1048). The concerns this causes for medical human-resource planning are outlined in a follow-up Task Force Two report:

> The debt loads of Canadian medical students at graduation are now at an all time high. Paying off debts as quickly as possible will become a high priority among medical graduates and new practising physicians. More students may feel compelled to maximize their earning potential by pursuing those specialties that generate high incomes, others may choose those specialties with short training periods so they can enter the workforce and start to pay off debts sooner. Debt load may also influence where graduating physicians choose to practise. The increasing willingness of American recruiters to pay off debts of new graduates provides tremendous incentive to practise in the US.
>
> (Task Force Two 2003: 50)

Kwong *et al.* (2002), for example, found that students facing higher tuition fees are more likely to report that financial considerations will influence their choice of specialty and location of practice.

Box 16.1 Background statistics on medical education in Canada

- Average medical school tuition costs were $6,654 for 2001–2002. This represents an increase of 39 per cent from their 1998–1999 levels.
- The average age of medical students has risen. Between 1977–1978 and 1999–2000, the proportion of applicants over 28 years old rose substantially from 7.4 per cent to 12.5 per cent. This trend has resulted in a higher average at graduation.
- There is a drop in the rate of entry by post-graduate trainee physicians into active practice. Between 1981 and 2000, there was an increase in the amount of time spent in post-graduate training. In particular, after rotating internships were eliminated in 1993, there was a large increase in those who enter practice after four or more years of training.
- Fewer students are interested in family medicine. Between 1981 and 1986, just over half of trainees entered practice as GPs or FPs. Between 1987 and 1992 this rose to almost two-thirds of all graduates. More recently, the proportion of Canadian medical-school graduates who studied in family medicine has shown a gradual decline, representing only 40 per cent of the total number of graduates in 2001. Over the same period, the proportion of graduates of medical laboratory/specialty programs went from 38.2 per cent to 42.8 per cent, while the proportion of those from surgical specialty programs remained more or less constant.
- Since 1995, more than 50 per cent of new medical students have been women,

and, by 2015, it is predicted that they will make up 40 per cent of the physician workforce. Women tend to work fewer hours and to be less present in specialty medicine than their male counterparts.

- The average age of physicians has risen to 47.5 years old. In 2000, 13 per cent of the physician workforce was under 35 years of age and 11 per cent were 65 or older. The number of physicians retiring each year in Canada has almost tripled from 295 in 1981 to 832 in 2000.

(Excerpted from Task Force Two 2003: 11, 21, 44)

Physician shortages and their relationship to changes in medical education

In the early 1990s, a report was prepared for the conference of the Federal, Provincial and Territorial Deputy Ministers of Health addressing issues regarding physician supply and demand in Canada – known as the Barer and Stoddart (1991) report. During this time period, it was perceived that Canada had a surplus of physicians. One of the many recommendations made in the report included a 10 per cent reduction in undergraduate medical school enrolment. Another recommendation was to increase efforts to control and monitor visa entry for IMGs. Indeed, during the mid-1990s, physician supply policies made it difficult for applicants who identified themselves as physicians to migrate to Canada (IMG Task Force 2004). Many of the report's other recommendations to stabilize health human resources, including the reorganization of services and shifting tasks to other health professionals, were not implemented.

Although the concern in the early 1990s was with a predicted physician surplus, towards the end of the 1990s, many professional associations, working groups and so on began to raise concerns about a shortage of physicians. As Grant states:

> After years of seeking to curtail the number of physicians, and foreign-trained physicians in particular, practising in the country, there is growing support for the view of an impending shortage. Despite a relatively high and stable physician/population ratio..., with an aging population increasing the demand for medical services, and demographic changes in the physician workforce (both in terms of aging and gender) resulting in a decline in the average hours worked by physicians, talk of a 'crisis' in Canada's health care system is more frequent.
>
> (2004: 7)

In 2007, a poll conducted by the CFPC found that as many as five million Canadians may not have a family physician. The Canadian Medical Association (CMA) has similarly estimated that Canada may be lacking up to 5,000 family physicians (Feasby 2008). The CMA and others (for example, Dauphinee and Buske 2006) further report that Canada ranks twenty-fourth among developed countries with respect to the number of physicians per capita: Canada has 2.1

physicians per 1,000 population compared to the OECD average of 2.8 (Task Force Two 2003). This is in contrast to Canada's fourth place ranking back in 1970.

Physician shortages were initially considered to be the result of a reduction in the investments made in medical education during the era of fiscal restraint in the 1990s. For example, the total number of post-graduate positions funded by provincial Ministries of Health has until most recently remained essentially static (Task Force Two 2003). Others argue that the changing gender demographics of the profession have exacerbated the shortages. According to this argument, women – who now make up over 30 per cent of practising physicians and over 50 per cent of medical students (Bowmer *et al.* 2008) – do not work at the same capacity as male physicians. Although this is true to a certain extent, particularly during childbearing and rearing years, we have witnessed an overall decline in the intensity that physicians practise regardless of gender (Chan 2002). Most agree that the single most important factor explaining the shortage has been the increased length of training (Chan 2002).

The shortage of physicians is most evident in the primary care sector with a lack of family physicians and general practitioners available. The shortage is particularly acute in rural or remote communities, where access to physicians and healthcare services in general is already scarce. The predominantly rural/ remote provinces of Saskatchewan and Newfoundland have the highest number of IMGs (Audas *et al.* 2005). The limited access to healthcare in such communities raises concerns over access to not only primary care, but also diagnostic services, chronic disease management and acute care (Padmos 2008). The goal of reducing shortages in these communities has been linked explicitly with international recruitment, which is regarded as a critical component of health human resource management schemes. Some provinces have recruited IMGs extensively, particularly from South Africa, to meet the needs of their rural communities, granting them either provisional or full licences to practice (Grant 2004). Some provinces have also resorted to interprovincial recruitment to meet their needs by using relocation and sign-on bonuses as incentives to move provinces, much to the dismay of 'source' provinces.

The issue of self-sufficiency

As the health human resource crisis reaches the forefront of health policy agendas, the issue of self-sufficiency is receiving increasing attention from different key players involved in workforce planning. As Little and Buchan describe:

> One major challenge for all countries is to establish workforce planning mechanisms that effectively meet the demands for health care and provide workforce stability. However, few nations have developed strategic plans ... that effectively address supply and demand. Instead, many developed countries choose to implement short term policy levers such as increased reliance

on immigration, sometimes to the detriment of developing countries. This has prompted calls for developed countries to employ a model of so-called 'self sufficiency/sustainability' in ... health human resource shortages.... There is broad agreement in the health professions regarding the need for developed countries to ensure an adequate domestic supply of health professionals, thereby lessening their dependency on developing countries.

(2007: 4)

In an effort to reduce the reliance upon other countries to address the health human resource shortages, the World Medical Association (WMA) developed a statement regarding the ethical guidelines for the international recruitment of physicians. It states:

Every country should do its utmost to educate an adequate number of physicians taking into account its needs and resources. A country should not rely on immigration from other countries to meet its need for physicians.

(WMA 2003)

Similarly, a 2005 international conference hosted by the British Medical Association (BMA), the Commonwealth Secretariat and representatives from Canada, the US, the UK and South Africa focused upon the issue of a global health workforce. Conference delegates agreed that all countries must seek to achieve self-sufficiency in their own workforce in an attempt to prevent the development of further problems for other countries that are depleted of their trained professionals (BMA 2005). Specifically in the Canadian context, the Health Action Lobby (HEAL), a coalition of more than 30 health professional and employer organizations, argues that self-sufficiency should be one of the ten principles that guide health human-resource planning (HEAL 2006).

Ethical arguments for self-sufficiency

A range of stakeholders, from medical associations and regulatory bodies to educators, express support for the notion of self-sufficiency and raise concerns about the morals of poaching internationally trained physicians. CMA Past-President Albert Schumacher (as cited in Sullivan 2005) emphasized the importance of achieving self-sufficiency in an effort to implement long-term solutions, while also preventing long-term consequences for donor countries: 'To continue to rely on and recruit IMGs in this way is both unsustainable and unethical, and we must overcome our reliance on them, particularly the active poaching from countries that can least afford it.' He places importance upon the fact that Canada must move towards a 'made in Canada' solution by being self-sufficient. Another Past-President of the CMA, Peter Barrett (as cited in Sullivan 2005) similarly raises questions about the appropriateness of relying upon other countries to fill our shortages: 'In the face of a global shortage of health care workers, can a country in which 24% of practicing doctors were educated outside its own borders continue to rely on physicians from countries that can least afford to lose them?' Representatives from the various medical associations and colleges do note that they must be a bit careful with this position. As noted by one of our informants: 'It's a sensitive issue. We certainly support our [IMGs] but at the same time we question the morals of bringing them in.'

While active recruitment of IMGs is a short-term solution until self-sufficiency strategies are developed and fully implemented, there remains a lack of agreement on some form of compensation for donor countries. Source countries invest funding in education and training for their healthcare professionals, yet this investment is lost when other countries actively recruit these individuals to practice. The IMG Task Force (2004: 4) has emphasized that, 'Improving Canada's lot, at the expense of healthcare delivery in countries who are less fortunate is not a Canadian healthcare policy goal.' Developed nations have a global responsibility to respect the needs of countries that are in need of physicians themselves. A member of one of the national professional accrediting bodies noted the following in our interview:

> I think the concern we have about international medical graduates is on the one hand we want to be open and receptive to individuals from around the world. On the other hand if we are seducing people away from countries that are in significant need of physicians themselves, then I think our global responsibility is a bit in peril.

This raises the issue of how best to achieve self-sufficiency without damaging the workforce of developing nations in the interim.

It is evident that key stakeholders have recognized both the poor long-term health human-resource planning and inappropriateness of active recruitment from other countries to satisfy our need for physicians. Developing countries face increasing challenges in managing the shortages of healthcare professionals. Active recruitment of physicians and other health professionals can lead to the collapse of healthcare infrastructure. Care must be taken to ensure that actions do not damage fragile health systems in low- and middle-income countries.

Self-sufficiency and health human-resource planning

With self-sufficiency increasingly being the ultimate goal of health human-resource policy agendas it is necessary to fully examine the issue in the context of evolving healthcare systems. Consideration must also be given to mechanisms to increase a nation's educational capacity, while also retaining professionals on a local level (Aiken et al. 2004; Little and Buchan 2007). A level of self-sufficiency can be achieved by developing, adapting and supporting the core educational capacity of healthcare professional training programs (Penn Consortium for Human Resources in Health 2006). There has, however, been a general lack of policy regarding self-sufficiency and its relationship to medical education. Working towards achieving self-sufficiency is dependent upon establishing sustainable educational infrastructure, yet also upon lending assistance to developing nations to educate and retain an adequate level of healthcare professionals to meet their own needs (Cooper and Aiken 2006: 66).

Medical schools are being challenged to move towards training the appropriate number and mix of physicians to meet the changing needs of Canadian society as a whole. Achieving the delicate balance will involve increasing undergraduate enrolment, while also providing adequate post-graduate positions to train the proposed intake of students following graduation. Furthermore, as Task Force Two (2006) identified, greater numbers of post-graduate positions are required to allow medical graduates the ability to change specialties when desired, to allow Canadian residents who were educated outside of Canada to practise in their home country, and to allow IMGs who reside in or migrate to Canada to join the healthcare workforce. It is believed that there are still inadequate positions available in post-graduate training programmes even in light of recent increases. Moreover, as the stakeholders in Task Force Two (2003) identified earlier, medical-education planning needs to be more closely linked to health human-resource planning rather than continue as a somewhat uncoordinated system.

Countries facing a shortage of physicians or healthcare professionals in general must implement workplace-planning mechanisms in order to meet the demands placed upon the system, while also establishing workforce stability. The issue of supply and demand is rarely addressed effectively because of a lack of strategic long-term planning, and this is not particular to Canada. While mechanisms to move towards self-sufficiency are developed and modified, existing health human-resource shortages must be resolved. Short-term solutions, such as the recruitment of IMGs, have been implemented to immediately address the issue at hand. While this tackles the problem in the developed country, the implications for the developing country noted above are not considered in the process. Necessary components of the move towards achieving self-sufficiency should also include policies addressing the ethical recruitment of internationally trained professionals, partnership agreements, and methods of compensation for 'donor' countries.

Although all stakeholders support the goal of self-sufficiency – indeed, to question it would be virtually unacceptable – there are two key difficulties in actually achieving this goal. The first is the lack of agreement on how to define self-sufficiency and the other difficulty arises from the limits to achieving self-sufficiency, which seem inherent to the health systems of destination countries.

The difficulty in defining self-sufficiency

There is ongoing debate of how to appropriately define self-sufficiency. It has been described as a sustainable supply of domestic professionals to meet service requirements (International Center on Nurse Migration (ICNM) 2007). But this in turn raises the question of how to define 'sustainable'. Essentially, there is no general agreement on the definition of self-sufficiency with respect to health human-resource planning, although the idea of 'growing our own' is critical to the argument for self-sufficiency. As aptly summarized in the Final Report of the Task Force on IMGs:

> To date, there has been no national consensus on the merits or meaning of physician self-sufficiency for Canada. This lack of consensus has contributed to a national physician workforce planning process that remains challenged to comprehensively address the health professional needs of the Canadian public.
>
> (Task Force Two 2006: 3)

Nor is there agreement surrounding how to measure self-sufficiency, or even if it is ultimately achievable (Little and Buchan 2007: 2). Achieving self-sufficiency draws attention to the need not only to recruit but also to retain through the reduction of student and professional attrition as well as through initiatives to increase the productivity of the existing workforce.

While it has been acknowledged that active recruitment from developing nations is unethical because it weakens their health infrastructure, the question becomes how best to manage those professionals who emigrate and seek employment independently. Immigrants have always formed a part of Canada's health workforce, historically at levels reaching nearly a third of all practising physicians (in the early 1970s) but more recently around 22 per cent. If the goal is to achieve self-sufficiency, *at what level* is self-sufficiency considered to be adequate? As one key government informant states: 'I mean self-sufficient doesn't mean every single one is accounted for. It just means you don't have to be in a gap situation that you have to go running out to other countries.'

The goal that the Canadian Medical Association has set out is to achieve at least 80 per cent self-sufficiency because it believes that Canada will benefit from some mobility and flexibility.

Therefore, the shift in health human-resource planning is to be from one of complete reliance upon immigration to one where a delicate balance is achieved between self-sufficiency and immigration. As noted in Task Force Two:

> It is also important to ensure that Canada balances its medical workforce needs without actively recruiting physicians from other countries, while recognizing the realities of international physician mobility. As such, Canada should achieve self-sufficiency by ensuring an adequate domestic production, together with the integration of ethical immigration policies to meet the evolving needs of society.
>
> (2006: 12)

Thus, there is a need for increased educational capacity in Canada, but there is also acknowledgement of the fact that immigration is a reality, and that such individuals are going to be active participants in the workforce. Any policy that encourages self-sufficiency needs also to include principles which support the fair and timely evaluation of IMGs and their integration into the Canadian Health System (cf., Society of Rural Physicians of Canada (SRPC) 2002 IMG Policy). An argument can be made that the migration of internationally trained medical professionals to Canada's workforce allows for the integration of knowledge from international practices.

Limits to achieving self-sufficiency

No doubt, achieving self-sufficiency is a challenge that encounters many obstacles. These primarily concern educational capacity and economics. First, with respect to capacity, there must be adequate resources in place, such as instructors and supervisors, to support an increasing enrolment in medical schools and in post-graduate training positions. As noted early on in Task Force Two (2003), medical schools are already facing a shortage of faculty, particularly clinical faculty, which challenges their ability to respond to calls for increased enrolment. Although the number of part-time faculty has kept pace with growing enrolments, the number of full-time faculty has not. The present system relies on the generosity of the largely unpaid part-time clinical faculty, a situation which is largely unsustainable. One of our informants in the province of British Columbia described the situation as follows:

> In British Columbia ... the university has doubled its class size ... which means they will have ... more medical students who will require clinical experience and they will have an equivalent number of post-graduate positions that they have to create to finish off that training.... They're overwhelmed. You know, to find training positions now for their students and their residents is almost impossible.

An additional barrier to achieving self-sufficiency in the short term is the length of time we must wait for these new students to enter practice.

Some of the educational capacity in Canadian medical schools is also limited by the needs of (largely wealthier) developing countries who send students for training in Canada. Ivison, for example, describes how Canada is collaborating with other countries to train physicians, who will ultimately return home to practice, in exchange for compensation:

> While university hospitals have been rejecting doctors who might have moved into towns and cities across Canada to provide the health care that Canadians expect and deserve, they have been accepting trainees from foreign countries in record-breaking numbers – all of whom come here at their governments' expense and then return home once fully trained. The numbers of foreign visa trainees rose to 2,082 in 2006–07, from 937 a decade ago, according to the Canadian post-MD Education Registry. The reason they are accepted in such numbers is that foreign governments (mainly from the Middle East) pay fees equivalent to the subsidy the

provincial government would stump up for Canadian students. In Ontario, this amounts to $25,000 per year. In addition, the foreign government pays a salary that ranges between $47,000–81,000 and a benefits package of around 12% of salary. In return for the potential outlay of $115,000 a year, the foreign government is guaranteed to have a fully qualified doctor return- ing home within five years.

(Ivison 2008)

This raises concerns about the arrangements being made with other countries to meet their needs, while Canada struggles to meet its own health human-resource demands.

The *economic* challenges to self-sufficiency are largely related to how high a cost is deemed acceptable. The rising costs of medical education in Canada create barriers to worthy students. When universities do provide financial aid, it limits their ability to expand their programmes unless alternative resources are made available. Some consider it more affordable to recruit IMGs than to train our own. As one of our stakeholders noted:

I don't know how much it costs to train a Canadian medical student but it's a big pile of money – well into six figures. The cost of an IMG assessment is probably somewhere around 30 to 40 thousand dollars. So if there are physicians out there who for 30 or 40 thousand dollars can be determined to be fully competent and able to practise, what a bargain. They're happier and the public should be happier because they get a trained physician for peanuts.

The active recruitment of physicians who are seen as nearly ready to practise is considered to be even cheaper than upgrading IMGs who are already in the country but may have trained under a very different system or some time ago. This argument is described by one of our key stakeholders: 'Until somebody makes it cheaper and easier for us to bring IMGs who are already in Canada into the system rather than dialling 1–800 South Africa, we're going to keep dialling 1–800 South Africa.'

The paradox of need and rejection

While Canada is struggling to achieve adequate numbers of physicians in its healthcare workforce, there is a perplexingly large number of seemingly quali- fied individuals who are eager to enter the medical profession yet are being denied acceptance into medical school. In the 2006–2007 application year, the Association of Faculties of Medicine of Canada (AFMC) reported that 10,673 people applied to enter Canada's 17 medical schools – the first time that greater than 10,000 applications were submitted. This number was a 10.5 per cent increase from the previous year and an increase of over 30 per cent from a decade ago (Sullivan 2008). As noted in the Task Force Two (2003: 49) report:

'Most provinces have a quota system for students who are residents in that province, with remaining entrance positions becoming part of a highly competitive pool.' Related to this increased competitiveness, although most medical schools require an undergraduate university degree for entrance, many successful candidates have already completed graduate work (Task Force Two 2003). As one of our key stakeholders noted:

> Canada is not very generous to its own students. I know at one time [a colleague] used to say the only country in Europe or North America and South America that takes fewer of its students than Canada was Albania. We've got over five students who probably are qualified to go to medical school for every one that's taken. And to me I think that's unethical.

Due to the limits placed on medical-school enrolments, it is estimated that more than 1,500 Canadian students attend medical school outside Canada. Canadians are currently studying medicine in countries such as Ireland, Australia, and even in the Caribbean and Mexico. Canadian attendance at schools in Ireland, for example, is facilitated by the Atlantic Bridge Programme, which was created by Ireland's medical schools in an attempt to attract North American students to their programmes. These schools have witnessed an increase in the number of applicants, paralleling the decline in the number of first-year positions available in Canada in the 1990s (Spurgeon 2000).

While these students may obtain a medical degree, it is very difficult for them to gain a residency position or a licence to practice in Canada, if they indeed intend to return, as they are considered IMGs. Some advocates have argued that many students ultimately seek residency training positions in the US because of its greater residency capacity (Spurgeon 2000). But it is also noted that undertaking residency training in the US is much more costly, putting already indebted students in even more debt:

> Students pay approximately three times more in tuition than in the most expensive Canadian medical school at a cost of approximately $30,000 per year. In addition, the cost of living is much greater, which contributes to their increasing debt.
>
> (2000: 136)

In order to accommodate the growing number of students studying medicine outside Canada, it has become necessary to expand the number of post-graduate training positions, something which has only recently begun to happen (Padmos 2008).

In addition to the problem of students leaving to pursue their training, there is concern that many of these rejected students may abandon their hopes of pursuing a career in medicine altogether (Sullivan 2008).

Discussion

Self-sufficiency is clearly a complex and multilayered issue that reflects and is influenced by several interlocking health human-resource problems leading to a mismatch between supply and demand: insufficient capacity for local medical students; too few students going into family medicine; changing demographics and practice patterns; too few physicians working in rural and remote areas and staying there when they do; and too much dependence on foreign countries to train physicians to fill the gaps in the system. Few of these problems are peculiar to the Canadian medical profession.

Proctor (2001), for example, describes how the situation in the US paralleled Canada in the early 1990s with many experts agreeing that they would experience an oversupply of physicians, yet this predicted situation did not materialize. Indeed, some experts forecast a shortage of physicians in the US similar to Canada's. It has been recommended that American medical schools should move quickly towards filling one-half of the residency gap with their own graduates, with a focus on being more self-sufficient (Mullan 2007). In Australia, the government is moving quickly towards self-sufficiency by dramatically increasing undergraduate medical-school enrolment through several newly established schools, but in the interim they continue to rely 'heavily on IMGs to supplement the medical workforce' (Spike 2006: 842). In the UK, the Department of Health (2007: 110) noted that 'the position from 2007 will be one of self-sufficiency, with the NHS developing its own workforce and placing less reliance on international recruitment'.

As Canada looks to the future with the goal of achieving self-sufficiency, it is necessary to balance the needs of both the home and donor countries as well as to balance the needs of self-sufficiency and immigration. Similar to the balanced immigration/self-sufficiency argument, the Penn Consortium for Human Resources in Health (2006) uses the terms 'core' and 'moderating the dependency', which implies some level of immigration is required and/or acceptable in the United States. Canada and other destination countries for IMGs must account for the circumstances of the donor country, while also respecting the right of individuals who seek work outside their home country. Canada and other destination countries must also recognize the investment lost on the part of the home country, provide some form of compensation and shift away from depleting another country of their required resources. Furthermore, it is important to acknowledge that a balance must be achieved in promoting awareness of opportunities for IMGs, while at the same time avoiding systematic targeting of vulnerable countries.

As Little and Buchan (2007) have argued in the case of nursing, achieving self-sufficiency must begin at the level of policy development and must clearly involve the medical-education and training policy community. This planning involves developing health human-resource workforce strategies that can make accurate forecasts and achieve a balance between supply and demand. In addition, strategies must be implemented to recruit and retain local professionals, in order to prevent loss of these individuals to other countries. Furthermore, as the healthcare system continues to evolve, an evaluation of skills of various healthcare professionals must be undertaken to ensure that each professional's skill set is used to its utmost potential in various clinical situations.

The challenge that lies ahead is achieving balance between immigration and self-sufficiency. This balance can be achieved via a collaboration of several partners involved in decision-making at the policy level. Government involvement and support will also play a critical role in working towards achieving greater self-sufficiency in the form of financial aid and policy development in expanding both undergraduate and post-graduate training programmes, while also increasing the faculty available to train and supervise students. Both short- and long-term workforce planning must be undertaken to meet demands in the interim period while working towards achieving workforce goals. In acknowledging that international recruitment is inevitable in the present time, it is important for both donor and recipient countries to collaborate to achieve solutions that satisfy the needs of both parties (Little and Buchan 2007: 12).

Notes

1 Although there are 56 accredited specialties, residency training is not available for all disciplines at all Canadian medical schools (Task Force Two 2003: 50).
2 CaRMS is a not-for-profit organization that provides an electronic application service and a computer match for entry into a variety of post-graduate medical residency positions throughout Canada. The CaRMS matching algorithm attempts to align the applicants with their most preferred programme, and the programme with the best fit. If the applicant's most preferred programme is not available, then the algorithm moves on to the next preferred programme and continues until a match is obtained or the applicant's choices have been exhausted. Over the past 13 years, over 90 per cent of applicants have been matched, with more than half receiving their first choice of programme and over three-quarters receiving a match in their preferred discipline (CIHI 2007: 33).
3 More recently there have been some residency programmes established specifically for IMGs, such as IMG Ontario, and some provinces allow IMGs to compete in the first CaRMS match

References

Aiken, L., Buchan, J., Sochalski, J., Nichols, B. and Powell, M. (2004) 'Trends in international nurse migration', *Health Affairs*, 23: 69–77.

Association of Faculties of Medicine of Canada (2007) *The Future of Medical Education in Canada*, online at www.afmc.ca/pdf/pdf_2007_future_exec_summary.pdf (accessed April 2008).

Audas, R., Ross, A. and Vardy, D. (2005) 'The use of provisionally licensed international medical graduates in Canada', *Canadian Medical Association Journal*, 173: 1315.

Barer, M. and Stoddart, G. (1991) *Toward Integrated Medical Resource Policies for Canada*. Report prepared for the Federal/Provincial/Territorial Conference of Deputy Ministers of Health.

Bowmer, M. I., Banner, S. and Buske, L. (2008) *Physician Self-Sufficiency*. Report prepared for the International Medical Workforce Collaborative Conference, Scotland, online at http://rcpsc.medical.org/publicpolicy/imwc/PAPERversionfinal.pdf (accessed April 2008).

British Medical Association (2005) *The Healthcare Skills Drain: a call to action*, online at www.bma.org.uk/ap.nsf/Content/skillsdrainOpenDocument&Highlight=2,self,suffici ency (accessed April 2008).

Canadian Institute for Health Information (2007) *Canada's Health Care Providers*, Ottawa: CIHI.

Chan, B. (2002) *From Perceived Surplus to Perceived Shortage: what happened to Canada's physician workforce in the 1990s?* Ottawa: Canadian Institute for Health Information, online at http://secure.cihi.ca/cihiweb/products/chanjun02.pdf (accessed April 2008).

Cooper, R. A. and Aiken, L. H. (2006) 'Health services delivery: reframing policies for global migration of nurses and physicians – a US perspective', *Policy, Politics, and Nursing Practice*, 7 (3 Suppl): 66S–70S.

Dauphinee, D. and Buske, L. (2006) 'Medical workforce policy-making in Canada, 1993–2003: reconnecting the disconnected', *Academic Medicine*, 81: 830–6.

Department of Health, UK (2007) *Departmental Report 2007*, online at www.dh.gov.uk/ en/Publicationsandstatistics/Publications/AnnualReports/DH_074767 (accessed April 2008).

Feasby, T. (2008) 'Medical schools are working hard to help cure the doctor shortage', *Globe and Mail Update*, 29 January, online at www.theglobeandmail.com/servlet/story/ RTGAM.20080129.wcomment29/EmailBNStory/specialComment/ (accessed April 2008).

Grant, H. (2004) *From the Transvaal to the Prairies: the migration of South African physicians to Canada*, Winnipeg: Prairie Centre of Excellence for Research on Immigration and Integration. Working Paper 02–04.

Health Action Lobby (HEAL) (2006) *Core Principles and Strategic Directions for a Pan-Canadian Health Human Resources Plan*, Ottawa: Health Action Lobby.

International Center on Nurse Migration (2007) *Nursing Self Sufficiency, Fact Sheet*, online at www.icn.ch/matters_Self_Sufficiency.pdf (accessed April 2008).

International Medical Graduate (IMG) Task Force (2004) *Report of the Canadian Task Force on Licensure of International Medical Graduates*, online at www.imgcanada.ca/ en/pdf/Forum2004English.pdf (accessed April 2008).

Ivison, J. (2008) 'Doctor shortage doesn't have to be. Glut of physicians who cannot earn accreditation', *National Post*, 29 April, online at www.nationalpost.com/news/story. html?id=478094 (accessed April 2008).

Joint Learning Initiative (2004) *Human Resources for Health: overcoming the crisis*, Cambridge, MA: Harvard University Press.

Kermode-Scott, B. (2000) 'Nurturing self-sufficiency', *Canadian Family Physician*, 46: 2352–3.

Kwong, J. C., Dhalla, I. A., Streiner, D. L., Baddour, R. E. and Johnson, I. L. (2002) 'Effects of rising tuition fees on medical school class composition and financial outlook', *Canadian Medical Association Journal*, 166: 1023–8.

Little, L. and Buchan, J. (2007) *Nursing Self-sufficiency/Sustainability in the Global Context*, developed for the International Centre on Nurse Migration and the International Centre for Human Resources in Nursing, Geneva, Switzerland, online at www. intlnursemigration.org/download/SelfSufficiency_US.pdf (accessed April 2008).

Maudsley, R. F. (1994) 'Canadian self-sufficiency in physician resources', *Canadian Medical Association Journal*, 150: 21–2.

Mullan, F. (2000) 'The case for more US medical students', *New England Journal of Medicine*, 343: 213–17.

—— (2007) 'The global medical village', *Medscape General Medicine*, 9: 6, online at www.pubmedcentral.nih.gov/articlerender.fcgi?artid=2234278 (accessed April 2008).

Padmos, A. (2008) 'Self-sufficiency', *CBC Radio Gander Morning Show*, 16 January.

Penn Consortium for Human Resources in Health (2006) *Conclusions of Human Resources for Health: national needs and global concerns. A research and policy retreat.* Philadelphia, PA: Penn Consortium for Human Resources in Health.

Proctor, J. (2001) 'Addressing the question of physician supply in America', *AAMC Reporter*, 10, online at www.aamc.org/newsroom/reporter/july01/physiciansupply.htm (accessed April 2008).

Reudy, J. and Gray, J. D. (1998) 'Undergraduate and postgraduate medical education in Canada', *Canadian Medical Association Journal*, 158: 1047–50.

Society of Rural Physicians of Canada (2002) *International Medical Graduate Policy: recommended strategies*, online at www.srpc.ca/librarydocs/IMG_SRPC.pdf (accessed April 2008).

Spike, N. A. (2006) 'International medical graduates: the Australian perspective', *Academic Medicine*, 81: 842–6.

Spurgeon, D. (2000) 'Canadian medical students are flocking to Ireland', *Student British Medical Journal*, 8: 136–9, online at http://student.bmj.com/issues/00/05/news/95a.php (accessed April 2008).

Sullivan, P. (2005) 'CMA challenges IMG facts before Commons committee', *Canadian Medical Association*, online at www.cma.ca/index.cfm?ci_id=10018542&la_id=1 (accessed April 2008).

—— (2008) 'Canada's medical schools attracting record number of applicants', *Canadian Medical Association*, online at www.cma.ca/index.cfm/ci_id/10042363/la_id/1.htm (accessed April 2008).

Task Force Two (2003) *A Physician Human Resource Strategy for Canada: a literature review and gap analysis*, online at www.effectifsmedicaux.ca/reports/literatureReview-GapAnalysis-e.pdf (accessed April 2008).

—— (2006) *A Physician Human Resource Strategy for Canada. Final Report*, online at www.physicianhr.ca/reports/TF2FinalStrategicReport-e.pdf (accessed April 2008).

World Health Assembly (2006) *World Health Organization Fifty-Ninth World Health Assembly Sixth Report Of Committee A (Draft)*, online at www.who.int/gb/ebwha/pdf_files/WHA59/A59_55-en.pdf (accessed April 2008).

World Health Organization (2006) *The World Health Report – Working Together for Health*, online at www.who.int/whr/2006/en/ (accessed April 2008).

World Medical Association (2003) *The World Medical Association Statement on Ethical Guidelines for the International Recruitment of Physicians*, online at www.wma.net/e/policy/e14.htm (accessed April 2008).

17 Innovations in medical education
European convergence, politics and culture

Fred C. J. Stevens[1]

Introduction

One of the milestones in the history of medical education in the second half of the twentieth century has been the introduction of problem-based learning (PBL). In the late 1960s PBL started at McMaster University in Canada. It was adopted as its basic teaching model by the new medical faculty in Maastricht, the Netherlands, in 1974, followed soon by the University of Newcastle, Australia, and the University of New Mexico in the US. From there it spread around, and still is spreading around, all over the world to many faculties in many developed and developing countries. The success and relative easiness of acceptance of the new problem-based model was not only due to its fashionable appeal. PBL as an educational strategy, and its later modifications, like self-directed learning, integrated learning, task-based learning, focal problems learning, community-based learning and project-based learning, appeared to foster adult learning, self-responsibility of students and early introduction of 'real' patient problems in a better way than any traditional teaching system up until that time. Instead of medical students playing a passive role, in PBL they needed to be active in shaping their own learning process through the curriculum. Problem-based learning was nothing less than a paradigm shift in students' learning and turned out to become the new 'belief system' in medical education. It conquered the world and became the modern standard for medical education, notwithstanding the fact that up to this day its superiority to traditional educational strategies has been difficult to prove in experimental designs (Dochy *et al.* 2003; Kirschner *et al.* 2006; Norman and Schmidt 1992). In particular in Northern Europe, PBL is the major teaching strategy in medical education, to be found in the UK, the Netherlands and the Scandinavian countries.

Looking back raises the question why PBL was launched in the first place, and then, why in some European systems innovations in medical education were more easily accepted and quickly adopted than in others. Studying the social dynamics of medical education in any country is to seize upon its social structure (Gallagher and Subedi 1995). So to answer the question of differences in medical education it is important to note that medical education goes along with the institution of medicine and mirrors the society in which it is embedded. In the next paragraphs we subsequently discuss, in a European context, the adoption of problem-based learning, the cultural impact in medical education, the European convergence in medical education, undergraduate medical education in the Netherlands, and finally, competence-based medical education. In dealing with these issues we further discuss the question of the institutionalization and professionalization of medical education. Why has PBL become such a big success in particular in the northern part of Europe, rather than fading away like so many fads in education? Finally, as this book is about the sociology of medical education, what has medical sociology gained from international innovations in medical education?

Problem-based learning

Problem-based learning is an active, student-centred learning strategy. It is grounded in small-group discussions on interdisciplinary problems with sufficient time for self-study and parallel training of skills (Dent and Harden 2005). In a medicine curriculum these problems are usually defined at the patient level and presented to students in an interdisciplinary way. In groups of 10–12 students a patient case is discussed. In several consecutive 'steps' the students try to solve this case. Students start by defining the problem(s) of the case (patient), after which they freely hypothesize ('brainstorm') on what might be the key problem(s) and discuss what they already know or have in their mind, whether correct or incorrect. From this, students organize their already present and tacit knowledge and translate missing knowledge into learning goals to work on at home. In the next meeting the students present to each other what they have read and learned from the literature, discuss differences in findings and views due to the use of different sources and, if necessary, try to clarify or correct incompatible results. A necessary ingredient is that a tutor guides the group's progress through the different steps.

   PBL came into existence at a time when there was urgent need for a new type of doctor. This new doctor would not only be an expert in the somatic aspects of a disease, but would also be able to integrate in his/her diagnosis, treatment and follow-up procedures the insights of different knowledge domains, including those of the social and behavioural sciences. The significance of an interdisciplinary, integrated view on medical problems, including social sciences insights for medical practice, was not really new, of course. Social medicine had already been an important springboard for the emergence of medical sociology. PBL, however, facilitated a smoother and more 'natural' integration of social and behavioural knowledge domains into the learning of medicine. In a traditional medical curriculum all the different disciplines are taught next to each other, by means of lectures and courses scheduled through the week, leaving little room for an interdisciplinary approach. By contrast, in PBL the patient is the starting point and therefore should better trigger students to learn about different domains, and to see their relevance in an integrated way. For example, in a problem case for students of a woman visiting her General Practitioner with suspected breast cancer, information can be included not only about growth of cancer cells, the lymph system and genetics, but also about screening, lifestyle risk factors, coping with illness, continuity of care, family impact and the importance of social networks in living with cancer. And so PBL would seem also to become the perfect carrier to introduce social sciences into medicine.

Not surprisingly, medical schools that embraced PBL had substantial departments of medical sociology, medical psychology, health economics and General Practice and, of course, distinctive departments focusing on educational development and research. For the training of physicians such departments were considered essential, even on a par with clinical departments. Departments of educational development and research in medical schools fostered first the introduction and then the use of PBL among staff and students, and collected the data needed for evaluation and scientific research. In doing so, medical-education research and development became a discipline in itself. National and international societies were founded, medical-education conferences were organized, peer-reviewed journals came into existence, textbooks were written. At present, there are at least 15 different peer-reviewed scientific journals for medical education, not to mention the many outlet opportunities for medical education in journals like *The Lancet, British Medical Journal, New England Journal of Medicine, Journal of the American Medical Association* and so on. There is a World Federation for Medical Education (WFME). In August 2007, the Association for Medical Education in Europe (AMEE) welcomed in Trondheim, Norway, 1,800 visitors to its annual conference (Segouin *et al.* 2007). On a national level the Dutch/Flanders organization for Medical Education (NVMO) attracts more than 600 people for its yearly conference.

Seen from the perspective of the sociology of the professions, there is no doubt that the coming into existence of the discipline of medical education since the 1970s must be considered a highly successful 'professional project', initiated by a 'new' profession that has been able to create a market for its own services (Sarfatti Larson 1978). As it stands now, medical education is a highly institutionalized and professionalized disciplinary field, for a substantial part thanks to the success of PBL and other educational innovations following in its slipstream. And where PBL was adopted, it has been a success. Medical curricula having a PBL format are ranked among the most popular ones by students as well as faculty staff.

This chapter, however, is not meant to be a tribute to the blessings of PBL. Notwithstanding the success story of medical education that accompanies PBL, it has not been a winner everywhere. A surface inventory, based on what is currently published in medical-education journals and presented at conferences in Europe, indicates that medical schools of the Scandinavian countries, the UK and the Netherlands are ahead in having adopted PBL as a basic educational strategy. In many other, mainly continental European countries, PBL has been less embraced. Many medical curricula in Germany, Belgium and France and in southern European countries still have 'traditional' ways of teaching medicine. This is even more so in Eastern European countries. But even in the Netherlands not all medical schools have adopted the PBL system wholeheartedly, although elements of it can be found everywhere (Ten Cate 2007). What may account for the adoption or rejection of PBL in continental Europe?

It seems that in the early 1970s PBL was launched at the 'right' time and at the 'right' spot, which was at the newly founded Medical Faculty of Maastricht, the Netherlands. At that time the Netherlands already had seven medical schools and there was not really a need for another. In contrast to the situation of a decade earlier, when first plans for a new medical school were launched, in the early 1970s the yearly national supply of physicians was considered sufficient. So the initial plans to start another medical school were nearly frozen, and established medical schools were not really happy when the efforts to found an eighth Dutch medical school persisted. But first, the national government and other stakeholders had to be convinced that Maastricht Medical School would have added value by doing something 'extra', or different from the other schools. One difference was that it would, more than the other medical schools, focus on the training of doctors for primary-care services (a kind of 'barefoot doctors for the modern world'). A second, more unique difference was the use of PBL as its basic teaching and learning strategy. Maastricht Medical School first adopted and then adapted the McMaster PBL system. In its first mission statement it proclaimed that PBL would respond to the challenges in western medicine and medical education in the light of changes in healthcare funding and delivery, and also to changes in patient demand. As it was argued, a new type of doctor was needed, who should be trained in a different way.

There were, of course, also local circumstances that facilitated the introduction of PBL. The local success was also due to the efforts of a handful of enlightened medical educators, physicians as well as behavioural scientists, who were eager to start something really new. Probably the most important factor, however, was that it was a new faculty with a new staff, and it goes without saying that it is always easier to start something fresh in a new situation, than trying to change an established one.

While in the beginning PBL was looked upon with suspicion, it was instantly embraced by faculty and students working with it. Gradually, however, a more substantiating characteristic of PBL came to the surface. When PBL started to gain a foothold in other medical schools too, nationally as well as internationally, it was seen as the panacea to problems with traditional curricula which allowed students to be passive, only memorize, and fail to learn how to apply knowledge in a clinical context. PBL fitted very well with the upcoming innovative, adult-learning theories, the constructivist approach and fostering students to become active learners. In this perspective, knowledge was not seen as absolute or stable, but rather as contextual and constructed on the basis of prior learning (Dent and Harden 2005).

As we know from the sociology of the professions, the optimal cognitive basis for any professional discipline is one whose claimed tasks are sufficiently distinctive to allow the drawing of clear jurisdictional boundaries so that standards of competent performance can be established (Abbott 1988). Such tasks, however, must not be standardized fully, because it would render discretionary professional judgement unnecessary (Freidson 2001; Stevens *et al.* 2007). In this light, the rise of PBL and of the discipline of medical education are strongly intertwined. And because of this relationship, many of the contentions earlier described by Robert Straus and others (Straus 1957) for the position of sociology *in* medicine apply here as well: distancing themselves by focusing narrowly on educational-theory development, educationalists risk their working relationships with medical practitioners (Albert *et al.* 2007). However, educationalists may also lose perspective and theoretical grounding when they identify too closely with the medical world (Dimitroff and Davis 1996). This contention, however, poses the interesting question for the sociology *of* medicine of why certain developments have taken place at a particular time, in a particular way, involving particular actors. Yet it is obvious that the training of physicians cannot be separated from the different perspectives on the position of professionals involved. In other words, the presence of academic departments of medical education fostered PBL and succeeded more and more in involving physicians in medical-education research and innovation. So the answer to the question of what accounts for the introduction of PBL goes beyond local facilitating circumstances. In the next section we will elaborate on this by introducing the international cultural perspective.

Cultural divergence and convergence in medical education

There is a tendency in medical-education literature and at conferences to propound that a set of shared values underlies the globalization of medical education (Phillips 2008). This, however, is only partly the case. Though there is a certain degree of consensus on the basics of educational programmes, methods and medical competence, fundamental differences underlie what educators believe to be effective and ethical in medical education (Hodges and Segouin 2008). Moreover, notwithstanding that to train medical professionals for the future, medical educators are working together more and more to construct global standards and methods for assessment, the perspective that modern medical education should be a vehicle to engage in and to improve global healthcare has not permeated everywhere (Hodges and Segouin 2008). 'Best evidence' medical education, universal standards and the training of health professionals for the future are not isolated from the context in which they take place. Health, healthcare and healthcare education are embedded in value systems. Cultures and nations can vary in value orientations to a considerable degree (Stevens 2001). Yet notwithstanding this notion, the cultural embeddedness of medical education in industrialized societies, or for that matter any society, is a rather under-researched topic. Except for a few cases, there is hardly any cross-cultural research that analyses core values underlying the organization of medical education in modern societies. Segouin and Hodges (2005), for example, describe the differences in medical education between France and Canada. Although both countries have a similar healthcare system, the authors point to significant differences in medical educational systems. The French basic medical curriculum is designed at the national level; the Canadian medical schools are freer, at least to a certain extent, to choose their own curricular format. In France it is assumed that standardization of the curriculum and the selection of students and teachers at the national level guarantees homogeneity and quality of medical education. In doing so, France adheres to the idea of elite education and the training of academics. By contrast, Canada's concept of medical education is more focused on training competent doctors for clinical practice, not necessarily academics. To do this, Canada's medical schools must meet standards at the national level. What these different principles of medical education between France and Canada show, however, is that national cultures underlie the choices made in medical education: in France elite education with major decisions at the central state level, versus education to practice and lower state involvement in Canada (Segouin and Hodges 2005).

Differences in national culture and value systems may also relate to the acceptance of PBL. Jippes and Majoor (2008), for example, explored the impact of national culture on the adoption of integrated and problem-based curricula in Europe, using four dimensions of culture as developed by Hofstede in his *Culture's Consequences: international differences in work related values* (Hofstede 1981). Hofstede surveyed employees of IBM plants in 40 different nations. He found that national cultures (societies) could be classified along four different value dimensions:

1   Individualism versus collectivism.
2   Large- versus small-power distance.
3   Strong versus weak uncertainty avoidance.
4   Masculinity versus femininity.

Individualism/collectivism refers to whether in a particular society the individual opinion and the individual interest is considered more important than collective opinions and collective interest, or vice versa. The second dimension, *power distance*, indicates the extent to which the less powerful members in a society expect and accept that power is unequally distributed. The third dimension, *uncertainty avoidance*, reflects the extent to which members of a society feel threatened by uncertain or unknown situations, and whether people are able to cope with these uncertainties. Finally, *masculinity/femininity* refers to the division of social roles between the sexes and indicates whether achievement and competitiveness (masculine behaviour) prevail above 'tender' relations and care for others (considered to be feminine behaviour). Hofstede's study was not designed to analyse medical-education systems, of course. But his work goes beyond the organizational settings and institutions subject to his research, and indeed may be applicable to educational systems as well (Hofstede 1991). As Jippes and Majoor (2008) observed in their analysis of the medical curricula of 17 European countries, in those with high scores on power distance and uncertainty avoidance, medical schools were less likely to adopt integrated curricula. As they hypothesize, power distance and uncertainty avoidance influence the

flexibility of the organizational structure of a medical school and thereby facilitate or impede the multidisciplinary cooperation between departments necessary
for implementing PBL. Medical schools in countries with high levels of power
distance and uncertainty avoidance may be more hierarchically and traditionally
organized, and may also lack the flexibility to innovate. By contrast, medical
schools in countries with lower levels of power distance and uncertainty avoidance may be flexible enough to innovate. But there may be alternative cultural
explanations for the acceptance of PBL, related to student–teacher interactions.

A few years ago, with many foreign (mainly German) students entering my
own university at Maastricht, colleagues made the following observations. Compared to Dutch students tutors felt that foreign students: (a) expected more initiatives from their teacher, instead of only being a learning facilitator; (b) expected
more instructions on what to do and how to study; (c) valued the opinion of the
group more than their own opinion; (d) considered maximal study efforts more
rule than exception; (e) were often annoyed by suboptimal study efforts of their
(Dutch) peers; (f) expected their teacher to act as the expert; and (g) did not
understand the Dutch student culture of leisure activities and student societies.
Very likely these differences between Dutch and foreign students, as observed
by colleagues, are culture-based. In *feminine* societies like in the Netherlands,
students do not exhibit much eagerness and prefer solidarity above individual
excellence (Hofstede 1991). By contrast, in typical *masculine* societies, like in
the US, for example, students are likely to want to act in a more 'visible' manner
and are more used to competing openly with each other. The uncertainty-
avoidance dimension may apply to the teacher–student relation (Hofstede 1981,
1991). When students grow up in a culture typified by high levels of uncertainty
avoidance they are likely to have more difficulties with uncertain situations and,
therefore, will rely more on the opinion of the teacher (the teacher as the
'expert') rather than on themselves or fellow students. In general, in large-
power-distance societies the educational process will be more *teacher*-centred
than in small-power-distance situations. Very likely, PBL will flourish more in
the latter situation, because students have learned to act more independently in
their learning process.

What we see in continental Europe is that problem-based learning has had a
much higher adoption rate in the group of *northern* European countries, consisting of Sweden, Norway, Finland, Denmark and the Netherlands. On Hofstede's
value dimensions these countries share high scores on femininity and low scores
on uncertainty avoidance. Alternatively, in the *southern* European countries with
high scores on masculinity and on uncertainty avoidance, specifically in France,
Italy, Spain and Greece, traditional educational systems seem to prevail (Mariolis *et al.* 2008; Palés and Gual 2008).

A further observation is that Hofstede's individualism–collectivism dimension points to the relationship between the individual and the group in learning.
In collectivist societies, the skills and virtues of a good group member are
stressed. In individualist societies one tries to provide skills to be able to discover new things, under the assumption that learning never ends, which is typical

of PBL. Again, northern European countries tend to be more individualist, while southern European countries seem to be more collectivist.

Finally, in societies typified by a high degree of uncertainty avoidance and a greater masculinity orientation, the physician has a dominant position in the healthcare system and consequently also in medical education (Stevens 2001; Stevens and Van der Zee 2007). This will make it more difficult for other disciplines to contribute to and to have an influence on medical education. In other words, in countries where the medical profession strongly dominates healthcare, medical education will be less innovative, a hypothesis also consistent with a north–south division in Europe regarding PBL.

Bologna and competency-based medical education

Education in Europe is subject to regulation through a set of vocational directives, stimulated by the European Community (Cumming and Ross 2007). The Bologna Declaration commits European Union (EU) member states to a process of harmonization and convergence in the higher education sector, resulting in a three-cycle system of degree qualifications, described as Bachelor's, Master's and Doctorate degrees. Key objectives include increased quality assurance, promotion of student mobility and cross-national comparability of degrees. Though it is a voluntary agreement, it extends far beyond the EU with 46 signatory nations, ranging from Norway to Azerbaijan. The Bologna process will make it easier for students to compare courses between countries, and to move between them. A framework for qualifications describes the typical learning outcomes for each cycle and discipline and is accompanied by a European Credit Transfer System (ECTS). Across countries ECTS points are interchangeable. So a German student who spends, say, half a year in Italy or Norway, gets a credit, a sort of Euro grade that has value at his home university. One ECTS point stands for 28 hours of study. While the Bologna process has no legal force behind it, it forces big changes. One is that adopting the international three-track system of a standard three- or four-year Bachelor's degree, a Master's and a PhD, makes Europe's universities more transparent. Students will be better able to choose between them, and whether universities or schools like it or not, it will compel more competition between universities to attract the most and the brightest students.

The new system may also have financial consequences. In the long run the Bologna principles will probably ditch the typical, but rather expensive continental style of a first degree, which takes five or six years of study. In many European countries admission to higher education is free or at least not expensive. So in a time of tightening budgets, offering shorter degrees to save money might be the next best thing to asking (higher) admission fees. As is well known, in medicine costs per student are high compared to other subjects. So the question is, will the new system apply to medical education too?

Applying the Bologna principles to undergraduate medical education in particular means splitting up the programme. Not surprisingly, the medical schools are the least enthusiastic. The majority of continental medical-degree programmes are considered as integrated, holistic five–six-year programmes, though tiered by a clinical and a non-clinical part. Medical institutions in Europe experience great difficulties in dividing their curriculum in Bachelor/Master's tracks. So there is broad consensus in the European community that the introduction of the two-cycle structure in medicine is problematic (Patrício *et al.* 2008). Across Europe (and elsewhere too) medical education seems to be moving in the other direction, towards more integrated curricula of basic and clinical sciences. In these integrated curricula it already appears to be difficult to incorporate the theoretical basis of medicine sufficiently. A first degree Bachelor would make this even more problematic.

Another problem is that medical education is oriented towards a strongly defined professional profile of a physician, who starts post-graduate training automatically after an undergraduate degree. Clinical medical education is further closely linked to teaching hospitals which have a mandate for healthcare and often for clinical education too. And EU directives require that a medical degree takes six years. All this shows that medical curricula are highly structured with relatively little freedom of choice. But while the subject matter of medical education compared to other professional programmes is perceived to be rather rigid and more or less identical in Europe and globally, the context and conditions in which the programme operates are very diverse. How the six years are filled and divided varies substantially between medical institutions in European countries. Moreover, the European region displays differences in disease patterns, healthcare-delivery systems and in the composition of the health workforce, which has consequences for the use of physicians and for the required qualifications of medical graduates. Even larger differences can be observed in the governance of medical education, in medical-curricula designs and in the resources allocated to medical education – as noted, differences firmly embedded in cultural traditions, political realities and economic development. So tensions exist between the global, uniform nature of medical education, the typical characteristics of professional education, the strong relations to national healthcare systems, and the European, trans-disciplinary nature of actions within the Bologna process.

A third problem is that at the labour market end there seems to be no real need for a Bachelor in medicine. At first glance, a Bachelor in medicine does not make much sense, though the EU countries of Portugal, the Netherlands and Denmark have adopted a two-tier system of 3+3 years, compliant with the mandate in Europe to have a six-year medicine curriculum. In Belgium (3+4 years) a Bachelor degree in medicine also exists, but this does not qualify the candidate for the labour market. Swiss medical faculties, however, have taken an alternative route in developing a flexible curriculum with a labour-market-relevant Bachelor degree, different Master's tracks and research opportunities. The Swiss model allows students to choose between different major and Master's programmes and to diversify in tracks such as research and medical practice (Probst *et al.* 2007). Because the Swiss model no longer results in one single type of graduate, paths to other professions in the healthcare area are opened up.

Though the Swiss model looks promising, many countries are further from putting into practice the Bologna principles in medical education.

A final problem that should be mentioned here is that the Bologna rules draw deeply on continental ideas of student achievement, measured in terms of activities undertaken and hours spent by students. As noted, French medical schools deliver the same, centrally created curriculum, based on normative guidelines for core content rather than for essential professional roles or key competencies of doctors. What matters more and more, however, and this is one of the guiding principles in modern medical education, is what the student has *learned* and/or the competencies s/he has gained. Seen from this perspective a European dimension to quality assurance and accreditation by means of the Bologna rules could be helpful to shift thinking from the acquisition of knowledge towards the achievement of solid learning outcomes and competencies. Not surprisingly, the latter is easier to realize in problem-based learning systems than in traditional ways of teaching. Up until now, the two/three-cycle system has not gained wide acceptance in European medical education, though elements of it are strongly supported. This regards the comparability of degrees, European credit systems (ECTS), student-mobility promotion, quality control and principles of lifelong learning. So it is probably only a matter of time before practical and financial advantages will emanate from the fundamental principles and that a Europe-wide programme of assessment, accreditation and certification will come into existence.

All in all, during the implementation of the Bologna process, diversities in Europe need to be taken into account, in particular when objectives include striving towards harmonizing the structure and function of European medical education. Harmonization, however, should not be seen as a process leading to uniformity but as convergence based on shared knowledge of best practices and respect for diversity and the autonomy of the medical institutions within nations.

Competency-based medical education

Educating physicians for new roles regarding societal needs and expectations has led to several innovative initiatives, of which the competency-based model is a major one. Very likely, competency-based medical education will be conducive to European convergence. Since the late 1990s medical educators have increasingly focused on the competencies in terms of knowledge, skills and attitudes, necessary for graduates to meet the needs of those they serve. The overall idea of competency-based education is that it is outcome-based, and that a physician must show that s/he has acquired the necessary competencies to practise as a doctor (Frank and Danoff 2007). The origins of competency-based medical education can be traced back to developments that have been described earlier and extensively, among others by medical sociologists, of the rise of consumerism, the need for physicians' professionalism and the lack of societal responsiveness in medicine. To be able to respond to new demands, medical education is more and more seen on a continuum of 'lifelong learning'. This starts at the undergraduate level, and it is the task of medical educators to help students to become lifelong learners. The competency-based model was first developed for specialist training and is now being used for undergraduate training too. Several initiatives have been taken to define required competencies for doctors. Well-known examples are to be found in *Tomorrow's Doctors* (GMC 2003) and the 'Scottish Doctor' (Simpson *et al.* 2002). The Dutch blueprint for medical education is another typical example of a competency/outcome-based framework, in which four physician roles are distinguished:

1   The physician as a medical expert.
2   The physician as a scientist.
3   The physician as a worker in healthcare.
4   The physician as a person (Metz *et al.* 2001).

German medical education also intends to move in this direction (Haage 2006).

While all these national documents more or less look alike, the Canadian CanMEDS Framework has the edge in defining the outcome-based key competencies needed for medical education and practice. CanMEDS focuses on the abilities needed by physicians to meet the healthcare needs of the patients, communities, and societies served. It is based on seven core roles:

1   Medical expert.
2   Communicator.
3   Collaborator.
4   Manager.
5   Health advocate.
6   Scholar.
7   Professional (Frank 2005; Frank and Danoff 2007).

The medical expert role is the central role, encircled by and overlapping with six other roles. In turn, these latter roles partly overlap each other outside the medical-expert domain. For another part, these roles are exclusive (non-overlapping).

The CanMEDS competency framework is rapidly becoming the worldwide standard. Synergetic collaborations have been started between the CanMEDS and the US Accreditation Council for Graduate Medical Education (ACGME), the Australian Medical Council, the Royal College of Surgeons of England and the central College of Medical Specialists of the Netherlands. Although CanMEDS is widely adopted in Canada and has been adapted around the world, there is still a long way to go. This is because competency-based medical education will intrude deeply into medicine's culture, as already became clear from our earlier example of the groundings of medical education in France. In many contexts medical education is marked by a similar tenacious conservatism. So the paradigm shift in implementing competency-based curricula and assessment programmes is in many countries perceived as nothing less than a 'culture shock'. To change medical curricula into competency-based ones needs ample faculty-development efforts, supported by frontline teachers, researchers and, in particular, educational leadership. There is progress, however. In 2004 the Tuning Project for Medicine started in Europe with its objectives being to formulate learning objectives, learning outcomes and competencies in medical education (Cumming and Ross 2007). Recently the International Federation of Medical Students' Associations (IFMSA), proposed an outcome-based curriculum, based on the Bologna principles, and consisting of nine domains of outcomes:

1   Clinical skills.
2   Communication.
3   Critical thinking.
4   Health in society.
5   Lifelong learning.
6   Professionalism.
7   Teaching.
8   Teamwork.
9   Theoretical knowledge (Hilgers *et al.* 2007; Rigby 2007).

From all this it becomes obvious that, notwithstanding (inter)national differences in phrasing and categorizing, the insight is growing that a good doctor is more than a medical expert. And because of this s/he needs also to be competent in other domains of practice. The near future will show how medical curricula in Europe will respond to this.

An example: innovative medical education in the Netherlands

In many of the innovations in medical education described above, the Netherlands is one of the forerunners. The Netherlands has a long tradition of research in medical education, in particular at the University Medical Centres (the equivalent of medical schools) of Groningen, Utrecht and Maastricht. The large output in scientific research also explains the prominent role in educational innovation.

The six-year medical undergraduate curriculum is the standard, historically anchored core within the sequence of educational links that constitutes the doctor-making process. All programmes of Dutch medical schools comply to a national blueprint of objectives with horizontal integration and a modular structure with unit periods of four–six weeks devoted to a coherent theme. So instead of teaching distinct disciplinary subjects like anatomy, physiology or epidemiology, bodily systems (for example the cardiovascular system) or life stages (such as 'adolescence' or 'adulthood') are focused upon. Parallel to these units, students are trained in physical examination skills, clinical reasoning and communication skills. At the end of every unit students have a unit test. But, alongside these unit tests, students of half of the Dutch medical schools participate four times a year in an inter-faculty progress test (Van der Vleuten *et al.* 1996). This progress test consists of multiple-choice questions on everything a doctor should know at graduation. Students of all years do this test, and in every progressive year students are expected to answer a larger part of the questions correctly. It should be noted, however, that this is not a national exam, as it is not meant to be used for central, national qualification (Van der Vleuten *et al.* 2004).

The traditional medical undergraduate curriculum in the Netherlands used to be H-shaped, with four years of non-clinical teaching, followed by two years of clinical rotations in different specialties. Currently, the distinction between basic-science teaching and clinical practice is not as strong as it was. Nearly all Dutch medical schools have introduced clinical practice early in the curriculum, facilitated by the participation of clinical departments. In other words, the H-shaped curriculum has been replaced by a Z-shaped curriculum, in which the clinical practice component preferably starts in year one and increases through the years. What made the transition from an H-shaped curriculum to a Z-shaped one possible is the change in teaching philosophy. Again, in modern medical education, a move has taken place from classroom teaching to small-group tutorials, from students as passive listeners to active creators of their own knowledge, from mono- to multidisciplinary approaches, and from learning in isolation to learning in an authentic context.

Most Dutch medical schools still have their clinical rotations in the last two years of the programme. Several medical schools deviate from this model in having the clinical rotation period in year four and five of the six-year curriculum. The early introduction of clinical practice, consistent with the principles of an integrated medical curriculum, is one of the reasons for choosing this curriculum format. The other reason is that it gives an opportunity to students in their sixth year to spend extra time on clinical practice and on clinical research. All students are obliged to spend six months of their final year as a 'semi-physician'/junior doctor in a clinical department, as well as six months in one of the faculty's research institutes to learn about the principles of scientific research. Some students combine research and clinical practice and spend a year in a hospital or primary-care department. The advantages of this medical curriculum format are obvious. It prepares students better for their post-graduate specialty training and makes the transfer from undergraduate student to medical resident much smoother. For some the sixth year may also be the start of their PhD track.

As can be imagined, the early organization of the clinical rotations has its consequences for the rest of the curriculum too. Students are not only one year younger when they enter the clinical rotations, they also 'miss' one year of basic-science preparation. So in Maastricht year three is used as a transitional year in which the teaching is organized in different, thematic and clinically based clusters (for example, lung and circulation, abdomen, psychomedical problems). In all these clusters students see and discuss in tutorial groups a lot of patients and clinical problems, which are the basis for studying the basic sciences (Diemers *et al.* 2007). Learning is most effective 'in context' and so the success of this third year is proved again and again in student programme evaluation. Though not all Dutch medical schools may go as far, all schools offer early clinical experiences. Several provide the opportunity to spend a substantial amount of time in one specialty in the final year. Early clinical experience is also being introduced in these innovative, vertically integrated undergraduate medical curricula. While on many occasions the early clinical experience is restricted to the presence of patients during lectures, in Utrecht students gain 'hands-on' experience of daily clinical practice during six-week clerkships (Ten Cate 2007). Less background knowledge and a lower age than is usual for the more traditional (later) clerkships, however, do not appear to hamper successful completion of an early clerkship. Indeed, early clerkships have several advantages, such as opportunities for early observation of the future profession, increased motivation for further study, contextual learning and the improvement of clinical skills (Kamalski *et al.* 2007).

Social sciences and competency-based medical education

What have the social sciences gained from all these innovations in medical education? It has always been difficult to successfully integrate social and behavioural sciences into a medical curriculum, whether this be a traditional one or a PBL one. But the move towards competency-based medical education and towards integrated medical curricula will have positive consequences for the position of the social sciences in medicine too. There is no doubt that social-and-behavioural-sciences insights are important for the development of a perspective – a view on medical work and medical reality – that medical students have to get a grip on in order to become competent doctors. Such an insight contrasts sharply with earlier days of traditional curricula when the social sciences were more often than not considered as 'add-ons' to the core medical curriculum. A recent survey conducted by the Tuning Project for Medicine ranked the assessment of the psychological and social aspects of a patient's illness, working effectively in a healthcare system and engagement with population health issues as (very) important (Cumming and Ross 2007).

One of the dilemmas, however, that still hasn't been solved is the timing, or the classic dilemma of too early versus too late (Gallagher and Searle 1989). To expose students to the social context of disease before they deal with patients seems too early, because there is no opportunity to understand the relevance. At the start of the course, students may be too young and lack a clinical context to be able to integrate social issues into their daily work practice. But to wait until they see patients may be too late, because by then, it may take second place to the students' anxieties about dealing with the patient's medical needs. As there is ample evidence that students learn most in context, experts are currently convinced that the social sciences are best integrated in a clinical context, when students have had at least some practical – which means clinical – experience, for example during clerkships. Notwithstanding this, at a later stage of their studies, during clerkships, students may lack the 'open mind' needed to be sensitive to and to develop new perspectives. In other words, it is important that students are not encouraged to develop a clinical gaze and to adopt a physician identity exclusively grounded in biological reductionism. As Hafferty notes, to begin with, medical students quickly find themselves enveloped by a culture and work climate typified by the 'hard' tracks of biosciences (Hafferty 1997). In turn, with increasing work pressure on students they quickly learn to devalue and resent the time they feel they must spend covering 'softer' issues such as physician–patient relationships, psychosocial factors in health and disease, ethics, and the organization and financing of healthcare.

The different European testing and 'tuning' activities in the light of the physician's competencies provide the social sciences with an 'earmarked' position in medical curricula (Cumming and Ross 2007). As part of a growing concern with what constitutes a good doctor and how such a person may best be trained, the role of the social sciences and other non-biological and non-clinical disciplines has been brought more to the foreground (Brähler et al. 2001). It is obvious that students should acquire an understanding of ethical standards and the social roles and responsibilities of the profession and that they should also find out for themselves what it means to be a 'professional', behaving 'professionally' in a professional environment (Harden et al. 1999; Jones et al. 2001). Medical professionals should not only have competitive biomedical knowledge and skills but should also be aware of their social responsibilities regarding patient care and be conscious of their role-modelling in healthcare and society (Davis and Harden 2003; Harden et al. 1999). Students start their critical thinking about what it means to become a doctor as soon as they enter medical school and continue this throughout the curriculum (Harden et al. 1999; Jones et al. 2001; Wear and Castellani 2000). This should be the guiding principle and a continuous and persistent part of their lifelong professional education. Innovations in medical education and the convergence of medical curricula will foster this.

Conclusion: the convergence and divergence in European medical education

In this chapter PBL and other innovations in medical education have been discussed from the perspective of European convergence in higher education. It was argued that medical innovations in Europe have spread unequally, and that northern European countries have been first to adopt them. Some of the European differences in medical education have cultural groundings. European national differences reflect variations in organizational flexibility, teacher–student relationships and the dominance of the medical profession in healthcare and medical education. Notwithstanding national differences in cultural traditions and the governance and resources allocated to medical education, there is no doubt that Europe will move towards even more convergence in medical education in the near future.

Medical education in Europe is oriented towards a rather uniform professional profile of a physician, to be accomplished within a defined period of six years. Yet the question is whether structural convergence on a European level will ultimately supersede national, culturally embedded customs and traditions in ways of teaching medicine and in assessment. The World Federation of Medical Education (WFME) has already developed standards to outline the minimum requirements for medical-education institutions. One of the aims is to judge on a national and international level the assessment and accreditation of medical schools, in order to assure minimum-quality standards for medical-school programmes. Currently, medical schools in the Netherlands and Flanders (Belgium) organize their accreditation together, but it will only be a matter of time before a European system of accreditation will be implemented. A logical next step would be the introduction of certifying medical exams on an international level. Outcome-based medical education will ultimately lead to uniform standards, and it does not need a fortune-teller to predict that a European system of accreditation and certifying exams on an international level will provide ample opportunities and pressure to catch up for those who lie behind. This, however, does not mean that cultural traditions in medical education will no longer play a role. A degree of national and institutional uniqueness is requisite, not only for the benefit of identity, but also for the advantage of continuing innovation. Institutions and national systems can learn from each other, and in this perspective it is remarkable how little comparative research has been done to underpin differences and similarities in the organization of medical education in Europe. More research effort is also needed, as it will be a major challenge for European medical education to find a healthy balance between European convergence, in the light of standardization and quality improvement, and divergence in the light of protecting national and institutional identity.

Note

1 The author wishes to thank Cees van der Vleuten and Albert Scherpbier for their comments on an earlier draft of this manuscript.

References

Abbot, A. (1988) *The System of Professions: an essay on the division of expert labor*, Chicago, IL: University of Chicago Press.

Albert, M., Hodges, B. and Regehr, G. (2007) 'Research in medical education: balancing service and science', *Advances in Health Sciences Education*, 12: 103–15.

Brähler, E., Bullinger, M., Gerber, W.-D., Meyer-Probst, B., Novak, P., Siegrist, J. and Tewes, U. (2001) 'Der neue Gegenstandskatalog "Medizinische Psychologie und Medizinische Soziologie"', *Sozial- und Preventivmedizin*, 46: 135–40.

Cumming, A. and Ross, M. (2007) 'The Tuning Project for Medicine – learning outcomes for undergraduate medical education in Europe', *Medical Teacher*, 29: 636–41.

Davis, M. H. and Harden, R. M. (2003) 'Planning and implementing an undergraduate medical curriculum: the lessons learned', *Medical Teacher*, 25: 596–608.

Dent, J. A. and Harden, R. M. (eds) (2005) *A Practical Guide for Medical Teachers*, Edinburgh: Elsevier.

Diemers, A. D., Dolmans, D. H., Van Santen, M., Van Luijk, S. J., Janssen-Noordman, A. M. and Scherpbier, A. J. (2007) 'Students' perceptions of early patient encounters in a PBL curriculum: a first evaluation of the Maastricht experience', *Medical Teacher*, 29: 135–42.

Dimitroff, A. and Davis, W. K. (1996) 'Content analysis of research in undergraduate medical education', *Academic Medicine*, 71: 60–7.

Dochy, F., Segers, M., Van Den Bossche, P. and Gijbels, D. (2003) 'Effects of problem-based learning: a meta-analysis', *Learning and Instruction*, 13: 533–68.

Frank, J. R. (2005) *The CanMEDS 2005 Physician Competency Framework*, Ottawa: Royal College of Physicians and Surgeons of Canada.

Frank, J. R. and Danoff, D. (2007) 'The CanMEDS initiative: implementing an outcomes-based framework of physician competencies', *Medical Teacher*, 29: 642–7.

Freidson, E. (2001) *Professionalism: the third logic*, Chicago: University of Chicago Press.

Gallagher, E. and Searle, M. C. (1989) 'Content and context in health professional education', in H. E. Freeman and S. Levine (eds) *Handbook of Medical Sociology*, 4th edn, Englewood Cliffs, NJ: Prentice Hall.

Gallagher, E. B. and Subedi, J. (eds) (1995) *Global Perspectives on Health Care*, Englewood Cliffs, NJ: Prentice Hall.

General Medical Council (GMC) (2003) *Tomorrow's Doctors*, London: General Medical Council.

Haage, H. (2006) 'Ausbildung zum Arzt: was ist erreicht, was bleibt zu tun? Eine Übersicht' [Medical education in Germany: past successes and future challenges. An overview], *Bundesgesundheitsblatt-Gesundheitsforschung-Gesundheitsschütz*, 49: 325–9.

Hafferty, F. W. (1997) 'To tell the truth: an in-class learning exercise for medical students', in B. Pescosolido, A. E. Figert and G. Weiss (eds) *A Handbook for Teaching Medical Sociology*, Washington, DC: American Sociological Association.

Harden, R. M., Cosby, J. R. and Davis, M. H. (1999) 'AMEE Guide No. 14: outcome-based education: Part 1 – An introduction to outcome-based education', *Medical Teacher*, 21: 7–14.

Hilgers, J., De Roos, P. and Rigby, E. (2007) 'European core curriculum – the students' perspective, Bristol, UK, 10 July 2006', *Medical Teacher*, 29: 270–5.

Hodges, B. and Segouin, C. (2008) 'Medical education: it's time for a transatlantic dialogue', *Medical Education*, 42: 2–3.

Hofstede, G. (1981) *Culture's Consequences: international differences in work related values*, London: Sage.

—— (1991) *Cultures and Organizations: software of the mind*, London: McGraw-Hill.

Jippes, M. and Majoor, G. D. (2008) 'Influence of national culture on the adoption of integrated and problem-based curricula in Europe', *Medical Education*, 42: 279–85.

Jones, R., Higgs, R., De Angelis, C. and Prideaux, D. (2001) 'Changing face of medical curricula', *Lancet*, 357: 699–703.

Kamalski, D. M. A., Ter Braak, E. W. M. T., Ten Cate, O. T. J. and Borleffs, J. C. (2007) 'Early clerkships', *Medical Teacher*, 29: 915–20.

Kirschner, P. A., Sweller, J. and Clark, R. (2006) 'Why minimal guidance during instruction does not work: an analysis of the failure of constructivist, discovery, problem-based, experiential, and inquiry-based teaching', *Educational Psychologist*, 41: 75–86.

Mariolis, A., Alevizos, A. and Mihas, C. (2008) 'Undergraduate medical education in Greece: a hostile environment for primary care', *Medical Education*, 42: 439–42.

Metz, J. C. M., Verbeek-Weel, A. M. M. and Huisjes, H. J. (2001) *Raamplan 2001 Artsopleiding* [Framework for training doctors in the Netherlands 2001]. Nijmegen: Mediagroep.

Norman, G. R. and Schmidt, H. G. (1992) 'The psychological basis of problem-based learning: a review of the evidence', *Academic Medicine*, 67: 557–65.

Palés, J. and Gual, A. (2008) 'Medical education in Spain: current status and new challenges', *Medical Teacher*, 30: 365–9.

Patrício, M., Den Engelsen, C., Tseng, D. and Ten Cate, O. (2008) 'Implementation of the Bologna two-cycle system in medical education: where do we stand in 2007? Results of an AMEE-MEDINE survey', *Medical Teacher*, 30: 597–606.

Phillips, S. (2008) 'Models of medical education in Australia, Europe and North America', *Medical Teacher*, 30: 705–9.

Probst, C., Weert, E. D. and Witte, J. (2007) 'Medical education in the Bachelor–Master structure: the Swiss model', www.bologna-handbook.com/docs/downloads/C_5_1_1. pdf.

Rigby, E. (2007) 'Taking forward aims of the Bologna declaration: European core curriculum – the student's perspective', *Medical Teacher*, 29: 83–4.

Sarfatti Larson, M. (1978) *The Rise of Professionalism: a sociological analysis*, Berkeley: University of California Press.

Segouin, C. and Hodges, B. (2005) 'Educating physicians in France and Canada: are the differences based on evidence or history?', *Medical Education*, 39: 1205–12.

Segouin, C., Hodges, B. and Byrne, N. (2007) 'World conference on medical education: a window on the globalizing world of medical education?', *Medical Teacher*, 29: 63–6.

Simpson, J. G., Furnace, J., Crosby, J., Cumming, A. D., Evans, P. A., Friedman Ben David, M., Harden, R. M., Lloyd, D., McKenzie, H., McLachlan, J. C., McPhate, G. F., Percy-Robb, I. W. and MacPherson, S. G. (2002) 'The Scottish doctor – learning outcomes for the medical undergraduate in Scotland: a foundation for competent and reflective practitioners', *Medical Teacher*, 24: 136–43.

Stevens, F. (2001) 'The convergence and divergence of modern health care systems', in W. C. Cockerham (ed.) *The Blackwell Companion to Medical Sociology*, London: Blackwell.

Stevens, F. and Van der Zee, J. (2007) 'Health care delivery systems', in G. Ritzer (ed.) *The Blackwell Encyclopedia of Sociology*, Malden, MA: Blackwell.

Stevens, F. C. J., Diederiks, J. P. M., Grit, F. and Van der Horst, F. (2007) 'Exclusive, idiosyncratic and collective expertise in the interprofessional arena: the case of optometry and eye care in the Netherlands', *Sociology of Health and Illness*, 29: 481–96.

Straus, R. (1957) 'The nature and status of medical sociology', *American Sociological Review*, 22: 200–4.

Ten Cate, O. (2007) 'Medical education in the Netherlands', *Medical Teacher*, 29: 752–7.

Van der Vleuten, C. P., Schuwirth, L. W., Muijtjens, A. M., Thoben, A. J., Cohen-Schotanus, J. and Van Boven, C. P. (2004) 'Cross institutional collaboration in assessment: a case on progress testing', *Medical Teacher*, 26: 719–25.

Van der Vleuten, C. P. M., Verwijnen, G. M. and Wijnen, W. H. F. W. (1996) 'Fifteen years of experience with progress testing in a problem-based learning curriculum', *Medical Teacher*, 18: 103–10.

Wear, D. and Castellani, B. (2000) 'The development of professionalism: curriculum matters', *Academic Medicine*, 75: 602–11.

Index

Milton Keynes UK
Ingram Content Group UK Ltd.
UKHW021621071024
44932 7UK00020BA/1138